MANAGING AND PREVENTING PANDEMICS

Using an evidence-based, critical, population health approach, this book provides a comprehensive analysis of the key errors and most effective interventions to contain the COVID-19 pandemic. It also examines the root determinants of pandemic risk on a global scale and addresses the policy changes to be implemented to prevent future health crises.

Part One of the book discusses the lethal errors in the management of the COVID-19 pandemic, focusing particularly on those countries that failed to limit the death toll caused by the health crisis. These mistakes include lack of preparation, disinformation, medicalization, adoption of a "laissez-faire the virus" approach and inequity. Part Two analyzes the vital actions that enabled "virtuous" countries to effectively limit the most deadly effects of the pandemic: prevention, immunization and support.

Part Three looks at what we should do to prevent the next pandemic. This part examines the proximal social and environmental causes of pandemic risk (e.g., deforestation, industrialized animal farming and climate change), as well as the "causes of the causes," which include our model of global economic development and its philosophical and ideological underpinnings.

Roberto De Vogli is an Associate Professor of Global Health and Psychology of Power, University of Padova, Italy.

MANAGING AND PREVENTING PANDEMICS

Lessons From COVID-19

Roberto De Vogli

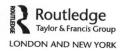

Routledge
Taylor & Francis Group

LONDON AND NEW YORK

First published 2025
by Routledge
4 Park Square, Milton Park, Abingdon, Oxon OX14 4RN

and by Routledge
605 Third Avenue, New York, NY 10158

Routledge is an imprint of the Taylor & Francis Group, an informa business

© 2025 Roberto De Vogli

British Library Cataloguing-in-Publication Data
A catalogue record for this book is available from the British Library

Library of Congress Cataloging-in-Publication Data
Names: De Vogli, Roberto, author.
Title: Managing and preventing pandemics : lessons from COVID-19 /
Roberto De Vogli.
Description: Abingdon, Oxon ; New York, NY : Routledge, 2025. |
Includes bibliographical references and index.
Identifiers: LCCN 2024015461 (print) | LCCN 2024015462 (ebook) |
ISBN 9781032842653 (hardback) | ISBN 9781032415550 (paperback) |
ISBN 9781003511977 (ebook)
Subjects: MESH: Pandemic Preparedness--methods |
COVID-19--prevention & control
Classification: LCC RA644.C67 D486 2025 (print) |
LCC RA644.C67 (ebook) | NLM WC 506.6 |
DDC 362.1962/4144--dc23/eng/20240430
LC record available at https://lccn.loc.gov/2024015461
LC ebook record available at https://lccn.loc.gov/2024015462

ISBN: 978-1-032-84265-3 (hbk)
ISBN: 978-1-032-41555-0 (pbk)
ISBN: 978-1-003-51197-7 ebk)

DOI: 10.4324/9781003511977

Typeset in Sabon
by KnowledgeWorks Global Ltd.

CONTENTS

List of figures   *ix*
Preface   *xi*

Introduction   1

Did they die with or due to COVID-19? 2
*The worst mortality crisis in the Western world
   since World War II 3*
*COVID-19 strategies: healthy nations and
   "failed" states 6*
References 8

PART I
Lethal errors   **13**

1 Unpreparedness   15

The white swan 15
Once upon a time there were pandemic plans 17
The "Italian job": a model to imitate? 19
Every time the pandemic "ended" 22
Trumping the World Health Organization 25
The "good virus" and pills of fatal optimism 28
References 30

2 Misinformation 37

    Seven myths about SARS-CoV-2 37
      The "health dictatorship" 38
      "It's flu-like" 39
      The "colding" of the virus 41
      "Masks are useless" 42
      "Asymptomatic people do not infect" 43
      The "tamponite" 44
      "The hidden cures they never tell us" 46
    Inoculation against evidence-free opinions 48
    References 52

3 Medicalization 61

    "Naked against the virus" 62
    The pandemic must be fought in the communities 64
    Prevention at the margins 67
    Sentinels "on the front line" against COVID-19? 71
    Italy is not a country for public health experts 73
    The United States' and United Kingdom's
      paradox 76
    References 77

4 "Laissez-faire the virus" 81

    Human sacrifices on the altar of the economy 82
    Herd immunity or social murder? 84
      Children as human shields 87
    Health for sale 89
    Economy or health is a false dichotomy 92
    The collapse of the Great Wall 95
    References 100

5 Inequity 107

    The announced suicide crisis that did not
      happen 107
    Psychodemia 110
    The unjust virus: it affects everyone, but it is not
      democratic 111
    Vaccine apartheid 114

*When the right to profit of a few wins over the
right to health of all 116
Bill Gates and how the ultra-rich can save the
world? 119
References 122*

PART II
Vital actions   **129**

6 Prevention   131

*Veneto: they called it "Northeast Korea" 132
Test, trace and isolate on time: how to save lives at
scale 134
Lessons from the East 135
Taiwan 135
South Korea 137
Vietnam 138
New Zealand 139
Singapore 141
Japan 141
Failures of the West: app flops 142
"Schools are safe, hands off the kids!" 145
References 148*

7 Immunization   157

*SARS-CoV-2 vaccines: killers or saviors? 157
"Natural" immunity? 162
Endemic but still lethal 167
Variants of concern and nation "super spreaders" 169
"Catapulting infections" 171
References 173*

8 Support   179

*To self-isolate or not to self-isolate? Inequity is the
problem 180
The antidote of solidarity 181
The myth of scarce resources 183
United we stand, divided we fall ill 187*

Lessons from the pandemic: letting the dead
   speak 189
References 193

PART III
Preventing future pandemics   **197**

9   COVID-19: A human-made pandemic   199

The Huanan horror market 200
Chinese shadows and the death of Li Wenliang 202
Pandemic risk amplifiers 204
Ecological crisis: sister to the pandemic one? 208
   "Greenwashing," "green wishing" and "green
   wishy-washy" 212
References 213

10 The economic fabric of zoonoses   220

Capital sins at the root of the pandemic 222
The neoliberal variant of capitalism 225
The liberalization of viruses 228
   Free markets "made in China" 232
Neoliberal unrealism: the viral utopia of global
   "disorder" 235
   The ideology beyond all ideologies 237
Economics: science or religion? 239
References 242

11 Humanitarian immune responses   248

Homo hubris 249
Collateral sustainability, healthy "de-growth" 252
Far beyond "One Health" 258
Progress or collapse: between the impossible and
   the unthinkable 261
Outcasts at the end of the world 265
Free radicals and the power of dissent 268
References 270

Index   276

FIGURES

0.1 The true death toll of the pandemic: estimated cumulative excess deaths vs. confirmed COVID-19 deaths in the world (Jan 1, 2020–Feb 4, 2024)   4

4.1 The surpassing: life expectancy at birth in China and in the United States (1930–2021)   95

5.1 Vaccine apartheid at the "end of the pandemic": share of people who had received at least one dose of COVID-19 vaccine on May 3, 2023   116

6.1 Lessons from the East, failures of the West: cumulative confirmed COVID-19 deaths per million people in the United States, United Kingdom, Italy, New Zealand, South Korea, Japan, Vietnam and Singapore (March 1, 2020 – February 4, 2024)   143

7.1 Lifesaving vaccination in the United States: COVID-19 weekly death rate by vaccination status (October 9, 2021 – April 1, 2023)   159

8.1 The revolution in reverse: income share of the richest 1% in the United States, the United Kingdom and Italy (1913–2021)   183

9.1 The (im)possible undertaking: carbon dioxide reductions needed to keep global temperature rise below 1.5°C   211

10.1 The longevity revolution: life expectancy at birth in the world, Italy, the United Kingdom and the United States (1543–2021)   221

10.2 Confronting historical pollution: per capita carbon dioxide emissions in the United States, China, Italy and the United Kingdom (1903–2022)   233

11.1 It takes a crisis: annual carbon dioxide emissions in the world and major economic recessions (1945–2022) 254

11.2A Long lives, low carbon: life expectancy at birth and carbon dioxide emissions per capita across countries (2019) 256

11.2B Happy lives, low carbon: life satisfaction and carbon dioxide emissions per capita across countries (2022) 257

PREFACE

On March 19, 2020, Lucetta and Carlo passed away just hours apart at the San Matteo Polyclinic in Pavia.[1] Married for many years, they lost their lives without even being able to exchange a final farewell. They surrendered to a cruel virus that had infected them both a few weeks earlier. Lucetta was a nurse, and in addition to having worked in some retirement homes in the area, every day she performed dozens of blood tests on behalf of an analysis laboratory. It is likely that she contracted the virus in this manner. After getting sick, she spent the first few days at home thinking she was treating bronchitis or a seasonal illness. However, her condition did not improve. She then turned to her family doctor, and, subjected to a swab, she tested positive for SARS-CoV-2. The next day, her husband also tested positive. Their conditions worsened, and both were admitted to the hospital where, however, the medical staff was unable to prevent their deaths a few days later. They died almost together, first he, then she. The same fate would befall two other spouses from Modena during the last days of 2020, when, within a few hours, they would leave us after fighting against the disease.[2]

These stories tell of a pandemic that took the lives of millions of people. The virus has not only left us breathless but also infected our minds and social relationships. It brought the world's economy to its knees, increased inequalities and put the social fabric of society to the test. SARS-CoV-2 proved to be a sneaky virus, often denying its victims even the chance to say goodbye. During the pandemic, we have listened to virologists, scientists and experts spouting statistics and their personal opinions about the virus, but rarely have we gotten to know the faces, personalities, emotions and experiences of those who lost their lives. Let us try to think for a moment about their names: it would take months to read them all. The question many have asked is, could we have saved them?

Some think everything possible has been done. Others believe that all measures adopted by governments to curb the virus and its impact on our health have been almost useless. Who is right? To find the answer, we must turn to the field of social epidemiology, the science that studies the distribution of deaths and diseases at the population level. Social epidemiology has a sister called public health, which is dedicated to the organized efforts of society to prevent diseases and prolong life. It is akin to saying that while social epidemiology counts the deaths, public health makes these deaths count. How? Through the systematic collection of information on the causes of mortality and its analysis to plan and guide lifesaving interventions. Mortality indicators are, indeed, our best informants on the pandemic. They clearly show which countries handled it well and those that failed. It seems paradoxical and perhaps even a little macabre but, amidst the confusion raised by virologists, journalists and self-styled experts, it is the information provided by those who died that best explains what really happened.

In the wake of a global pandemic that shook the world, this book embarks on a journey to uncover the mistakes made, to explore what could have been done differently and to discuss how to avoid future health crises. The first part addresses the ways in which we could, as a global society and individual countries, slow down the spread of the virus and avoid its most lethal effects. Why have some countries been hit hard by the pandemic and others less so? While the role of factors that have exposed countries to various degrees of danger but that do not depend on their national strategies must also be recognized, there are five categories of lethal errors that distinguished failure from success:

Unpreparedness
Misinformation
Medicalization
"Laissez-faire the virus" approach
Inequity

The analysis of errors in the management of the pandemic is not intended to trigger a sterile witch hunt or pointlessly blame some politicians or experts but to communicate a criticism at the heart of societies unprepared to prevent and face a crisis of this scale. The pandemic has laid bare the constraints of health systems overly focused on disease management and their unpreparedness in the realm of population health, often relegated to a secondary position in comparison to the more "dominant" biomedical disciplines. Unlike the latter, public health is transdisciplinary, a no man's land within the social sciences that deal with health. It studies the determinants of morbidity, mortality and longevity by synthesizing knowledge from a wide range of disciplines including sociology, economics, political science, psychology and anthropology, as well as medicine and biology. Yet, it is not comparable to any of them.

After analyzing the lethal errors in the management of the pandemic, the second part of the book investigates the vital actions that saved human lives on a large scale. Some nations have had huge success in limiting the number of COVID-19 deaths. What were their secrets? The book analyzes key national strategies of proven scientific effectiveness in reducing mortality and hospitalizations, which can be summarized in three major dimensions:

Prevention
Immunization
Support

Although a substantial portion of this book's content concerns Italy, ground zero of the health crisis in Europe, this work examines the merits and limits of several national strategies and talks about the pandemic at a global level. Globalization has created enormous challenges for modern society, including the need to conceive of and manage health problems across geographical borders. In this book, I examine strategies that could have allowed a better management of the pandemic through international cooperation and solidarity. One of the lessons we should have learned from the crisis is that to effectively manage a pandemic, a global health approach is not a choice but a necessity.

After analyzing the lethal errors and vital actions in managing COVID-19, the third part of the book focuses on what can be done to prevent future health emergencies. Since the beginning of the crisis, the scientific world has mobilized to understand where the virus came from. Most scientists are inclined to support the "natural" origin of the virus, even though the most important amplifiers of pandemic risk are anthropogenic:

Consumption and excessive exploitation of wildlife
Industrialization and intensification of animal production
Deforestation
Population explosion
Urbanization
International travel
Climate change

These pandemic risk factors share some common causes. At their root is a hubristic view of nature and a model of development that prioritizes economic growth, profit and markets before any other value of society. The collective desire to "return to normal," without dealing with the "causes of the causes" of this health crisis and the social, economic and ecological factors that determined it, is a serious obstacle to our capability to prevent future pandemics. Worse, there is an even more serious global health threat to confront: ecological collapse. If not addressed in time, it could cause consequences far worse than COVID-19.

This book advocates for an alternative approach to human progress to avoid future global health disasters and foster greater harmony among people, animals and the environment. An effective strategy against future crises requires not only a new paradigm that extends beyond the biomedical approach to comprehend global health but also profound changes to our economy, policies, behaviors and philosophy of human development. We need a powerful antidote, a humanitarian immune response to protect ourselves against future pandemics and the ecological crisis.

I'm not sure what the moment was when I decided to write this book. I had never dealt with pandemics before, even though I have dedicated almost my entire working life to the study of global health. Being stuck at home during a lockdown and realizing that almost everyone on TV had something to say on a topic familiar to me made me ponder and wonder. I felt the need and perhaps the duty to make use of what I had studied and researched in different parts of the world, in the hope of contributing to a debate too often dominated by misinformation, fake news and evidence-free opinions.

This book is aimed not only at global health experts and researchers but also at decision makers who can influence the management of new global health crises and may contribute to adopting policies capable of reducing their onset or impact. The book is also written for those who dream of a healthier and fairer world, those who dissent and those who oppose policies harming health. It is a tribute to the healthcare personnel who worked tirelessly to save the lives of others. It is aimed at those who have been directly or indirectly affected by the pandemic, those who have lost their jobs, those who have had to shut down their companies and those who have suffered the psychological and social consequences of the crisis. A thought also goes to those who ended up in intensive care and those who are still suffering from the long-term effects of the disease. Finally, the book is dedicated to the people who have left us, suffocated by a cruel virus and our collective inability to protect them.

The Italian slogan "everything will be fine" was repeated very often during the pandemic, yet without the necessary groundwork to ensure its actual happening, it failed to prevent the death of hundreds of thousands of Italians. From the regret for the lives we couldn't defend, however, emerges the hope to understand what can save others in the future, to ensure that the million victims of this pandemic did not leave us in vain.

Parleranno i morti
Di tutto quello che non siamo riusciti a capire
Di battaglie perse
Costi umani del nostro fallire

Parleranno i morti
Non chiederanno perché a loro è toccato partire
Se ne andranno in silenzio
Senza colpo ferire

**

The dead shall speak
Of what we couldn't grasp
Of lost fights
Human costs of our oversights

The dead shall speak
They won't ask about their fate
They will quietly go
Without hate

References

1. Redazione La Repubblica. Coronavirus, a Garlasco marito e moglie muoiono a poche ore di distanza: anche la figlia è positiva. La Repubblica. Published online Mar 23, 2020. https://www.repubblica.it/promo/zeropubblicita/?wt_g=ATP_OV-LFUNDC.fundchoice.0adv.TERM…&source=ATP_OVLFUNDC&ref=fndgc (accessed Jan 17, 2024).
2. Redazione ANSA. Coronavirus: marito e moglie muoiono a poche ore distanza – Notizie. Agenzia ANSA. Published online Mar 22, 2020. https://www.ansa.it/lombardia/notizie/2020/03/22/coronavirus-marito-e-moglie-muoiono-a-poche-ore-distanza_15e82b45-4abe-46a1-af99-b3c5c41a0e51.html (accessed Jan 17, 2024).

INTRODUCTION

On March 19, 2020, as Italy grappled with an alarming death toll of over 6,000 COVID-19 fatalities, a prominent virologist, a familiar face on Italian television and newspapers, reassured everyone: "Do you know how many people died only because of the coronavirus? All right. Until yesterday, do you know how many there were [while using two fingers indicating the number 2]? Today I think I have read there are 17."[1] During those same days, a well-known nanopathologist frequently featured on Italian television asserted: "there have been [only] three confirmed deaths from coronavirus."[2] Such downplaying was not isolated to "*il belpaese*." A world-renowned figure and professor of epidemiology at the University of Stanford argued that the reaction to the virus was exaggerated. On March 23, 2020, he explained: "many of these people probably would have had very limited life expectancy in the absence of such infection, and it still remains to be decided how many of these infections are deaths with SARS-CoV-2 versus deaths by SARS-CoV-2."[3]

These types of assertions may have contributed to widespread skepticism over the actual health effects of the virus. A survey of approximately 26,000 people in 25 countries conducted at the beginning of the pandemic showed that about 38% of Americans and 30% of Italians thought that the death rate of the virus has been "deliberately and greatly exaggerated."[4] The claims of experts who frequently appeared on TV casting doubt on the official death toll of the pandemic influence public discussions even today. In fact, many still wonder: was there an overestimation in reported COVID-19 fatalities? Or were these claims of inflated numbers themselves a misrepresentation of the pandemic's true death toll?

DOI: 10.4324/9781003511977-1

Did they die with or due to COVID-19?

The data capable of clearing the fog raised by these questions was already available during the first months of the health crisis. On March 28, 2020, the Italian National Institute of Statistics (ISTAT) published the mortality data of over a thousand Italian municipalities, to compare the deaths that occurred in March 2019 against those ascertained in March 2020. These numbers showed that the municipalities most affected by the coronavirus experienced a 300% increase in deaths compared to the previous year. The city of Bergamo, for example, had gone from 123 to 597 deaths, Brescia from 177 to 460, Cremona from 78 to 311 and Piacenza from 97 to 399.[5] The publication of these figures did not deter some commentators who continued to state that official data was "inflated."[6] A medical doctor argued that the numbers were "misleading" and we will have no way of knowing the real cause of these deaths because "they were all cremated and autopsies were prohibited."[7] We have also heard another expert say that "death certificates have always been inaccurate, but COVID-19 maximizes the challenge of prioritizing multiple comorbidities."[8]

In addition to some renowned health professionals, journalists and politicians, the bandwagon of skepticism was joined by famous artists and public figures. A successful US guitar player, for example, just before testing positive, observed: "They claim five hundred thousand people have died from COVID-19. Bullshit."[9] A worldwide acclaimed Italian singer swore that he had never met a person who ended up in intensive care due to the virus.[10] In July 2020 in Rome, a conference entitled "COVID-19 in Italy, between Information, Science and Rights" brought together the Italian elite of skeptics who stigmatized any preventive action by the government as "alarmist" or a symptom of a "health dictatorship." On November 19, 2020, amid the second wave, a well-known physician explained: "we made a mistake in counting the deaths, even those who had a heart attack with a positive swab were recorded as having died from COVID."[11] In October 2021, an Italian newspaper even dedicated its front page to the topic with the headline "Deaths of Everything, Not COVID." The author of the article was convinced he had produced a journalistic scoop and cited a "sensational" report by the Italian Institute of Health (ISS) which, according to the journalist, demonstrated that "only 2.9% of the deaths recorded since the end of February 2020 were [caused] by COVID-19." The corollary was that all the other people who lost their lives due to COVID-19 (96.1%) had little hope to survive anyway due to old age and pre-existing conditions.[12] In reality, the ISS report said none of this.[13] Instead, its analyses were consistent with previous research that showed COVID deaths, far from being overcounted, were vastly underestimated.[14]

Undoubtedly, advanced age and pre-existing pathologies have played an important role in these deaths. However, the most common "diseases" in patients who died due to SARS-CoV-2 include health risk factors such as hypertension and type 2 diabetes mellitus, which do not necessarily lead to premature death.[15] The same Stanford University epidemiologist quoted earlier, who also became famous for having launched a crusade against the reproducibility crisis in science, claimed: "it is very likely that many of them would have died anyhow, if not immediately within a very short period of time, because of these other causes of death that they had."[3] These claims were preposterously wrong: an analysis conducted by Scottish scientists showed that males who died of COVID-19 would have lived on average another 14 years, while women would have lived on average another 12.[16] Further research from the United States estimated that each person who died due to COVID-19 lost an average of 10 years of life expectancy.[17, 18] Another study involving 81 countries estimated a total of 16 years of life lost on average.[19]

The worst mortality crisis in the Western world since World War II

In early February 2022, I found myself participating in two Italian radio broadcasts, where the main topic of discussion revolved around what some journalists called a "controversy": the potentially inflated numbers of COVID-19 deaths.[20, 21] In the preceding days, Italian newspapers and television programs had featured commentators who were eagerly heralding the "end of the pandemic" and what they perceived as the "colding off" of the virus.[22] It was disheartening to note that during the same period, Italy recorded an average of 400 deaths per day due to SARS-CoV-2. In the previous month, the pandemic had claimed the lives of over 10,000 Italians and caused the highest number of pediatric hospitalizations ever recorded since the beginning of the pandemic not only in Italy but also in the United Kingdom and the United States. These statistics painted a grim picture of a virus that some had previously described as "mild." When called to address the age-old debate over whether individuals had "died with or from coronavirus," I simply presented the official statistics and provided an interpretation of the key findings from studies already published in international scientific literature. What did these data reveal?

They showed, very clearly, that official COVID-19 deaths were not "inflated" but, in fact, vastly underestimated. The day before my first interview, Italy reported a cumulative number of 149,512 COVID deaths. However, excess mortality amounted to 203,094 fatalities.[23, 24] Globally, the underestimation of the pandemic's true impact on mortality was even more pronounced. Estimates published in *The Lancet*[25] and *The Economist*[26] highlighted that the "true" death toll from COVID was roughly three to four times the official death toll. An editorial in *Nature* explained how epidemiologists managed to estimate the impact of the pandemic by examining excess mortality indicators in

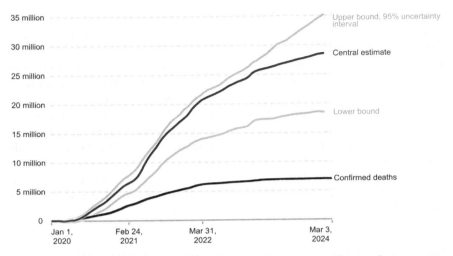

FIGURE 0.1   The true death toll of the pandemic: estimated cumulative excess deaths vs. confirmed COVID-19 deaths in the world (Jan 1, 2020–Feb 4, 2024)

Source: The Economist (2023) – processed by Our World in Data. "Central estimate." [original data]. World Health Organization – processed by Our World in Data. "Confirmed deaths" [dataset]. World Health Organization [original data]. Retrieved Feb 14, 2024 from https://ourworldindata.org/grapher/excess-deaths-cumulative-economist-single-entity

each country. In addition to considering official COVID-19 deaths, researchers compared the total number of deaths during the pandemic years to the annual average of deaths recorded over the previous five years.[27, 28] These analyses revealed that in most countries, although not universally, the official COVID-19 data fell notably short of the excess deaths recorded during the corresponding period. As of March 3, 2024, while the official worldwide COVID-19 death count was around 7 million fatalities, excess mortality figures indicated that the pandemic may have killed over 27 million people (Figure 0.1).[29]

These large discrepancies can be attributed to a multitude of factors. In numerous countries, only COVID-19 deaths that occurred within hospital settings were officially reported, and a significant portion of individuals who succumbed to the virus went untested. This issue is particularly pronounced in low-income nations with limited medical and scientific resources. However, it is essential to acknowledge that the pandemic has also exerted a profound impact on other causes of death. Various studies, for instance, have demonstrated marked increases in mortality attributed to cardiac arrest.[30–32] The most likely reasons for the escalation in deaths from other causes are the strain on emergency healthcare systems, resulting in significant delays in arranging and providing care, along with hesitation to seek hospital treatment due to fears of contracting the virus. Additionally, there has been a reduction in preventive activities, such as screening tests for potential neoplasms.

There may be other factors indirectly influenced by the pandemic that contributed to the overall increase in deaths, including health-related behaviors like increased alcohol consumption and health effects of psychosocial factors such as stress,[33] anxiety and concerns regarding one's health, economic instability and employment prospects. It's worth noting that excess mortality needs to be viewed in a broader context, and there have even been some unintended positive consequences as well. For instance, during the pandemic years there has been a decrease in the number of deaths from road accidents and workplace accidents compared to previous years, which served as counterbalances to the overall increase in mortality.

In scientific debates, areas of disagreement and uncertainty are commonplace, and it is precisely for these reasons that considerable caution is exercised before making public statements. However, what became evident from these data and studies is that assertions like "almost everyone died with the coronavirus, but not due to the coronavirus" were entirely unfounded. Nonetheless, during both of my radio interviews, the interviewers' surprise at my statements regarding the "true" death toll of the pandemic was palpable. In the days leading up to the interviews, the Italian media discourse had been dominated by fake news on COVID-19 data, and some even claimed that data were manipulated. The undersecretary of health of the Italian government, for example, expressed doubts about the authenticity of COVID-19 deaths. A virologist argued that it no longer made sense to count COVID positives[34] and added: "enough with the evening bulletin. The way we count patients must be changed."[35] Even an epidemiologist, whose discipline is founded on the systematic collection and interpretation of mortality data, joined the chorus, launching a bizarre proposal: "recording infections? Let's stop counting them!"[36]

Scientific information and data have been pivotal in helping us comprehend the true extent of the pandemic's impact on public health. As highlighted in the World Health Statistics 2021, COVID-19 has led to the worst mortality crisis in Europe and in the United States since World War II.[37] In the hardest-hit nations, the pandemic has become one of the leading causes of death, significantly reducing life expectancy,[38] with enduring effects that are not yet fully understood. In addition to millions of deaths and hospitalizations, the virus has given rise to a range of long-term symptoms called "long COVID,"[39] along with psychological problems, psychiatric illnesses and neurological conditions.[40] It is thanks to the dedication of those who analyze data, develop statistics and interpret them based on solid theoretical and scientific knowledge that we have acquired information essential to comprehend and contain the pandemic. Depriving ourselves of this information is unwise. Instead of advocating for the cessation of data collection, wouldn't it have been more appropriate if some virologists had simply stopped "spouting numbers"?

COVID-19 strategies: healthy nations and "failed" states

The pandemic has left no continent untouched. Yet, its impact has been vastly divergent across nations. Countries that failed to adopt effective prevention interventions, such as Italy, the United States, and the United Kingdom, have witnessed significant reductions in life expectancy at birth. The mortality crisis has left particularly tragic imprints on several other European nations, including Bosnia, Bulgaria, Romania, Spain, and France. The health emergency has also taken a heavy toll in Latin America, where Peru, Chile and Brazil have been hit very hard. The Russian Federation too has grappled with the overwhelming impact of the pandemic. While official statistics of some developing countries, like India, seem to indicate that they have been only minimally affected, it's important to note that epidemiological data in these regions have been disproportionately biased by underreporting issues.[41]

Not all countries have succumbed to the full impact of the health crisis. There are nations, such as New Zealand, Australia and Norway, that experienced a reduction, rather than an increase, in mortality during the pandemic.[42] Several other countries in East Asia, like Taiwan, Vietnam, Singapore, Japan and South Korea, have also effectively limited the most devastating effects of the virus.[25] Among European nations that experienced a lower than average mortality crisis due to COVID-19, there are Denmark and, to some extent, Germany. In the Americas, Canada stands out as a country that has been able, to some degree, to mitigate the impact of the health emergency.

What did more successful countries do to achieve more favorable results? This book aims to investigate this question in detail, but before doing so, it's important to acknowledge the presence of national characteristics that can explain differences in COVID-19 mortality which cannot be attributed to the merits or demerits of preventive interventions. Comparing nations in terms of their responses to the pandemic is indeed a challenging task. Numerous risk and protective factors determine a country's vulnerability or capability to reduce the health effects of the pandemic. One of the most obvious is the average age of the population. For example, Italy, with the oldest population in Europe and over 22% of its residents aged 65 and above, started from a position of clear disadvantage when facing a virus that disproportionately affects older individuals. There are countries like Japan, however, with a higher proportion of elderly residents than Italy, which have achieved relatively favorable COVID-19 mortality indicators.

Geographical location can also play a crucial role as a protective factor against the pandemic. Countries that are geographically isolated or are islands have a distinct advantage in controlling the virus within their borders. Notable examples include Taiwan, New Zealand and Iceland. Nevertheless, being surrounded by the sea does not guarantee automatic success in virus control, as evidenced by the abysmal COVID-19 failure of the United Kingdom.

Population density is another significant characteristic influencing a country's capability to manage a pandemic. There is a strong and positive correlation between population density and mortality due to COVID-19 among European nations. Countries with low population density, like Iceland, Finland and Norway, managed the crisis better. Conversely, countries with high population density, such as Belgium, Slovenia, Italy and the United Kingdom, have had very high COVID-19 mortality rates per million inhabitants. This dimension, however, doesn't seem to be significant for East Asian countries with the highest population density in the world, such as Singapore, Vietnam, Japan and South Korea. These nations have experienced some of the lowest COVID-19 death rates per million inhabitants globally.

To understand why different countries have responded differently to the pandemic, it is relevant to also scrutinize the quality of care and support provided by national healthcare systems. It's undeniable that the pandemic has laid bare various weaknesses and limitations of national healthcare systems. Safeguarding the health of a population from a pandemic necessitates a universal healthcare system, public administration of the hospital network and the timely implementation of health protection, such as the provision of personal protective equipment (PPE) for healthcare workers. In the effort to explain the high levels of COVID-19 mortality, some have turned to the hypothesis that hospital bed saturation is a key indicator for assessing a healthcare system's response to COVID-19. However, among the countries that have best managed the pandemic, we find nations with a modest number of intensive care beds per capita, such as New Zealand, Japan, Denmark and Norway.

Additionally, researchers have attempted to account for different countries' vulnerability to COVID-19 mortality by exploring genetic heritage. A study published in *Nature* suggested that a primary genetic risk factor for severe COVID-19 symptoms and hospitalization is a gene cluster prevalent in approximately 50% of people in southern Asia and around 16% of people in Europe. It is nearly absent in eastern Asia, however. This genetic trait's high prevalence in countries like Australia, which has seen relatively few COVID-19 deaths compared to other nations, weakens this hypothesis considerably.[43] Moreover, this genetic factor does not align with the scientific evidence showing higher COVID-19 mortality rates among people of African ancestry than among those of other ethnic backgrounds, even after considering geographic and socioeconomic factors.[44] As some authors explained, "social inequality and its consequences appear to explain a greater proportion of the risk of death from COVID-19 than Neanderthal-derived DNA."[45]

Other factors that influenced a country's capability to attenuate SARS-CoV-2's death toll include temperature, climate, humidity, people's mobility, the proportion of workers in informal sectors and socioeconomic conditions. All these factors may have played a significant role in explaining cross-national differences in COVID-19 mortality indicators. Yet, there are some even more important dimensions capable of explaining why some countries succeeded or failed in controlling the deadly impact of the virus: the lethal errors and vital actions of their COVID-19 containment strategies. The first part of the book deals with the former, the second with the latter.

References

1. Marco Montemagno. Quattro chiacchiere con Ilaria Capua (Director One Health Center of Excellence, University of Florida). YouTube. https://www.youtube.com/watch?v=z9WsX3hdCyU&ab_channel=MarcoMontemagno (accessed Jan 17, 2024).
2. Gerbella M. Coronavirus? Una bufala, i morti sono 3. C'è dietro un business di Big Pharma. Affaritaliani.it. Published online Mar 21, 2020. https://www.affaritaliani.it/cronache/coronavirus-una-bufala-660556.html (accessed Jan 17, 2024).
3. Perspectives on the pandemic: Dr John Ioannidis of Stanford University, Episode 1. Dailymotion. Published online June 5, 2020. https://www.dailymotion.com/video/x7ubcws (accessed Jan 19, 2024).
4. Henley J, McIntyre N. Survey uncovers widespread belief in 'dangerous' Covid conspiracy theories. *The Guardian*. Published online Oct 26, 2020. https://www.theguardian.com/world/2020/oct/26/survey-uncovers-widespread-belief-dangerous-covid-conspiracy-theories (accessed Jan 27, 2024).
5. Istituto Nazionale di Statistica. Decessi e cause di morte: cosa produce l'Istat. https://www.istat.it/it/archivio/240401 (accessed Jan 19, 2024).
6. Pagella Politica. "I numeri dei morti in Italia sono gonfiati!": così gli argomenti (sbagliati) di Sgarbi alla Camera sono stati ripresi in tutto il mondo. https://pagellapolitica.it/articoli/i-numeri-dei-morti-in-italia-sono-gonfiati-cosi-gli-argomenti-sbagliati-di-sgarbi-alla-camera-sono-stati-ripresi-in-tutto-il-mondo (accessed Jan 19, 2024).
7. Avvenire. Gismondo: "Fuorvianti i numeri sui morti da Covid-19." https://www.avvenire.it/attualita/pagine/linfluenza-non-banale-ma-quelli-forniti-dal-governo-rimangono-numeri-fuo (accessed Jan 19, 2024).
8. Ioannidis JPA. Over - and under-estimation of COVID-19 deaths. *European Journal of Epidemiology* 2021; **36**: 581–8.
9. Mel Q, Brogan K, Ioannidis J "What exactly did the virus do to all these people?" Reflections on Ted Nugent,. Science-Based Medicine. Published online June 18,

2021. https://sciencebasedmedicine.org/what-exactly-did-the-virus-do-to-all-these-people-reflections-on-ted-nugent-mel-q-kelly-brogan-and-john-ioannidis/ (accessed Jan 27, 2024).

10. Repubblica TV. Convegno dei 'negazionisti del Covid', Bocelli: 'Io, umiliato e offeso dalla privazione della libertà durante il lockdown'. Published online July 27, 2020. https://video.repubblica.it/politica/convegno-dei-negazionisti-del-covid-bocelli-io-umiliato-e-offeso-dalla-privazione-della-liberta-durante-il-lockdown/364715/365267 (accessed Jan 19, 2024).

11. Corriere TV. Bassetti: "Abbiamo sbagliato a contare i decessi, anche chi aveva un infarto con un tampone positivo veniva registrato come morto per Covid". Published online Jan 19, 2024. https://video.corriere.it/cronaca/bassetti-abbiamo-sbagliato-contare-decessi-anche-chi-aveva-infarto-un-tampone-positivo-veniva-registrato-come-morto-covid/3ec83d10-2a5d-11eb-a3fb-78126c23822f (accessed Jan 19, 2024).

12. Roberto De Vogli. Morti con o per il coronavirus? L'apice degli errori sul tema è stato raggiunto in questi giorni. *Il Fatto Quotidiano*. Published online Oct 25, 2021. https://www.ilfattoquotidiano.it/2021/10/25/morti-con-o-per-il-coronavirus-lapice-degli-errori-sul-tema-e-stato-raggiunto-in-questi-giorni/6366640/ (accessed Jan 19, 2024).

13. Istituto Superiore di Sanità. Pubblicato il quinto Rapporto sui decessi ISTAT-ISS. https://www.iss.it/news/-/asset_publisher/gJ3hFqMQsykM/content/pubblicato-il-quinto-rapporto-sui-decessi-istat-iss (accessed Jan 19, 2024).

14. Rizzo M, Foresti L, Montano N. Comparison of reported deaths from COVID-19 and increase in total mortality in Italy. *JAMA Internal Medicine* 2020; **180**: 1250–2.

15. Istituto Superiore di Sanità. Caratteristiche dei pazienti deceduti positivi all'infezione da SARS-CoV-2 in Italia. EpiCentro. Published online Mar 30, 2021. https://www.epicentro.iss.it/coronavirus/bollettino/Report-COVID-2019_30_marzo_2021.pdf (accessed Jan 19, 2024).

16. Hanlon P, Chadwick F, Shah A, *et al.* COVID-19 – Exploring the implications of long-term condition type and extent of multicomorbidity on years of life lost.l Wellcome Open Research. https://wellcomeopenresearch.org/articles/5-75 (accessed Jan 19, 2024).

17. University of South Florida. Death counts fail to capture full mortality effects of COVID-19, study finds. Science Daily. https://www.sciencedaily.com/releases/2020/09/200923124557.htm (accessed Jan 19, 2024).

18. Woolf SH, Chapman DA, Lee JH. COVID-19 as the leading cause of death in the United States. *JAMA* 2021; **325**: 123–4.

19. Pifarré i Arolas H, Acosta E, López-Casasnovas G, *et al.* Years of life lost to COVID-19 in 81 countries. *Scientific Reports* 2021; **11**: 3504.

20. Zapping Radio 1. RaiPlaySound. Published online Feb 8, 2022. https://www.raiplaysound.it/audio/2022/02/Zapping-Radio-1-del-08022022-91d44b6f-ebe6-46a4-bafd-08ac79137884.html (accessed Jan 19, 2024).

21. Prisma di mer. Radio Popolare. Published online Feb 9, 2022. https://www.radiopopolare.it/podcast/prisma-di-mer-09-02-22/ (accessed Jan 19, 2024).

22. Il Fatto Quotidiano. Covid, l'epidemiologo Icardi: 'Con Omicron e vaccinazioni ci aspettiamo che il virus in un paio di mesi si autolimiti e ci porti fuori da pandemia'. Published online Jan 4, 2022. https://www.ilfattoquotidiano.it/2022/01/04/covid-lepidemiologo-icardi-con-omicron-e-vaccinazioni-ci-aspettiamo-che-il-virus-in-un-paio-di-mesi-si-autolimiti-e-ci-porti-fuori-da-pandemia/6444185/ (accessed Jan 19, 2024).

23. The Economist – processed by Our World in Data. Estimated cumulative excess deaths during COVID. Our World Data. https://ourworldindata.org/grapher/excess-deaths-cumulative-economist?country=~ITA (accessed Jan 19, 2024).

24. Istituto Nazionale di Statistica. Andamento dei decessi 2015–2022. https://public.tableau.com/views/Andamentodeidecessi2015-2021_/Andamentodeidecessi?%3Adisplay_static_image=y&%3AbootstrapWhenNotified=true&%3Aembed=true&%3Alanguage=en-US&:embed=y&:showVizHome=n&:apiID=host0#navType=0&navSrc=Parse (accessed Jan 19, 2024).
25. Wang H, Paulson KR, Pease SA, *et al*. Estimating excess mortality due to the COVID-19 pandemic: a systematic analysis of COVID-19-related mortality, 2020–21. *The Lancet* 2022; **399**: 1513–36.
26. The Economist. The pandemic's true death toll. Published online Oct 25, 2022. https://www.economist.com/graphic-detail/coronavirus-excess-deaths-estimates (accessed Jan 19, 2024).
27. Adam D. The pandemic's true death toll: millions more than official counts. *Nature* 2022; **601**: 312–5.
28. Islam N, Shkolnikov VM, Acosta RJ, *et al*. Excess deaths associated with Covid-19 pandemic in 2020: age and sex disaggregated time series analysis in 29 high income countries. *BMJ* 2021; **373**: n1137.
29. The Economist – processed by Our World in Data. Estimated cumulative excess deaths during COVID-19. https://ourworldindata.org/grapher/excess-deaths-cumulative-economist-single-entity (accessed Jan 19, 2024).
30. Chan PS, Girotra S, Tang Y, Al-Araji R, Nallamothu BK, McNally B. Outcomes for out-of-hospital cardiac arrest in the United States during the coronavirus disease 2019 pandemic. *JAMA Cardiology* 2021; **6**: 296–303.
31. Eloi M, Nicole K, Daniel J, *et al*. Out-of-hospital cardiac arrest during the COVID-19 pandemic in Paris, France: a population-based, observational study. *The Lancet Public Health*. 2020; **5**: e437–43.
32. Baldi E, Sechi GM, Mare C, *et al*. Out-of-hospital cardiac arrest during the Covid-19 outbreak in Italy. *The New England Journal of Medicine* 2020; **383**: 496–8.
33. Wadhera RK, Shen C, Gondi S, Chen S, Kazi DS, Yeh RW. Cardiovascular deaths during the COVID-19 pandemic in the United States. *Journal of the American College of Cardiology* 2021; **77**: 159–69.
34. La Repubblica. Il report quotidiano diventa un caso, Bassetti: 'Non ha più senso, anche i dati dei deceduti sono falsati'. Published online Jan 11, 2022. https://genova.repubblica.it/cronaca/2022/01/11/news/bassetti_basta_con_il_report_quotidiano_sui_contagi_non_ha_piu_senso_il_sottosegretario_alla_salute_costa_ha_ragione_-333431697/ (accessed Jan 19, 2024).
35. Agenzia Dire. Covid, Bassetti: 'Basta col bollettino serale. Il conteggio dei malati va cambiato'. Published online Jan 11, 2022. https://www.dire.it/11-01-2022/697938-covid-bassetti-basta-col-bollettino-serale-il-conteggio-dei-malati-va-cambiato/ (accessed Jan 19, 2024).
36. Il Fatto Quotidiano. Omicron, Lopalco a La7: 'Record di contagi? Smettiamo di contarli. Non è assolutamente un raffreddore ma vanno abbassati i toni'. Published online Jan 5, 2022. https://www.ilfattoquotidiano.it/2022/01/05/omicron-lopalco-a-la7-record-di-contagi-smettiamo-di-contarli-non-e-assolutamente-un-raffreddore-ma-vanno-abbassati-i-toni/6446069/ (accessed Jan 19, 2024).
37. World Health Organization (WHO). World health statistics 2021: monitoring health for the SDGs, sustainable development goals. 2024. https://www.who.int/publications-detail-redirect/9789240027053 (accessed Jan 19, 2024).
38. Huang G, Guo F, Zimmermann KF, *et al*. The effect of the COVID-19 pandemic on life expectancy in 27 countries. *Scientific Reports* 2023; **13**: 8911.
39. Davis HE, McCorkell L, Vogel JM, Topol EJ. Long COVID: major findings, mechanisms and recommendations. *Nature Reviews Microbiology* 2023; **21**: 133–46.

40. Xie Y, Xu E, Al-Aly Z. Risks of mental health outcomes in people with Covid-19: cohort study. *BMJ* 2022; 376: e068993.
41. Taylor L. Covid-19: true global death toll from pandemic is almost 15 million, says WHO. *BMJ* 2022; 377: o1144.
42. Woolf SH, Masters RK, Aron LY. Effect of the Covid-19 pandemic in 2020 on life expectancy across populations in the USA and other high income countries: simulations of provisional mortality data. *BMJ* 2021; 373: n1343.
43. Zeberg H, Pääbo S. The major genetic risk factor for severe COVID-19 is inherited from Neanderthals. *Nature* 2020; 587: 610–2.
44. Irizar P, Pan D, Kapadia D, *et al*. Ethnic inequalities in COVID-19 infection, hospitalisation, intensive care admission, and death: a global systematic review and meta-analysis of over 200 million study participants. *eClinicalMedicine* 2023; 57.
45. Luo Y. Neanderthal DNA highlights complexity of COVID risk factors. *Nature* 2020; 587: 552–3.

PART I
Lethal errors

1

UNPREPAREDNESS

"If you fail to plan, you are planning to fail."

Benjamin Franklin

Former Italian Prime Minister Giuseppe Conte was not entirely wrong when he defined the pandemic as "an unprecedented crisis."[1] Similarly, there is some degree of truth in the words of the former Director of Health Planning of the Italian Ministry of Health, Andrea Urbani, when he compared the pandemic to a "tsunami that hit Italy as the first country in Europe."[2] The virus really caught the world off guard, and most countries, even the most economically advanced, were ill prepared.[3] The pandemic has often been compared to a black swan, drawing from the metaphor popularized by Nicholas Taleb's best-selling book. In the upgraded version of the Italian pandemic preparedness plan, for example, zoonoses are described as random, accidental events of a "capricious nature."[4] But is this really the case?

The white swan

Those who called the pandemic a "black swan" may not have fully considered Taleb's opinion. For the Lebanese-American essayist, the COVID-19 health crisis did not have the characteristics of an exceptionally unpredictable event.[5] Experts on emerging infectious diseases share a similar view: even though SARS-CoV-2 appeared suddenly and seemingly without prior warnings, it was largely predictable. While the proximal factors capable of triggering pandemics are very hard to foresee, the historical factors that influence these phenomena are relatively easy to recognize. Many scientists

DOI: 10.4324/9781003511977-3

have repeatedly explained where these pandemic dangers originate and expressed their disappointment with their governments' unpreparedness. None predicted the exact timing of the COVID-19 pandemic, but many have, for years, warned of its possible occurrence. The words of David Quammen, written in black and white in *Spillover* back in 2013, are astonishing: "there is no reason to believe that AIDS will remain the only global disaster of our time caused by a strange microbe that jumped out of an animal. Some well-informed Cassandras even speak of the Next Big One, the next big event, as an inevitable fact. Will it be caused by a virus? Will it manifest itself in the rainforest or in a city market in southern China?"[6] Michael Osterholm, author of *Deadliest Enemy: Our War Against Killer Germs*, written almost 20 years before the outbreak of the health crisis, sounded prophetic too: "this is a tipping point in history. Time is running out to prepare for the next pandemic. We must act now with decision and determination." He also added: "The arrival of a pandemic flu would trigger a reaction that would change the world overnight. A vaccine would not be available for a number of months after the start of the pandemic and there are very limited supplies of antiviral drugs … Foreign trade and travel would be reduced or even ended in an attempt to prevent the virus from entering new countries … The global, regional and national economies would come to a screeching halt, something that has never happened because of HIV, malaria or tuberculosis despite their dramatic impact on the developing world."[7] In a similar vein, Larry Brilliant, a physician with experience in epidemiology and one of the leaders of the anti-smallpox campaign, explained in 2009 that "the threat of deadly new viruses is increasing due to population growth, climate change, and increased contact between humans and animals. What the world needs to do is prepare."[8]

The growing pandemic risk could also be observable from the increasingly frequent crises caused by viruses such as HIV, SARS-CoV-1, MERS and Ebola and the exponential growth of social and environmental factors that increase their likelihood.[9] Among scientists, there was significant concern regarding the arrival of a respiratory pathogen with a short incubation period that could be transmitted without symptoms.[10] In short, public health researchers who devoted their entire careers to studying emerging infectious diseases knew very well that a global health event like the COVID-19 pandemic was not only predictable but inevitable. The question was not whether a new pandemic could happen but when.[11]

Scientists' concerns about the risk of new global pandemics had generated numerous warnings that were never taken too seriously. As noted by the Independent Commission on Pandemics at the World Health Organization (WHO), "since the 2009 H1N1 influenza pandemic, at least 11 high-level committees and commissions have made specific recommendations in 16 reports to improve global pandemic preparedness … However, most recommendations were ignored."[12] A question that will probably remain un-answered is whether the SARS-CoV-2 disaster could have been averted. The authors of another WHO report on national and global responses to the health crisis believe so: "the COVID-19 pandemic could have been avoided. [But] a toxic cocktail of denial, poor choices and lack of coordination have thrown the world into a catastrophe."[13] It is extremely difficult to estimate the consequences of the initial inaction by so many governments and the delayed response by China during the early phases of the crisis. Yet, many experts share the sentiment that initiating preventive strategies earlier could have fundamentally altered the course of the pandemic. As one of them noted, "outbreaks are inevitable, pandemics optional."[14]

An important first step to better control future health emergencies is to understand that as all risk factors increase, so does the likelihood of their occurrence. If they have a high likelihood to occur, they are just another "white swan." In an attempt to highlight the great successes of modern society in reducing mortality, some intellectuals may have taken for granted that there has been a "conquest of infectious diseases in Europe and America."[15] Unfortunately, most infectious diseases have not been "conquered." They remain serious threats that we must keep preparing for.

Once upon a time there were pandemic plans

One of the most critical features of effective pandemic management is time-liness. Public health scientists explain that, if preventive actions are carried out early, their effectiveness significantly increases.[16] If they are adopted late, however, controlling the spread of the virus becomes problematic. Once the window of opportunity to stop a pandemic in its early stages has closed, it becomes difficult, if not impossible, to reopen it. When prevention fails due to a delayed response, the remaining options are unappealing, such as adopting a national lockdown. Of course, timeliness depends on the level of preparedness, as well as the capability of national and global epidemiological surveillance systems to identify and target outbreaks in an effective manner. As Jeremy Farrar, the author of the book *Spike: The Virus vs the People – the Inside Story,* observed, smarter surveillance is key because "if you don't look, you don't see. If you don't see, you will always respond too late."[17]

In recent decades, major institutions responsible for global health protection have urged governments to prepare for new pandemics. For instance, the WHO Global Influenza Strategy 2019–2030 encouraged nations to improve surveillance and early response capabilities to pathogenic events through models aimed at estimating the risk of influenza pandemics, using tools such as the Tool for Influenza Pandemic Risk Assessment (TIPRA).[18] Alongside the World Bank, the WHO also established the Global Preparedness Monitoring

Board, another body responsible for assisting countries in their preparation for global health crises.[19] Since 2005, the WHO has also been asking governments to establish, implement and maintain a national action plan to respond promptly and effectively to public health risks of international concern.[20] It also persuaded many of them to update their plan every three years.

To assess the readiness of nations, researchers at Johns Hopkins University developed the Global Health Security Index. Unfortunately, this index failed to assess the effectiveness of national responses to the COVID-19 crisis. Based on this indicator, the United States ranked number one out of 195 countries in terms of pandemic preparedness. Yet, the American death toll proved that the country completely failed to manage the health emergency. While this index has shown clear limitations in predicting countries' response effectiveness,[21] it's crucial to recognize that national governments' response to a pandemic largely depends on the political willingness to "follow the (public health) science." Regrettably, this was not the case for numerous economically rich nations that, in theory, possessed advanced public health knowledge and solid scientific expertise to combat the pandemic. In practice, however, such an advantage ended up being inconsequential.

Despite repeated warnings, when the COVID-19 crisis broke out, many countries were completely unprepared, and only a few had updated their pandemic plans. After initially underestimating the problem, governments finally began adopting prevention interventions, but did so late and in an improvised manner. The United States serves as a stark example of a nation where the idea of preventing pandemics was not taken seriously. In the years before the emergence of COVID-19, the Trump administration not only disregarded recommendations for global health preparedness but also fired the entire team of researchers and experts tasked with monitoring pandemic outbreaks, including Prof. Alexander Azar, the so-called Global Health Czar. As Jeffrey Shaman of Columbia University pointed out, the dissolution of the entire unit responsible for global health and security in the country is "not just ineptitude. It's sabotage."[22] The complete disregard of prevention by the Trump administration and former Vice President Mike Pence is destined to be remembered as one of the most embarrassing instances of mismanagement in the field of public health. However, as noted in an editorial in the *Journal of Epidemiology and Community Health*, the lack of preparedness and reluctance to take decisive actions against the virus were prevalent not just in the United States but throughout the Western world.[23]

Most likely, leaders of economically advanced countries did not expect a virus so dangerous to be capable of spreading by air, through commercial and tourist travel, thereby posing a threat to even the most privileged segments of the global society. There may have been an assumption that viruses capable of triggering health crises like Ebola, SARS and MERS would predominantly afflict poor countries, perhaps in some remote rural areas.

SARS-CoV-2 indeed represented a unique virus, notably distinct from previous ones, particularly in its severity and impact on affluent, interconnected cities like Milan, London, Madrid and New York, especially during the early stages of the pandemic. Perhaps, as Taiwan's Minister of Health, Chen Shih-chung, pointed out, Western countries seemed to downplay the virus in its initial phases maybe because they were driven by their unwavering belief in their advanced medical technologies and healthcare system.[24]

The "Italian job": a model to imitate?

In the summer of 2020, the Italian government was widely praised in the international press, as well as by the WHO, for its apparently effective strategy in containing COVID-19.[25,26] Some journalists wrote that the nation deserved particular admiration for having taught the rest of the world how to "defeat" the virus. Others considered Italy even as a model to emulate. Indeed, according to a research analysis published in *Nature*, Italy's lockdown, one of the longest and strictest in the world, did save the lives of hundreds of thousands of people.[27] Riding on the wave of these flattering reviews, the then Minister of Health, Roberto Speranza, decided to share the details of the Italian pandemic response by writing a book titled *Why We Will Heal: From the Toughest Days to a New Concept of Health*. The book, which lauded the actions directed by the minister himself, stated that the country had "bent the curve of infection with … courageous choices, with the fundamental collaboration of citizens … and a serious teamwork by the entire government." The book also emphasized that we should all remember July 2020 as "the moment when everything changed." The former minister elaborated on the elements that, in his opinion, were key for the "defeat" of the pandemic: "The country essentially doubled the number of intensive care units in just a few months … Today, we are better able to control the course of infections because we have increased the number of tests conducted."[28]

But what really changed in July 2020? Perhaps Speranza's *speranza*, which in Italian means hope, was that the pandemic had already ended. Unfortunately, the virus did not cooperate. The image of Italy as a model to emulate was completely shattered by the death toll of the second wave. The situation was almost as dire as in the first wave. In November 2020, Filippo Anelli, President of the National Federation of Medical Doctors, made an appeal for a new lockdown, stating that the healthcare system was on the verge of collapse.[29] The presentation of the book *Why We Will Heal*, supposed to be released on October 22, 2020, was suspended, and the copies already in circulation disappeared from Italian bookstores. Minister Speranza had one thing right, though: July 2020 was indeed a date when everything could have truly changed. In theory, it was the right moment to adopt a truly effective prevention strategy capitalizing on the results achieved after the lockdown.

In practice, it did not happen. During the summer of 2020, the opinions of those virologists who declared that "the emergency is over" prevailed. The country practically "went back to normal." By the beginning of the fall, it was overwhelmed by the virus again.

Italy suffered a staggering death toll because of COVID-19. It is among the hardest-hit nations in the Western world, not a model to emulate. The Italian government did partly redeem itself later, thanks to an excellent immunization campaign that achieved one of the highest vaccination rates with boosters in Europe.[30] However, the goal of limiting the damage and saving as many lives as possible until the arrival of pharmaceutical measures had failed. Preventive interventions were poorly implemented, adopted late and not based on the best available evidence and global practices that required early testing, effective contact tracing and isolation with support.

The country's lack of preparedness to fight the pandemic was evident. In line with the technical recommendations of the WHO, Italy had developed a national plan for preparedness and response against influenza in 2006.[31] However, most of the actions aimed at preparing the nation to adequately address new emerging infectious diseases such as COVID-19 did not take place. Worse, from 2006 until the outbreak of the health crisis, the pandemic plan was not updated and remained based on outdated technical know-how. Such unpreparedness was not even recognized as a problem by most Italian health institutions. According to an editorial that appeared in *The Guardian*, Italy had even tried to "deceive ... the WHO [and] the EU [as well as itself] ... by claiming to have capabilities that, in light of the facts, it did not have."[32]

The controversy over Italy's real preparedness to handle the pandemic turned into a full-blown diplomatic crisis after the publication of a report by the European division of the WHO based in Venice, titled "An Unprecedented Challenge: Italy's First Response to COVID-19." The report not only highlighted that the pandemic plan had not been updated for 14 years but also described Italy's pandemic management as "creative, chaotic, amateurish, and improvised."[33] It was the last nail in the coffin of the myth that depicted the Italian COVID-19 management strategy as a "success." Like Speranza's book, shortly after its release, the WHO report was swiftly removed from public scrutiny and even disappeared from the organization's website. This time, however, the retraction was not triggered by a decision of the author but was an effect of political pressure. Predictably, the document had created considerable embarrassment not only for the Italian government but also for the WHO's Deputy Director, Ranieri Guerra, who had previously served as the Director of Prevention of the Italian Ministry of Health from 2014 to 2017. In fact, he was one of the top officials in charge of updating the 14-year-old pandemic plan.

The media storm turned into a hurricane after an Italian TV program published some internal email exchanges between Ranieri Guerra and a representative of the Italian Ministry of Health. Two statements stood out. The first regarded the need to hide the lack of updates to the pandemic plan from the public to avoid tarnishing Minister Speranza's image. This happened after a 10-million-euro contribution from the Italian government in favor of the WHO. The second pointed fingers at some "disastrous decisions" such as the "scrapping" of the Italian National Center for Epidemiology, Surveillance, and Health Promotion (CNESPS).[34] The decision to shut down the center, just a few years before the outbreak of the pandemic, was taken unilaterally without proper consideration of the effects such an action could entail in terms of the country's expertise in prevention capability to confront health crises. The closure of CNESPS had sparked numerous protests. Many health professionals strongly opposed the center's elimination, and hundreds of them had written a public letter published by the Italian magazine *Quotidiano Sanità*.[35] According to the authors of the appeal, the CNESPS played a strategic role in supporting local public health functions such as the prevention and control of infectious and chronic diseases as well as the analysis of behavioral risk factors and health promotion. The signatories of the letter also argued that it was thanks to the initiatives of the CNESPS that local access to information and monitoring systems for many preventable diseases was possible. These data collection and surveillance systems allowed for not only national but also regional planning and evaluation of public health activities and elaborated information aimed at increasing citizens' ability to make virtuous decisions about their health.[34]

The shutdown of the CNESP was indeed an ill-conceived decision. Pandemic plans are of little use if there are no institutions capable of coordinating epidemiology and health protection activities in the communities. Nations that have better contained the pandemic established effective epidemiological surveillance systems, in addition to investing in infrastructure and technologies to coordinate prevention actions such as testing and contact tracing. In April 2020, I asked Ranieri Guerra (who contacted me via social media) why the Italian office of the WHO he directed, as well as the COVID-19 Italian Technical Scientific Committee (CTS) of which was a member of, had not tried to adopt more vigorous prevention policies, perhaps learning from the lessons offered by countries such as South Korea, Taiwan and Vietnam.[36] He basically told me not to raise "useless polemics." The "polemic" was anything but "useless": timely prevention activities such as testing, contact tracing and isolation with support proved to be crucial in saving lives, especially before the arrival of vaccines, but also after. As noted in an editorial by Alessandro Mantovani, however, Ranieri Guerra seemed more interested in his political power than in public health interventions that could have avoided the deaths of tens of thousands of Italians.[37] The scandal caused by the leaked emails, the forced withdrawal of the WHO report and the outrage derived from the failure to update the pandemic plan, together with the involvement of the city of Bergamo prosecutor's office, was followed by Ranieri Guerra's resignation from the position of Deputy Director of the WHO.

At the beginning of 2021, after so much political and media heat, the Ministry of Health finally decided to quickly move on the process of updating the Italian pandemic plan. On that occasion, a colleague and I co-authored an editorial in the magazine *Il Sole 24 Ore* to comment on its strengths and weaknesses. The updated version of the plan emphasized the importance of using masks and personal protective equipment and increasing the number of intensive care beds. It also envisaged the provision of national stocks of antiviral drugs and the continuous training of healthcare workers.[38] The plan contained significant improvements in terms of preparedness and better protection of healthcare workers. However, even the updated version of the plan did not sufficiently enhance the importance of preventive strategies at a community level such as network testing and contact tracing. It did not sufficiently emphasize activities aimed at reducing the danger of infections in schools, workplaces and other closed environments and did not even mention the role of social inequalities in determining different vulnerability and exposure to contagion between different social classes. The approach used was firmly anchored to a biomedical, reductionist model of health which viewed health as the "absence of disease." The upgraded plan does not adequately prepare the nation to face new pandemics. Moreover, as mentioned in the editorial, the actions outlined in it may enable Italy to respond to emerging health crises, but not to predict and prevent them.[39]

Every time the pandemic "ended"

"I said some time ago, and I repeat it, that as of May 31 [2020] the virus is clinically dead."[40] When these words were uttered by a renowned Italian physician and personal doctor of former Prime Minister of Italy Silvio Berlusconi, many believed them. After one of the strictest lockdowns ever, Italians were anxious to consider the health crisis gone and done. Regrettably, the virus disagreed. Since the day these words were uttered, Italy buried more than 100,000 corpses because of COVID-19. Berlusconi's personal physician, now president of the soccer team I have been supporting since childhood, Genoa, will probably be remembered for this shining blunder. However, his foreign counterparts didn't hesitate to publicly share similar failed predictions, either. In March 2020, an American pediatrician specialized in infectious disease argued: "I can't imagine, frankly, that it would cause even one-tenth of the damage that influenza causes every year in the United States."[41] In May 2020, a professor from the University of Oxford assured that "the epidemic is going away."[42] In a similar vein, a well-known Italian academic working at Emory

University echoed an analogous refrain: "the virus is going away, at a rapid pace, and we are happy to accompany it to the door."[43]

An Italian medical doctor ventured to provide an explanation as to why the virus would have gone away so quickly: it was "emptying itself."[44] A similar but less weird argument was presented by another expert: "Here is a fact that we were all waiting for and that some of us had widely predicted already three months ago. After the reduced viral load, here is the demonstration that SARS-CoV-2 has mutated."[45] There was no shortage of these types of "contributions" even from members of the team in charge of directing the pandemic containment strategy, the Italian Technical Scientific Committee (CTS), a body made up of 20 experts. During the same period, one of them explained: "There is growing and clear evidence ... that the virus has lost strength, as happens in the history of epidemics."[46] Later, in October 2020, another CTS member downplayed a clear exponential curve of new infections and intensive care unit admissions by stating that it was not "exponential."[47] Perhaps he was misled by what some experts call the "exponential growth bias," or underestimated the growth speed of an exponential curve due to too much focus on the linear growth of cases before the threshold beyond which infections tend to increase faster.[48]

Absolutely convinced of the "weakening" of the virus, in June 2020 a dozen Italian experts signed what some Italian journalists called "the end of the emergency" report.[49] One of the authors labeled those who feared a new increase of infections as "catastrophists."[50] As another virologist argued, "I don't believe in a second wave; we just have to apply the criteria of surveillance and control of the territory to start living again."[51] In the opinion of these experts, the priority was not to prepare for a new resurgence of infections, as predicted by many public health experts, but just to "stop the fear."[52] "There will not be a second wave," another expert assured.[53]

During the same summer, some optimistically celebrated "the end of the pandemic" in Sweden as well. Anders Tegnell, a physician specialized in infectious diseases and top Swedish government' epidemiologist, gave reassurances that there wouldn't be a second wave.[54] As for Italy and the United States, the stark reality revealed by the data ruthlessly contradicted his claims. The underestimated second wave in Sweden ultimately resulted in a higher number of deaths than the first one.

After the litany of outbursts, many harbored the illusion that a meticulous gathering of solid scientific evidence regarding the true danger posed by the virus would eliminate baseless claims and technical inaccuracies. Unfortunately, they were mistaken. Efforts to downplay the virus's threat, even prior to any substantial reduction in its dangers, persisted unabated throughout subsequent waves. The summer of 2021 saw a resurrection of the idea of "the end of the pandemic." The embarrassment of having been publicly proven wrong did not dent the egos of those experts who, after having totally failed to foresee the impact of the virus the year before, ventured to declare the pandemic "over" a second time. "Italy will be out of the pandemic in the autumn," explained a physicist in August 2021.[55] He was joined by two well-known experts in the country. In September 2021, the first explained that the pandemic was over and that "the new emergency risks becoming virus anxiety."[56] The second, a couple of weeks later, stated: "we have put [COVID-19] in a pen like the flu."[57]

Even abroad there were those who organized an early funeral for the virus without making sure it had actually passed away. On February 8, 2021, a US expert argued: "I do not think variants are going to cause a third wave of COVID-19 in the coming weeks or months across Northern Europe or North America." In the year following such wrong predictions, nearly 1,000 American children died of COVID-19.[58] On July 21, 2021, a world-renowned expert announced that "The disease has been defanged. We actually should be declaring victory. We have done a fantastic job." Since that day, the United States registered more than half a million COVID-19 deaths.[59] In June 2021, one of the heads of Norway's health organization stated: "the country has the lowest number of infections ever and almost half of the population vaccinated." On the basis of these data, he confidently asserted, "the pandemic is over."[60]

Along with the first two phases of the pandemic, the waves of misinformation continued, and come winter 2022, with the spread of the Omicron, some virologists "made" the pandemic end prematurely for a third time. In January 2022, an expert explained: "The numbers are clear ... the scientific community agrees that we are moving towards the end of the pandemic." The virologist was joined by other experts inclined to treat Omicron as a virus "in an endemic phase" – that is, a mild infection constantly present in the territory but not very dangerous. It's a shame that, as highlighted in an editorial in *Nature*, a disease can be endemic but not at all harmless.[61] In fact, in January 2022 in Italy, during the high prevalence of Omicron, over 10,000 people died of COVID-19 and almost 3,000 children were hospitalized, the highest number of pediatric hospitalizations ever observed since the start of the pandemic.

As observed by the UN global health body's Head of Emergencies, Mike Ryan, in addition to SARS-CoV-2, the world found itself facing a pandemic of "epidemiological stupidity."[62] Pandemics do not end when some virologists decide to make them end on television talk shows. They do when cases approach zero or when indicators of hospitalizations and mortality become acceptable. Omicron has been shown to be inherently less lethal than previous variants, as its danger has been significantly limited by vaccines and previous infections. However, virus mutations do not necessarily lead to lower lethality. For instance, the Delta variant was more dangerous than the Alpha variant, which, in turn, was more dangerous than previous ones, including the original Wuhan virus. As predicted in an article in *Nature Medicine*, SARS-CoV-2 would have become a seasonal infection and circulated in humans indefinitely,[63] but as stated by the authors of another editorial in *The Lancet*, it is important to remain vigilant, encourage maximum transparency in reporting cases, hospitalizations and deaths and accelerate collaborative surveillance of variant testing and vaccinations.[64] In January 2024, after more than three years since the beginning of the pandemic, about 1,500 Americans were still dying from COVID-19 every week.[65]

A study published in *JAMA* found that in fall-winter 2023-2024, the risk of death in patients hospitalized for COVID-19 continued to be significantly greater than the risk of death in patients hospitalized for seasonal influenza. Moreover, COVID-19 caused nearly twice as many hospitalizations.[66] As American scientist Eric Topol observed, in an opinion piece published in the *Los Angeles Times* in early 2024, SARS-CoV-2 proved to be very resilient and although some may want us to believe that it has been transformed into a common cold, in reality this is not the case and "the pandemic is far from over."[67]

Trumping the World Health Organization

To effectively prepare for future pandemics, updated national pandemic plans alone are insufficient. A supranational strategy capable of coordinating prevention efforts among countries is also necessary. Therefore, the WHO, whose mission is to "promote health for all," plays a fundamental role in managing a global pandemic. After the outbreak of SARS-CoV-2, the organization urged governments not to underestimate the virus and to adopt timely preventive strategies to contain the spread of the virus. It's hard to forget the words of Director Tedros Adhanom Ghebreyesus when, during the early months of the pandemic, he cautioned, "Test, test, test: you can't fight a fire blindfolded."[68]

The WHO, however, is not exempt from criticism. One particularly contentious issue revolves around a significant and prolonged delay in acknowledging the crucial role of aerosol transmission in the diffusion of SARS-CoV-2, a matter examined in a *Nature* editorial titled "Why It Took the WHO Two Years to Say That COVID Is Transmitted through the Air."[69] Throughout this period, the WHO consistently asserted that the primary mode of virus transmission was through respiratory droplets expelled from the mouth, infecting individuals in close proximity or via contact with contaminated surfaces. However, the hypothesis that the virus can also be transmitted through the air had already been introduced in a letter published in the *New England Journal of Medicine* as early as April 2020.[70] At the end of June 2020, it had been substantiated by the publication of a meta-analysis and systematic review in *The Lancet*.[71] Later, compelling scientific evidence supported the hypothesis.[72]

The effects of the delayed acknowledgment of aerosol-based transmission were significant, leading to a misallocation of scarce resources and implementation of ineffective or even irrelevant interventions. In Italy, for instance, the initial months of the pandemic witnessed a frenzied pursuit of scapegoats that included joggers and a solitary sunbather on an empty beach, chased by a police helicopter dispatched to confront the violator. By neglecting the pivotal role of airborne transmission, preventive efforts for months failed to adequately focus on enclosed spaces – be they private homes, public venues or workplaces – where the majority of infections occur.[72] A systematic review published in the *Journal of Infectious Diseases* revealed that less than 10% of global SARS-CoV-2 infections occurred outdoors, highlighting that the risk of infection indoors is nearly 19 times higher than the risk of contracting the virus outdoors.[73]

The downplayed significance of aerosol transmission may have also impeded the timely implementation of crucial modernization and ventilation measures in both public and private facilities.[74] Furthermore, this oversight may have affected messaging in prevention campaigns. Rather than emphasizing directives like "maintain a two-meter distance," "frequently wash your hands," "use gloves" and "ensure premises are disinfested," campaigns could have had an emphasis on "consistent mask-wearing," "avoiding crowded indoor spaces" and promoting "adequate ventilation through open windows" and advocated for the use of carbon monoxide detection and air filtration tools.

In defense of the WHO, it's crucial to acknowledge that the organization's primary responsibility lies in changing policies after there is solid and widely recognized scientific consensus, not just new provisional knowledge. WHO guidelines evolve following the solidification of evidence in the international scientific literature. However, criticisms have been leveled at the organization for perceived rigidity, slow updates to guidelines and a tendency to disregard empirical analyses and guidance that fell outside its expectations on the subject. As Trisha Greenhalgh, a professor at the University of Oxford and author of "Ten Scientific Reasons for Airborne Transmission of SARS-CoV-2," emphasized, in public health science it is important to recognize that "the absence of evidence is not evidence of absence."[75]

The WHO has also faced criticism for another shortcoming: advising against the widespread use of masks in the general population during the initial months of the pandemic. Until June 2020, the institution recommended "the use of masks only by those with symptoms and health workers."[76] According to a review published in the *British Medical Journal (BMJ)* on the topic, however, given the serious threat posed by COVID-19, masks had to be used even in the absence of definite evidence, applying the principle of precaution.[77] A subsequent meta-analysis, drawing on evidence from the previous SARS epidemic, supported the recommendation to use face masks. To be fair, the WHO faced extenuating circumstances, notably the scarcity of masks during the early stages of the pandemic. Prioritizing healthcare personnel, who were disproportionately exposed to contagion, was crucial. Subsequently, the WHO corrected its stance by updating guidelines to recommend mask usage for the entire population.

Another misstep was underestimating the significance of asymptomatic cases and advising against swab testing for asymptomatic individuals. For months, the WHO asserted that the rate of asymptomatic COVID-19 infections was minimal and not a major factor in transmission. However, studies published early in the pandemic in the *BMJ*, *New England Journal of Medicine* and *Science* suggested otherwise. Subsequent analyses in the literature affirmed the accuracy of these studies, assigning a role to asymptomatic transmission in the spread of the pandemic.

The WHO faced additional criticism, as highlighted in a *BMJ* editorial, for delays in declaring an international health emergency and recognizing person-to-person transmission of SARS-CoV-2.[78] Critics point out that by the end of December 2019, the WHO had received reports of atypical pneumonias in China, yet it did not act promptly. In contrast, the Taiwanese government swiftly implemented quarantine measures for travelers from Wuhan, acting even before the WHO comprehended the potential global threat. By December 31, 2019, several weeks ahead of the WHO's pandemic declaration, Taiwan had initiated health screening for airline passengers arriving from Wuhan.[79] News from China triggered suspicions among experts of Taiwan's established health surveillance systems and prompted an immediate and comprehensive response, integrating data from immigration records and national health insurance databases in real time. In the subsequent weeks, Taiwan's proactive measures demonstrated foresight, validating their concerns. However, two weeks after Taiwan's actions, the WHO continued to assert that there was no definitive evidence of person-to-person transmission of the SARS-CoV-2 virus.[80] It took another week for the WHO to declare an international emergency.

While some criticism directed at the WHO for delays in intervening to prevent the crisis may be acceptable, it's crucial not to oversimplify the situation. Before a pandemic, the WHO finds itself in a difficult position: economic and political factors have historically influenced against declaring international emergencies because they can harm economies and trade. Moreover, despite the WHO's communication to world political leaders on January 4, 2020, about a potentially dangerous new virus, the most powerful Western nations disregarded the warnings. By the end of February 2020, almost a month after the international health emergency declaration, Western governments exhibited indifference, denial and minimization of the virus's danger. Even much later, the repeated WHO warnings were largely ignored.

During the pandemic, the WHO became the focus of conspiracy theories and wild political attacks, the most notable one coming from former US President Donald Trump. In 2021, after prolonged threats to withdraw funding, Trump formally notified the American Congress and the United Nations of the United States' exit from the international organization. Most of Trump's accusations against the WHO were not just totally unfounded but potentially intended to divert attention from the abysmal failure of his administration in handling the health crisis. Recall that on February 2, 2020, Trump believed he had already defeated the "Chinese" virus, and on February 25, he declared that those who had contracted the virus were already getting better. Two days later, he optimistically stated that the virus would disappear "like a miracle."[81] As one of the participants in one of the Zoom meetings of the Covid Crisis Group, a team of 34 experts who published "Lessons from the COVID War," put it, "Trump was a comorbidity."[82]

Weakening the power of the WHO, as Trump and his supporters have attempted to do, is a misguided and self-defeating strategy. In an interconnected world grappling with health challenges extending beyond geographical borders, a global health organization is not just important but indispensable. Errors happen. Rather than withdrawing funding and support for the WHO, the world needs to foster a stronger and more independent WHO in a spirit of international collaboration, solidarity and cooperation between countries. The alternative is unilateralism, nationalism and populist self-interest, which create a perfect recipe for not preventing future global health crises and fostering even more international tensions and conflicts.

The "good virus" and pills of fatal optimism

Have you ever seen a cartoon character named Mr. Magoo? He embodies a lovable elderly man, completely myopic and prone to finding himself in perilous situations due to his peculiar and involuntary aversion to perceiving any risk. Mr. Magoo stands as a symbol for those individuals who, despite their inability to see beyond their nose, miraculously navigate countless dangers unscathed, thanks to a series of extraordinary strokes of luck. In the whimsical world of cartoons, Mr. Magoo thrives. However, the real world operates under different rules: relying solely on luck and persistently defying danger, fueled by an unyielding optimism and disregard for risk, doesn't always lead to favorable outcomes. Those who continue down this path are destined to eventually confront their destiny.

During the pandemic, we heard a litany of experts accusing anyone who defended the importance of public health interventions as being a spreader of "gloom and doom" or "corona-phobia." Instead of fostering humility and caution, some influential figures in medicine and public health recommended facing the virus with some "pills of optimism." Some have repeatedly highlighted that the priority was to communicate reassuring messages (e.g., "be cheerful," "take a deep breath and step back from the hysteria" or "listen to all the optimism and phase out the doom"), even in the most dramatic months of the crisis when hospitals and morgues grappled with overwhelming surges of COVID-19 deaths. A renowned Italian academic who teaches in a prestigious American university even characterized SARS-CoV-2 as a benign phenomenon and published a book titled *The Good Virus*.[83]

The need to adopt positive and proactive tones in public communication campaigns to foster trust and increase persuasiveness is understandable. As Italy faced the harsh lockdown and saw sharp increases in infections, the slogan "everything will be fine" tried to reassure millions of children and adults stuck at home, some of them panicking about the surreal situation. But reassuring the public by depicting a deadly pathogen as a "good virus" distorts reality and induces people to ignore key scientific evidence related to its danger. In the early and most critical weeks of the pandemic in Lombardy, reports emerged from the Pio Albergo Trivulzio, a residential facility for old people, indicating that staff and nurses faced "veiled threats" pressuring them to not wear masks to "prevent scaring the patients."[84]

Even amid significant surges in hospitalizations in intensive care units during winter peaks, optimistically inclined virologists offered benign explanations for the pandemic's impact. According to one of them, hospitals were overwhelmed not due to a surge in demand for pandemic-related care but rather "because of those who were sowing panic."[85] The deaths of millions seemingly failed to shake the steadfast determination of some to paint an overly optimistic picture of the pandemic. Even the presentation of public health data has been unwelcomed by some because "people can't take it anymore." Such criticism extended to warnings from organizations such as the WHO and the Centers for Disease Control and Prevention (CDC), with their alerts labeled as "apocalyptic." Those advocating for vigilance, aiming to save lives, found themselves accused of adhering to a "catastrophist narrative" supposedly fueled by sensationalist media and opportunistic politicians.[86]

Of course, encouraging people to avoid overly pessimistic views of reality during a pandemic is a commendable activity. As demonstrated by a significant amount of research in social psychology, optimism is a healthy human quality. Motivational messages from positive psychology are widely sensationalized and glorified in part for some good reasons: optimism is associated with a long list of physical and mental health benefits. And life should be inspired by dreams, not fear. Visualizing positive prospects helps one not only to feel better but also to achieve them. Mentally reframing a potentially stressful event by focusing on the positive aspects of it, ignoring overly painful details, is a potentially valuable skill. This mode of thinking is widely used, for example, in psychotherapy, in what is called "cognitive restructuring." Psychologist Shelley Taylor, author of *Positive Illusions*, explained that if we didn't have a certain number of positive illusions about our day, we wouldn't even leave the house for fear that a roof tile might fall on our head.[87]

Science, however, also shows that even positive thinking has its dark side.[88] While optimism motivates people to live better and longer, it can lead to a form of cognitive distortion akin to mental myopia. The spread of slogans like "Milan doesn't stop" and "we are not afraid of the virus" certainly did not help protect the lives of nearly 200,000 people who died in Italy due to the virus. On the contrary, unrealistic collective optimism, a characteristic often associated with "wishful thinking," may have led many of them to an avoidable death. This is not healthy positive psychology but toxic positivity. Deceitful positive slogans, in fact, carry the risk of causing errors in judgment typical of a cognitive modality called confirmation bias, which consists of fixating on a pre-established hypothesis and selectively ignoring the evidence and facts that contradict it. Also, as explained by Lancelot Pinto, an epidemiologist at the Hinduja National Hospital, optimism may have "lowered the guard" of citizens regarding preventive measures.[89] An online cross-sectional study conducted in 2021, based on nearly 300 participants, showed that people with high scores on the optimistic bias scale had a distorted perception of the risk of contracting COVID-19. Their unrealistic optimism reduced their motivation to take precautions and protective behaviors, exposing them to a higher risk of hospitalization and death.[90]

A virus like COVID-19 does not respect our wishes. It does not care whether we are optimistic or pessimistic. But we are realistic, we have a better chance of understanding its true danger.

References

1. Quotidiano Sanità. 73ᵃ Assemblea mondiale Oms. Conte: "Ammettiamolo, non eravamo preparati per una crisi globale così grande come il Covid". Published online May 20, 2020. https://www.quotidianosanita.it/governo-e-parlamento/articolo.php?articolo_id=85390 (accessed May 28, 2024).
2. Huffington Post. "Piano Italia segreto, per non spaventare gli italiani. Rischiavamo 800 mila morti". HuffPost Italia. Published online Apr 21, 2020. https://www.huffingtonpost.it/politica/2020/04/21/news/piano_italia_segreto_per_non_spaventare_gli_italiani_rischiavamo_800_mila_morti_-5184357/ (accessed Jan 21, 2024).
3. Boyd I. We practised for a pandemic, but didn't brace. *Nature* 2020; 580(7801): 9. https://www.nature.com/articles/d41586-020-00919-3
4. Ministero della Salute. Piano pandemico antinfluenzale (PanFlu) 2021–2023. Ministero della Salute, Direzione Generale della Prevenzione Sanitaria. Published online Jan 21, 2021. https://www.certifico.com/news/274-news/12568-piano-pandemico-antinfluenzale-panflu-2021-2023 (accessed Jan 21, 2024).

5. Avishai B. The pandemic isn't a black swan but a portent of a more fragile global system. *The New Yorker*. Published online Apr 21, 2020. https://www.newyorker.com/news/daily-comment/the-pandemic-isnt-a-black-swan-but-a-portent-of-a-more-fragile-global-system (accessed Jan 21, 2024).
6. Quammen D. Spillover: animal infections and the next human pandemic. New York, NY: WW Norton & Co, 2013.
7. Osterholm MT. Preparing for the next pandemic. *Foreign Affairs* 2005; **84**. https://www.foreignaffairs.com/articles/2005-07-01/preparing-next-pandemic
8. Brilliant L. The age of pandemics. Wall Street Journal. Published online May 3, 2009. https://www.wsj.com/articles/SB124121965740478983 (accessed Jan 21, 2024).
9. Centers for Diseases Control. National pandemic influenza plans | Pandemic influenza (flu). Published online June 2, 2023. https://www.cdc.gov/flu/pandemic-resources/planning-preparedness/national-strategy-planning.html (accessed Jan 21, 2024).
10. Johns Hopkins Center for Health Security. Preparedness for a high-impact respiratory pathogen pandemic. Published online Sep 10, 2019. https://gpmb.org/reports/m/item/preparedness-for-a-high-impact-respiratory-pathogen-pandemic (accessed Jan 21, 2024).
11. Webster RG, Peiris M, Chen H, Guan Y. H5N1 outbreaks and enzootic influenza. *Emerging Infectious Diseases* 2006; **12**: 3–8.
12. The Independent Panel for Pandemic Preparedness and Response. The Co-Chairs' presentation of the second report on progress to the WHO executive board. Published online Jan 19, 2021. https://theindependentpanel.org/the-co-chairs-presentation-of-the-second-report-on-progress-to-the-who-executive-board-19-january-2021/ (accessed Jan 21, 2024).
13. Artiaco I. "La pandemia di Covid poteva essere evitata": gli esperti indipendenti Oms contro i leader mondiali. *Fanpage*. Published online May 12, 2021. https://www.fanpage.it/esteri/la-pandemia-di-covid-poteva-essere-evitata-gli-esperti-indipendenti-oms-contro-i-leader-mondiali/ (accessed Jan 21, 2024).
14. Brilliant L. Sometimes brilliant in conversation with Stewart Brand. *The Interval*. https://theinterval.org/salon-talks/02017/feb/21/sometimes-brilliant-conversation-stewart-brand (accessed Jan 21, 2024).
15. Pinker S. Enlightenment now: the case for reason, science, humanism, and progress. New York, NY: Viking, an imprint of Penguin Random House LLC, 2018.
16. Kretzschmar ME, Rozhnova G, Bootsma MCJ, van Boven M, van de Wijgert JHHM, Bonten MJM. Impact of delays on effectiveness of contact tracing strategies for COVID-19: a modelling study. *Lancet Public Health* 2020; **5**: e452–9.
17. Maxmen A. Has COVID taught us anything about pandemic preparedness? *Nature* 2021; **596**: 332–5.
18. World Health Organization. Global influenza strategy 2019–2030. Geneva, 2019. https://www.who.int/publications-detail-redirect/9789241515320 (accessed Jan 21, 2024).
19. World Health Organization. A World in Disorder: Global Preparedness Monitoring Board annual report 2020. 2020 (accessed Jan 21, 2024). https://www.gpmb.org/docs/librariesprovider17/default-document-library/annual-reports/gpmb-2020-execsum-annualreport-en.pdf?sfvrsn=b3eca80f_30.
20. World Health Organization. WHO global influenza preparedness plan: the role of WHO and recommendations for national measures before and during pandemics. Published online 2005. https://iris.who.int/handle/10665/68998 (accessed Jan 21, 2024).
21. Alhassan RK, Nketiah-Amponsah E, Afaya A, *et al*. Global health security index not a proven surrogate for health systems capacity to respond to pandemics: the case of COVID-19. *Journal of Infection and Public Health* 2023; **16**: 196–205.

22. Tollefson J. How Trump damaged science—and why it could take decades to recover. *Nature* 2020; **586**: 190–4.
23. Saracci R. Prevention in COVID-19 time: from failure to future. *Journal of Epidemiology and Community Health* 2020; **74**: 689–91.
24. Shridar D. Preventable: how a pandemic changed the world & how to stop the next one. Viking, 2023.
25. Horowitz J. How Italy turned around its coronavirus calamity. *The New York Times*. Published online July 31, 2020. https://www.nytimes.com/2020/07/31/world/europe/italy-coronavirus-reopening.html (accessed Jan 21, 2024).
26. Financial Times. Italy's harsh lessons help keep second wave at bay. Published online Sep 23, 2020. https://www.ft.com/content/6831be3e-2711-4ea3-8f62-daa82cf9ca11 (accessed Jan 21, 2024).
27. Flaxman S, Mishra S, Gandy A, *et al.* Estimating the effects of non-pharmaceutical interventions on COVID-19 in Europe. *Nature* 2020; **584**: 257–61.
28. Andrea Capocci. Il giallo delle illusioni di Speranza. Il manifesto. Published online Oct 27, 2020. https://ilmanifesto.it/il-giallo-delle-illusioni-di-speranza (accessed Jan 21, 2024).
29. La Repubblica. 'Covid, negli ospedali situazione fuori controllo': medici e infermieri chiedono subito il lockdown. Published online Nov 9, 2020. https://www.repubblica.it/cronaca/2020/11/09/news/l_allarme_di_medici_e_infermieri_situazione_fuori_controllo_serve_il_lockdown_-273696431/ (accessed Jan 21, 2024).
30. Our World in Data. COVID-19 vaccine boosters administered per 100 people. https://ourworldindata.org/grapher/covid-vaccine-booster-doses-per-capita?tab=map (accessed Jan 21, 2024).
31. Ministero della Salute. Piano pandemico influenzale 2021–2023. https://www.salute.gov.it/portale/influenza/dettaglioContenutiInfluenza.jsp?lingua=italiano&id=722&area=influenza&menu=vuoto (accessed Jan 21, 2024).
32. Giuffrida A. Italy 'misled WHO on pandemic readiness' weeks before Covid outbreak. The Guardian. Published online Feb 22, 2021. https://www.theguardian.com/world/2021/feb/22/italy-misled-who-on-pandemic-readiness-weeks-before-covid-outbreak (accessed Jan 21, 2024).
33. Borrelli SS, Johnson M. WHO pulled report on Italy's 'chaotic' first response to Covid-19. Published online Dec 5, 2020. https://www.ft.com/content/7c8633ea-87b3-4aa1-90b6-a15a089bc1c2 (accessed Jan 21, 2024).
34. Ciccolella C, Valesini G. I somarelli di Venezia. Rai Report. Published online Apr 12, 2021. https://www.rai.it/programmi/report/inchieste/Gli-asinelli-di-Venezia-334c14f0-a917-48df-ae1a-7ff1bc49d022.html (accessed Jan 21, 2024).
35. D'Alessandro M. Storia del Centro di Epidemiologia che venne depotenziato da Ricciardi. AGI. https://www.agi.it/cronaca/news/2020-12-11/centro-epidemiologia-depotenziato-walter-ricciardi-istituto-superiore-sanit-10631421/ (accessed Jan 21, 2024).
36. Roberto De Vogli. Coronavirus, i test di massa contrastano davvero la pandemia? Ecco le voci più autorevoli. *Il Fatto Quotidiano*. Published online Apr 22, 2020. https://www.ilfattoquotidiano.it/2020/04/22/coronavirus-i-test-di-massa-contrastano-davvero-la-pandemia-ecco-le-voci-piu-autorevoli/5776811/ (accessed Jan 21, 2024).
37. Mantovani A. Oms, l'email di Guerra: "Non suicidiamoci, adesso blocco tutto". *Il Fatto Quotidiano*. https://www.ilfattoquotidiano.it/in-edicola/articoli/2020/12/01/lemail-di-mr-oms-non-suicidiamoci-adesso-blocco-tutto/6022199/ (accessed Jan 21, 2024).
38. La Repubblica. Mascherine, farmaci antivirali e terapie intensive: pronto il piano pandemico 2021–2023. 'Se risorse sono scarse scegliere chi curare prima'. Jan 11, 2021. https://www.repubblica.it/cronaca/2021/01/11/news/mascherine_farmaci_antivirali_e_terapie_intensive_pronto_il_piano_pandemico_2021-2023_se_risorse_sono_scarse_scegliere_c-282122918/ (accessed Jan 21, 2024).

39. De Vogli R, Gawronski P. Il piano pandemico bis non è all'altezza. Il Sole 24 Ore. Published online Mar 4, 2021. https://www.ilsole24ore.com/art/il-piano-pandemico-bis-non-e-all-altezza-ADCgPYNB (accessed Jan 21, 2024).

40. Mari L. Coronavirus, al Senato il convegno dei 'negazionisti'. Salvini: 'Non metto la mascherina'. Sgarbi: 'In Italia non c'è più'. La Repubblica. Published online July 27, 2020. https://www.repubblica.it/politica/2020/07/27/news/cornavirus_sgarbi_insiste_in_italia_non_c_e_piu_il_governo_ci_ascolti_-262991120/ (accessed Jan 21, 2024).

41. Szabo L. Many US health experts underestimated the coronavirus … until it was too late. KFF Health News. Published online Dec 21, 2020. https://kffhealthnews.org/news/article/many-us-health-experts-underestimated-the-coronavirus-until-it-was-too-late/ (accessed Feb 2, 2024).

42. Sayers F. Sunetra Gupta: Covid-19 is on the way out. UnHerd. Published online May 21, 2020. https://unherd.com/2020/05/oxford-doubles-down-sunetra-gupta-interview/ (accessed Jan 21, 2024).

43. Palma A. Silvestri: "Virus via a passo veloce, ma non è ancora KO". *Fanpage*. Published online May 10, 2020. https://www.fanpage.it/attualita/il-virologo-silvestri-il-virus-se-ne-sta-andando-a-passo-veloce-ma-non-e-ancora-ko/ (accessed Jan 21, 2024).

44. Roberto De Vogli. Covid-19, da pandemia a crisi economica e sociale. E i migranti come capro espiatorio. *Il Fatto Quotidiano*. Published online Aug 3, 2020. https://www.ilfattoquotidiano.it/2020/08/03/covid-19-da-pandemia-a-crisi-economica-e-sociale-e-i-migranti-come-capro-espiatorio/5887380/ (accessed Jan 21, 2024).

45. Bassetti M. Svolta coronavirus: 'C'è stata una mutazione, ora abbiamo un nuovo ceppo'. https://www.liberoquotidiano.it/news/scienze-tech/24279349/matteo-bassetti-coronavirus-mutazione-nuovo-ceppo-piu-contagioso-meno-letale.html (accessed Jan 21, 2024).

46. De Bac M. Covid ora meno contagioso? L'epidemiologo Greco: "In alcune Regioni mascherine inutili". *Corriere della Sera*. Published online June 24, 2020. https://www.corriere.it/cronache/20_giugno_24/coronavirus-l-epidemiologo-donato-greco-in-alcune-regioni-mascherine-non-servono-piu-9388c214-b647-11ea-9dea-5ac3c9ec7c08.shtml (accessed Jan 21, 2024).

47. Fatto Quotidiano. Coronavirus, Locatelli: 'C'è accelerazione, non crescita esponenziale. Niente panico. La scuola resti aperta, controlli sugli assembramenti'. *Il Fatto Quotidiano*. Published online Oct 18, 2020. https://www.ilfattoquotidiano.it/2020/10/18/coronavirus-locatelli-ce-accelerazione-non-crescita-esponenziale-niente-panico-la-scuola-resti-aperta-controlli-sugli-assembramenti/5970752/ (accessed Jan 21, 2024).

48. Robson D. Exponential growth bias: the numerical error behind Covid-19. BBC. Aug 13, 2020. https://www.bbc.com/future/article/20200812-exponential-growth-bias-the-numerical-error-behind-covid-19 (accessed Jan 21, 2024).

49. De Bac M. 10 esperti dicono che "l'emergenza Covid è finita". Ma è scontro nella comunità scientifica. Corriere della Sera. Published online June 24, 2020. https://www.corriere.it/cronache/20_giugno_24/coronavirus-10-esperti-emergenza-finita-ma-scontro-comunita-scientifica-f457226e-b5f4-11ea-9dea-5ac3c9ec7c08.shtml (accessed Jan 21, 2024).

50. Primocanale.it. Coronavirus, Bassetti: "Difficile un aumento dei contagi misti a influenza". https://www.primocanale.it/archivio-news/223155-coronavirus-bassetti-difficile-un-aumento-dei-contagi-misti-a-influenza-.html (accessed Jan 21, 2024).

51. Il Messaggero. Coronavirus, il virologo Clementi (San Raffaele): "Seconda ondata non ci sarà e vi spiego il perché". Published online Aug 6, 2020. https://www.ilmessaggero.it/salute/focus/seconda_ondata_coronavirus_covid_ci_sara_o_no_virologo_clementi_motivi-5390382.html (accessed Jan 21, 2024).

52. Imarisio M. Remuzzi: "I nuovi positivi non sono contagiosi". Corriere della Sera. Published online June 19, 2020. https://www.corriere.it/cronache/20_giugno_19/coronavirus-remuzzi-nuovi-positivi-non-sono-contagiosi-stop-paura-bf24c59c-b199-11ea-842e-6a88f68d3e0a.shtml (accessed Jan 21, 2024).

53. Sablone L. La previsione del virologo Palù: 'Non ci sarà la seconda ondata'. *Il Giornale*. Published online Aug 31, 2020. https://www.ilgiornale.it/news/cronache/previsione-virologo-pal-non-ci-sar-seconda-ondata-1886647.html (accessed Jan 21, 2024).

54. Vogel G. Critics slam letter in prestigious journal that downplayed COVID-19 risks to Swedish schoolchildren. Science. Mar 2, 2021. https://www.science.org/content/article/critics-slam-letter-prestigious-journal-downplayed-covid-19-risks-swedish (accessed Jan 21, 2024).

55. Maggio G. Covid, i tre motivi che ci dicono perché l'Italia in autunno potrà essere fuori dalla pandemia. *La Stampa*. Published online Aug 15, 2021. https://www.lastampa.it/topnews/primo-piano/2021/08/16/news/covid-i-tre-motivi-che-ci-dicono-perche-in-autunno-saremo-fuori-dalla-pandemia-1.40603196/ (accessed Jan 21, 2024).

56. Il Mattino. La pandemia "è finita, la nuova emergenza rischia di diventare l'ansia da virus". L'affondo di Antonella Viola. Published online Sept 18, 2021. https://www.ilmattino.it/primopiano/sanita/pandemia_finita_antonella_viola_ansia_virus_ultime_notizie-6203628.html (accessed Jan 21, 2024).

57. Peretti G. "Covid nel recinto come un'influenza". Ilaria Capua esulta: la vita può tornare alla normalità. Il Tempo. Published online October 5, 2021. https://www.iltempo.it/attualita/2021/10/05/news/ilaria-capua-covid-come-influenza-recinto-virus-inverno-vita-ritorno-normalita-dimartedi-28944488/ (accessed Jan 21, 2024).

58. Howard J. Chapter 2: 'It was an unimaginable hell to be quite honest.' In: Howard J. We want them infected: how the failed quest for herd immunity led doctors to embrace the anti-vaccine movement and blinded Americans to the threat of COVID. Hickory, NC: Redhawk Publications, 2023: 38–9.

59. Kalen Hill Z. Stanford doctor calls vaccine mandates 'unethical': patients can choose. *Newsweek*. Published online July 21, 2021. https://www.newsweek.com/stanford-doc-jay-bhattacharya-calls-vaccine-mandates-unethical-says-patients-can-choose-1611938 (accessed Jan 29, 2024).

60. Frezza G. La Norvegia è la prima a dire 'la pandemia è finita'. Sanità Informazione. Published online June 8, 2021. https://www.sanitainformazione.it/sanita-internazionale/la-norvegia-e-la-prima-a-dire-la-pandemia-e-finita/ (accessed Jan 21, 2024).

61. Redazione Adnkronos. Variante Omicron fine pandemia? Cosa dicono Oms e esperti. Adnkronos. Published online Jan 24, 2022. https://www.adnkronos.com/Archivio/cronaca/variante-omicron-fine-pandemia-cosa-dicono-oms-e-esperti_4Skg3ABOBamUiwvO5FLXc5 (accessed Jan 21, 2024).

62. Beaumont P. WHO warns of 'epidemiological stupidity' of early Covid reopening. *The Guardian*. Published online July 7, 2021. https://www.theguardian.com/world/2021/jul/07/countries-should-not-relax-covid-rules-too-quickly-says-who-official-mike-ryan (accessed Jan 21, 2024).

63. Chen J-M, Chen Y-Q. China can prepare to end its zero-COVID policy. *Nature Medicine* 2022; 28: 1104–5.

64. The Lancet. The COVID-19 pandemic in 2023: far from over. *The Lancet* 2023; 401: 79.

65. Kekatos M. Why are 1,500 Americans still dying from COVID every week? ABC News. https://abcnews.go.com/Health/1500-americans-dying-covid-week/story?id=106237143 (accessed Jan 30, 2024).

66. Yan X, Choi T, Al-Aly Z. Mortality in patients hospitalized for COVID-19 vs influenza in fall-winter 2023–2024. *JAMA* 2024: e247395.

67. Topol E. Opinion: The U.S. is facing the biggest COVID wave since Omicron. Why are we still playing make-believe? *Los Angeles Times*. Jan 4, 2024. https://www.latimes.com/opinion/story/2024-01-04/covid-2024-flu-virus-vaccine (accessed May 28, 2024).
68. United Nations. 'You cannot fight a fire blindfolded': WHO chief blasts slow virus testing response. UN News. Published online March 16, 2020. https://news.un.org/en/story/2020/03/1059552 (accessed Jan 22, 2024).
69. Lewis D. Why the WHO took two years to say COVID is airborne. *Nature* 2022; 604: 26–31.
70. van Doremalen N, Bushmaker T, Morris DH, *et al*. Aerosol and surface stability of SARS-CoV-2 as compared with SARS-CoV-1. *New England Journal of Medicine* 2020; 382: 1564–7.
71. Chu DK, Akl EA, Duda S, *et al*. Physical distancing, face masks, and eye protection to prevent person-to-person transmission of SARS-CoV-2 and COVID-19: a systematic review and meta-analysis. *The Lancet* 2020; 395: 1973–87.
72. Weed M, Foad A. Rapid scoping review of evidence of outdoor transmission of COVID-19. MedRxiv. 2020. https://doi.org/10.1101/2020.09.04.20188417.
73. Bulfone TC, Malekinejad M, Rutherford GW, Razani N. Outdoor transmission of SARS-CoV-2 and other respiratory viruses: a systematic review. *The Journal of Infectious Diseases* 2021; 223: 550–61.
74. Lewis D. COVID-19 rarely spreads through surfaces. So why are we still deep cleaning? *Nature* 2021; 590: 26–8.
75. Greenhalgh T, Jimenez JL, Prather KA, Tufekci Z, Fisman D, Schooley R. Ten scientific reasons in support of airborne transmission of SARS-CoV-2. *The Lancet* 2021; 397: 1603–5.
76. World Health Organization. Updated WHO recommendations for international traffic in relation to COVID-19 outbreak. Feb 29, 2020. https://www.who.int/news-room/articles-detail/updated-who-recommendations-for-international-traffic-in-relation-to-covid-19-outbreak (accessed Jan 22, 2024).
77. MacIntyre CR, Chughtai AA. Facemasks for the prevention of infection in health-care and community settings. *BMJ* 2015; 350: h694.
78. Mahase E. Covid-19: WHO and China acted too slowly in early days of pandemic, says report. *BMJ* 2021; 372: n172.
79. Watt L. Here's what Taiwan told the WHO at the start of the virus outbreak. Time. Published online May 19, 2020. https://time.com/5826025/taiwan-who-trump-coronavirus-covid19/ (accessed Jan 22, 2024).
80. Givas N. WHO haunted by old tweet saying China found no human transmission of coronavirus. Fox News. Published online March 20, 2020. https://www.foxnews.com/world/world-health-organization-january-tweet-china-human-transmission-coronavirus (accessed Jan 22, 2024).
81. Pilkington E. Six months of Trump's Covid denials: 'It'll go away ... It's fading'. *The Guardian*. Published online July 29, 2020. https://www.theguardian.com/world/2020/jul/29/trump-coronavirus-science-denial-timeline-what-has-he-said (accessed Jan 22, 2024).
82. Covid Crisis Group. Chapter 1: From tragedy to possibility. In: Lessons from the COVID war: an investigative report, 1st ed. New York, NY: Public Affairs, 2023: 7.
83. Leggo. Il virologo Silvestri: "Virus in ritirata, chi lo nega dice sciocchezze". La risposta sulle torri 5G. Published online June 19, 2020. https://www.leggo.it/italia/cronache/il_virologo_silvestri_virus_ritirata_nega_dice_sciocchezze_la_risposta_sulle_torri_5g-5297248.html (accessed Jan 21, 2024).
84. Rai News. Rsa, le testimonianze al Trivulzio: 'Non dovevamo spaventare i pazienti'. rainews. Published online Apr 20, 2020. https://www.rainews.it/dl/rainews/articoli/milano-trivulzio-inchiesta-deposizione-infermieri-0c7283bd-a1e0-4c33-b102-c68435cb3af2.html (accessed Jan 21, 2024).

85. Bassetti M. 'Ospedali al collasso per colpa di chi semina il panico', dice Bassetti. AGI. Nov 9, 2020. https://www.agi.it/cronaca/news/2020-11-09/covid-bassetti-ospedali-collasso-per-panico-10225266/ (accessed Jan 21, 2024).
86. Adnkronos. Coronavirus, Silvestri: 'Numeri ok, andiamo verso la fine'. Adnkronos. Published online Dec 12, 2020. https://www.adnkronos.com/Archivio/cronaca/coronavirus-silvestri-numeri-ok-andiamo-verso-la-fine_1EPAaBgw0qq5md0YZkVrPQ (accessed Jan 21, 2024).
87. Taylor SE. Positive illusions: creative self-deception and the healthy mind. New York, NY: Basic Books, 1989.
88. Ehrenreich B. Bright-sided: how the relentless promotion of positive thinking has undermined America, 1st ed. New York, NY: Metropolitan Books, 2009.
89. Falcioni D. Perché in India i contagi sono esplosi: "A gennaio credevamo che il Covid-19 fosse scomparso". *Fanpage*. Published online Apr 27, 2021. https://www.fanpage.it/esteri/perche-in-india-i-contagi-sono-impennati-a-gennaio-credevamo-che-il-covid-19-fosse-scomparso/ (accessed Jan 21, 2024).
90. Park T, Ju I, Ohs JE, Hinsley A. Optimistic bias and preventive behavioral engagement in the context of COVID-19. *Research in Social and Administrative Pharmacy* 2021; **17**: 1859–66.

2

MISINFORMATION

"A lie can travel halfway around the world while the truth is putting on its shoes."

Anonymous source (often attributed to Mark Twain)

During the spring of 2021, I received a phone call from one of the organizers of the 13th National Conference of the Italian Society of Palliative Care, inviting me to be a guest speaker. I was flattered, but I raised a concern on the phone: "Thank you, but there might be a mistake. Truthfully, I have never delved into palliative care." The response was surprising: "We don't want you to deal with palliative care. We would like to invite you to give a lecture on COVID-19 misinformation." The purpose of their invitation had eluded me initially, but it was straightforward: many healthcare professionals had faced attacks from relatives of patients who had been misinformed by fake news on SARS-CoV-2. In Italy, there has been an embarrassing amount of false information spread during prime time on TV and in major national newspapers, and unfortunately, many listeners, readers and journalists bought it all. Pleasantly surprised, I replied, "Yes, I gladly accept." They needed someone who could debunk the litany of errors and lies that have been circulating during the pandemic. "It's me," I thought.

Seven myths about SARS-CoV-2

We've all fallen victim to it: from comparisons with a regular flu to the crusades against vaccines, the pandemic inundated us with an enormous amount of misinformation and technical inaccuracies. Unfortunately, wrong

DOI: 10.4324/9781003511977-4

information was propagated not solely by influencers posing as epidemiologists but also by eminent scientists, doctors and virologists who made misleading statements in the media. A study in *JAMA* concluded that doctors in the United States played a significant role in misinforming the public about key pandemic issues, often through erroneous messages on social media.[1] If this misinformation had not resulted in lethal consequences, it might have been overlooked, sparing embarrassment for those who provided false statements and predictions. However, scientific evidence indicates that exposure to misinformation and a distorted perception of the actual danger of the virus influence behaviors such as vaccination, mask-wearing, and adherence to distancing measures.[2,3] If implemented appropriately, these measures could not only reduce infections but also save lives. While it's very challenging to estimate how many deaths can be attributed to misinformation, the scientific literature suggests a link: if preventive behaviors save lives, wrong health information can kill.[4]

Unveiling the main myths spread during the health crisis is vital to raise the bar of civic responsibility of those who make statements in the media, ensuring that scientific information promotes public health rather than causing harm. It's not just about holding commentators, journalists and experts on media and social platforms accountable. It's also about learning lessons to avoid similar mistakes in the future. Any fact or reference to events or individuals in this chapter is not casual. It's causal.

The "health dictatorship"

Ideas that the virus was intentionally created and deliberately disseminated by powerful esoteric entities like "The Illuminati" or ultra-rich individuals such as Bill Gates, possibly through 5G networks, microchips under the skin or contact tracing apps, stand out as the most egregious hoaxes of the health crisis. Those spreading this misinformation often assert a conspiracy, suggesting that the pandemic served as a pretext to curtail freedoms. This was claimed even by a prominent Italian philosopher.[5] Some conspiracy theories went so far as to claim that the implemented restriction measures and alarmism were part of a covert plan to establish a "healthcare dictatorship." Remarkably, the abundance of data and scientific evidence on the severe consequences of SARS-CoV-2 has failed to sway supporters of these unfounded speculations. According to a survey conducted at the onset of the pandemic, one in four Italians believed that COVID-19 was engineered to control or manipulate citizens.[6] Toward the end of 2021, another survey revealed that 31.4% of Italians thought COVID-19 vaccines were "experimental," while 10.9% deemed them useless and harmful. Additionally, 12.7% believed that science had caused more harm than good, and nearly one in five people embraced the baseless belief that 5G networks were employed as a tool to control citizens' minds.[7]

In the United States too, COVID-19 hoaxes have ensnared numerous victims and garnered followers. A Pew Research Center survey released at the onset of the pandemic revealed that nearly a third of Americans believed the coronavirus was concocted in a lab.[8] Former President Donald Trump, asserting the same hypothesis, blamed the WHO for being too "China-centric" in its tackling of the coronavirus pandemic.[9] Certainly, the possibility that the virus could have accidentally escaped from a lab shouldn't be dismissed outright,[10] but as of now, there is no evidence supporting this assumption. Moreover, the idea that the virus has been strategically created for geopolitical purposes, in the context of a biological war or as an attempt to create a "health dictatorship," is totally unfounded.

Trump, no stranger to hyperboles and outbursts, previously spread preposterous fake news on Obama (that he was born in Kenya),[11] global warming (that it was "created by and for the Chinese in order to make U.S. manufacturing non-competitive")[12] and Mexicans (that "most … are rapists").[13] Trump's prolific fake news – he made at least 20,000 false or inaccurate statements during his first 440 days in office[14] – led to the creation of an artwork called "The Wall of Lies," showcasing his "impressive achievements." Trump also topped a special BBC ranking of those who spread the worst COVID-19 hoaxes, followed by Zhao Lijian, Jair Bolsonaro, Subramanian Swamy and Matteo Salvini.[15] Of course, false theories about the pandemic have also been widely disseminated in Vladimir Putin's Russia[16] and in China.[17]

"It's flu-like"

February 26, 2020: "It seems crazy to me. An infection slightly more serious than influenza has been mistaken for a lethal pandemic," explained the director of a well-known clinical microbiology, virology and diagnostics laboratory in Italy.[18] Also in February 2020, a head physician and director of an infectious diseases clinic in a hospital in Northern Italy complained about "much ado about nothing" in reference to the virus. He added: "outside China it is not that contagious."[19] In the same weeks, during an interview on prime-time Italian TV, another well-known virologist said: "In Italy the risk is zero. The virus does not circulate. This doesn't happen by chance: it happens because precautions are being taken."[20] A week later, he reiterated the message, assuring the public, "[In Italy] we can rest assured … the virus is not there … we are not impressed by the 2% mortality … the data from China can be very unreliable … our country has been able to defend itself from this threat … Italy is one of the few countries that have blocked flights from China."[21] Another figure frequently appearing on Italian TV predicted optimistically that "the best predictive models for Italy estimate that we will have a maximum of 4,000 COVID-19 deaths at the end of the epidemic."[22] At the end of February 2020, a well-known and respected Italian professor from the University of Florida explained: "The fact that there are hundreds of people who … have caught this flu-like infection should reassure. My impression is that this virus has actually been really overhyped."[23] Then she added: "I believe that there is media alarm that is not justified by the actual behavior of the infection. And I think that, within a week, a lot of things will become clear."[24] What became clear shortly after, however, was the rapid rise of COVID-19 deaths.

During the same period, voices of experts ready to downplay the risk and compare SARS-CoV-2 to a normal flu were also heard in other countries, In the United States, an epidemiologist recognized worldwide claimed that the lethality of the COVID-19 disease was even lower than that of seasonal flu.[25]

It is crucial to emphasize that these misjudgments did not occur in the total absence of warnings or scientific findings on the actual danger of the virus. On January 24, 2020, the first analysis on the consequences of COVID-19 was published in *The Lancet*. The authors wrote: "we must be aware of the challenge and concerns brought by 2019-nCoV to our community. Every effort should be made to understand and control the disease, and the time to act is now."[26] These words did not particularly impress the scientific director of the Spallanzani National Institute for Infectious Diseases in Rome who, more than a week later, predicted a certain "attenuation of the virus." In the same period, two members of the Istituto Superiore di Sanità assured that the dangers of COVID-19 were "comparable to those of the flu."[27] Exactly one month later, an empirical analysis that appeared in *JAMA* clearly demonstrated that COVID-19 had a lethality rate much higher than that of the normal flu, along with a much more rapid propagation capacity.[28] However, in Italy, wrong messages continued. In the middle of summer 2020, a CTS member stated on television that COVID-19 was "a normal disease."[29] A few months later, a well-known emeritus professor from the University of Padova analyzed COVID lethality by saying: "it fluctuates between 0.3% and 0.6%; it means a relatively low lethality, lower than other infectious diseases, certainly lower than road accidents and suicides."[30] There is no such thing as a lethality rate for road accidents and suicides. In this passage, the expert probably confused lethality (number of deaths from a disease divided by the number of subjects affected by the disease) with cause-specific mortality (number of deaths due to a certain cause out of the total population). But even mortality data contradicted the virologist's claim: while on that day Italian statistics showed that the coronavirus had already caused over 36,000 deaths, in recent years annual deaths caused by suicides and road accidents in Italy did not exceed 4,000.

The "colding" of the virus

In the summer of 2020, after the catastrophic death toll caused by the virus and the dissemination of tragic images such as military trucks transporting coffins near Bergamo, some naively hoped that attempts to minimize the danger of the virus had finally ceased. However, the disinformation continued unabated. The propagation of inaccuracies about SARS-CoV-2 took a peculiar turn with the arrival of the Omicron variants and the hypothesis of the "colding" of the virus. An Italian expert in molecular virology assured: "Omicron [is] weak … we are moving towards the 'colding' of the virus."[31] Another virologist reiterated the same idea: "[Omicron] has colded down COVID."[32] Similarly, another expert argued: "the symptoms are absolutely mild. In Europe we could be more than calm."[33] Then, a member of the CTS chimed in: "Omicron … no longer appears to be as transmissible as initially thought and is certainly less pathogenic."[34] The colding of SARS-CoV-2 gained followers in the United States too. A professor at Johns Hopkins University School of Medicine explained that the virus was "dumbing down" and coined the term "Omi-cold."[35] Since the date of this interview, the United States has experienced more than 400,000 deaths due to COVID-19.

Some experts also complained that media outlets were just causing unnecessary "alarmism"[36] or an unjustified "contagion paranoia."[37] During the early appearance of Omicron, the number of patients hospitalized in intensive care reached record levels in several countries. Early analyses published by Imperial College,[38] the UK Health Security Agency, and the *New England Journal of Medicine* indicated that what worried experts the most about the first Omicron variant was the speed of spread.[39] As Neil Ferguson of Imperial College London pointed out, "This level of immune evasion means that Omicron represents a serious and imminent threat to public health."[40] The first analyses on the dangers of Omicron were published in the *New England Journal of Medicine*, estimating that it was only 25% less likely than Delta to cause hospitalization in an unvaccinated person with no history of SARS-CoV-2 infection. Further studies confirmed the lower severity of Omicron[41] compared to Delta, but no reputable scientific article in a well-established journal has ever entertained the idea that SARS-CoV-2 has been "colding down."

The confusion of many experts may have been perhaps facilitated by the complexity of extrapolating the intrinsic severity of a virus while accounting for the effects induced by vaccines and previous infections.[39] Omicron variants' ability to kill and send people to hospitals has been substantially attenuated by the large proportion of citizens vaccinated or immunized due to previous infections.[42] Yet, Omicron is not a simple cold. Epidemiological analyses from Massachusetts showed that during the first eight weeks of the "Omicron period," excess mortality from all causes was higher than that observed during the "Delta period."[43] Moreover, the rapid increases in mortality after the relaxation of restrictions in countries such as Hong Kong and China confirmed the danger of Omicron. Mistaking a weak virus for a virus that causes attenuated effects due to vaccinations was a serious misstep. As a comment on social media put it, "Omicron didn't shoot rubber bullets at us instead of metal ones: it only seems that way because we're wearing bulletproof vests."

"Masks are useless"

Even the use of masks has been subject to embarrassing falsifications. A systematic review and meta-analysis revealed a significant gap between the effectiveness of masks in preventing respiratory diseases and the public's perception of their effectiveness.[44] The lack of adherence to their use has been fueled in part by the spread of false information on social media,[45] but not only that. A renowned American expert contributed to the confusion by initially stating that "in the United States, people should not be walking around with a mask."[46] In Italy, on January 30, 2020, a well-known virologist from the State University of Milan declared that the mask "makes no sense in Italy. It may serve to reduce the influence we have a little, but it is not in the style and habits of Italians." And then he explained: "citizens must remain calm. The institutions, in Italy in particular, in my opinion are moving to manage and organize the treatments of the many suspected cases, precisely because there is great confusion with the flu."[47] Even the Italian representative of the WHO board, in a TV interview on March 10, 2020, advised against the use of masks: "they are of absolutely no use to healthy people; they give no protection against the viruses that penetrate through those sheets of gauze. It's just paranoia that people misuse."[48] The official WHO position was different and had no reference to any "paranoia." Yet, in April 2020, WHO guidelines recommended the use of masks only for those with COVID-19 symptoms and healthcare workers. The error was obvious, but a few months later the guidelines were amended, and masks were recommended for all.

This change did not stop masks from being targets of wrong information even after that. During the summer of 2020, a CTS member underlined: "Today it makes little sense to wear masks, gloves and keep distanced in certain areas of the country."[49] Already in spring of 2020 there were studies and scientific literature supporting the importance of masks in reducing the possibility of contracting respiratory infections.[50-52] In April 2020, a review published in the British Medical Journal argued that "the precautionary principle states that sometimes we should act without definitive evidence, just in case. Because COVID-19 is such a serious threat, wearing masks in public should be recommended."[53]

In line with these recommendations, in the first months of 2020, countries such as Hong Kong, Japan, South Korea, Thailand and Taiwan ignored the WHO recommendations and suggested or required their citizens to use masks.[54] In July 2021, a meta-analysis and systematic review of the literature was released, concluding that the use of masks was associated with a significant reduction in the risk of COVID-19 infection.[54] Further reviews supported similar findings.[55,56] Analogous results were observed in another review, emphasizing that inhalation protection via masks is particularly important in reducing aerosol transmission of COVID-19.[57] Another study that appeared in the Centers for Disease Control and Prevention journal underlined the importance of using masks to reduce exposure to infections, especially in closed environments.[58] This sentiment was echoed by a randomized experiment involving over 300,000 people, demonstrating the effectiveness of wearing masks in reducing COVID-19 infections in rural areas of Bangladesh.[59]

In June 2022, a professor of clinical pathology at La Sapienza University of Rome insisted that "there is no international study which can demonstrate that the massive use of masks has had any effect in containing the spread of Sars-Cov-2."[60] Two editorials appearing in *Forbes* and *The New York Times* suggested that masks worked only individually, not when adopted as a preventive political measure on a collective level.[61] Contrary to this, a study published in the *New England Journal of Medicine* showed that COVID-19 infections increased substantially in Massachusetts schools just as mandatory mask policies were lifted.[62] Unfortunately, the abolition of the obligation to use masks during the most dangerous weeks of the pandemic exposed many children, adolescents and adults to re-infections, with serious effects on long COVID.[63,64]

"Asymptomatic people do not infect"

As previously mentioned, in the summer of 2020, Italy adopted one of the longest and most rigid lockdowns in the world. During those months, infections significantly decreased, creating a false sense of security. According to a well-known professor who has labelled prevention measures as "terrorism." the pandemic was already "under control" adding that "90% of positive cases [were] asymptomatic."[65] A few months later, another expert with a prestigious scientific background asserted that "95% of positive cases [were] asymptomatic."[66] Even the deputy director of the WHO in an earlier interview said that "for every 5 clinically relevant cases, there are 15 mildly symptomatic and 80 completely asymptomatic."[67] Was this truly the case?

Not even a single scientific analysis supported the hypothesis that 90–95% of those infected by COVID-19 were asymptomatic. An Italian study conducted during the summer of 2020 indicated that positive cases without symptoms were around 55.9%.[68] Another contribution published in *Nature* estimated 42.7% of asymptomatic individuals.[69] Furthermore, a meta-analysis and systematic review of 94 studies published in *PloS One* reported an asymptomatic rate of about 20%.[70]

The exaggerations on the proportion of asymptomatic cases often coincided with denialism regarding the effective capability of asymptomatic individuals to spread the virus. At the end of February 2020, one of the main leaders of the CTS highlighted "the futility of swabbing asymptomatic people."[71] Unfortunately, even the WHO initially shared this view. On February 24, 2020, a WHO official wrote: "The proportion of truly asymptomatic COVID-19 infections is unclear, but appears to be relatively rare and does not appear to be a major channel of transmission."[72] Yet, during those same days, credible scientific information on their danger was already available.[73,74] Months later, another WHO representative insisted that contagion from people without symptoms was "very rare." She ignored a growing number of studies that suggested the opposite.[75] The statement attracted criticism from numerous public health experts.[76] The risk posed by asymptomatic individuals in terms of virus transmission was subsequently highlighted and supported by additional studies[77–79] as well as a systematic review of 94 articles. The CDC confirmed previous findings[77] suggesting that asymptomatic individuals were responsible for about one-fourth of infections.[80]

Scientific evidence, however, seemed totally irrelevant to some Italian experts who had preemptively decided that "asymptomatic people are not contagious."[81] While this might appear just as another academic debate, it was, in fact, a crucial matter. Understanding the contagiousness of asymptomatic individuals was essential for shaping preventive strategies and determining whether to use tests to diagnose potential contagion in those without symptoms.

The "tamponite"

The front page of the main Italian sports newspaper *La Gazzetta dello Sport* on September 29, 2020, declared, "Genoa shock!," referring to the Serie A match between Naples and Genoa, which ended 6-0 for Naples, with 10 Genoa players testing positive for SARS-CoV-2. However, the real shock, according to the director of the infectious disease clinic at San Martino Hospital in Genoa, was not the widespread outbreak of the virus in Italian football but the unreliability of the tests used to establish COVID-19 cases. As he put it, "what is happening to Genoa football could represent the Waterloo of swabs."[82] In another interview, he explained: "what's the point of saying that we have 250,000 people who have a positive swab? ... these are numbers that make us look bad towards the rest of the world, because it seems like everything is going badly ..."[83]

The incapability to grasp the significance of preventive strategies based on mass testing is a recurring theme in Italy's pandemic management. During the first tragic weeks of the pandemic, while dozens of patients and health workers were dying of COVID-19 in local hospitals, an Italian company based in Brescia exported half a million swabs to the United States. Investigations by the Bergamo prosecutor's office revealed that top officials in charge of the Italian COVID-19 strategy misunderstood both the role of asymptomatic individuals in the pandemic and the usefulness of widespread testing. On March 15, 2020, the deputy director of the WHO remarked that "doing swabs for everyone is now the bullshit of the century" and advised another expert to refrain from proposing "nonsense such as swabs for everyone." Another expert underscored that "the problem is that everyone thinks that the test is useful for something."[71]

Some Italian experts even argued that the country's main problem was not the overwhelming number of infections but the excessive use of swabs. Despite scientific evidence supporting the critical importance of widespread testing to manage outbreaks, a prominent epidemiologist claimed there was an "epidemic of swabs" in Italy. He explained in a critical tone: "for the first time in human history, a pandemic sees diagnostic confirmation with direct research of the presence of the virus as a cornerstone of infection control."[84] These words echoed those of the governor of the Campania region, who explained that the real disease of Italy was not COVID-19 but excessive testing that had become a disease itself: the "tamponite."[85]

These statements may sound remarkably absurd, but they merely scratch the surface of the outlandish criticisms surrounding the use of swabs during the health crisis. The crusade against testing commenced early in the pandemic's unfolding. On March 17, 2020, the WHO deputy director explained that mass swabs were "scientifically useless" and "logistically impossible."[86] Almost simultaneously, the representative for Italy on the WHO executive council claimed that excessive swab testing in the pandemic's early stages had unfairly labeled Italy as a nation of "infectors," as positive cases were erroneously inflated.[87] An epidemiologist from the State University of Milan asserted that swabs should not have been administered to asymptomatic individuals.[88] In a notable television appearance, another renowned virologist added fuel to the fire, suggesting that swabs could lead to severe injuries by breaching the blood-brain barrier. This assertion was supported by a single case study involving only one individual, albeit one with an "extremely rare" event triggered by an anatomical defect and pre-existing clinical conditions, a detail conveniently downplayed by the expert criticizing the excessive use of testing.[89]

While the term "tamponite" has gained traction mainly in the Italian discourse, the notion of vilifying swab usage has found echoes in other countries. In the United States, Donald Trump, facing pressure to test millions of

Americans, argued that the surge in COVID-19 cases resulted from testing itself rather than the actual spread of infections. The logic was "flawless": the fewer swabs, the fewer infections. This represents an unusual turn in the discussions about swabs, where the focus seemed to change from implementing effective infection control measures to waging a peculiar fight against the very tool to detect the virus and aid in prevention interventions.

The accusations of excessive testing run counter to authoritative analyses published in international scientific journals, which unequivocally endorse the swab as a reliable and indispensable diagnostic tool for guiding preventive strategies.[90] As underlined by an article in *Nature Medicine*, testing early during an outbreak is key to interrupting chains of contagion. The authors remarked: "...the main tool (to prevent cases) will remain the swab, to be done as soon as possible to all suspected infected people and their contacts."[91] The significance of testing was further underscored by cross-national comparisons and case studies of countries that excelled in containing the pandemic.[92] Other articles that appeared in scientific journals such as *Science*,[93] *JAMA*[94] and *Nature*[95] emphasized that mass testing strategies adopted by countries like South Korea, Taiwan, Singapore and Hong Kong played a pivotal role in limiting mortality rates.

Contrary to assertions about the uselessness of swabs, numerous experts in epidemiology and public health expressed their full support for the mass testing policy. As Devi Sridhar, author of *Preventable* and professor of global health at the University of Edinburgh, explained at the beginning of the spread of SARS-CoV-2, "without mass testing, the coronavirus pandemic will continue to spread."[96] In Italy, the most vocal supporters of this policy were healthcare workers. At the pandemic's onset, a letter from 100,000 doctors spanning all specialties and services across Italy, addressed to Minister Speranza, emphasized, "mapping these patients, whether asymptomatic or minimally symptomatic, along with all family members of confirmed cases, is extremely essential to prevent falling into a vicious circle, with waves of recurring infections once the lockdown ends."[97]

"The hidden cures they never tell us"

Since the onset of the pandemic, healthcare workers have displayed heroic dedication in the face of an unprecedented health crisis. However, instead of receiving the gratitude they deserved, they have become targets of numerous attacks and acts of violence. As underlined in an editorial that appeared in *The Lancet*, misinformation and conspiracy theories have contributed to their demonization.[98] Some misguided relatives of severely ill patients (or those who succumbed to the virus at home) in particular firmly believed in the existence of effective treatments that were never administered to their family members. This misperception led to violent repercussions against healthcare professionals already grappling with immense stress from years of the pandemic.

Compounding the issue is the ambiguity surrounding the virus's effects. A considerable portion of COVID-19 patients experienced spontaneous recovery without specific treatments, merely relying on drugs to alleviate symptoms. Unfortunately, this has fueled the misconception that a cure exists. Some journalists and commentators, lacking the ability to decipher scientific literature, have exacerbated the situation by sensationalizing false beliefs. An emblematic example is the misinterpretation of a study published in *Lancet Infectious Diseases* entitled "Home as a New Frontier for the Treatment of COVID-19: The Case of NSAIDs (Non-Steroidal Anti-Inflammatory Drugs)."[99] Based on its results, some media reporters claimed that NSAIDs, if adopted in time, would have been capable of "saving" about 90% of COVID-19 deaths.[100] In the following days, all hell happened. Social media platforms were inundated with insults directed at the Italian government and the health minister, accusing them of deception and even demanding legal action. Had readers scrutinized the original study and delved into the scientific literature, they would have discovered that the purported lifesaving effects of NSAIDs were not supported by any solid evidence. Moreover, the "90% effect" was not reflected on any page of the article widely misquoted in the media.[101] A systematic review and meta-analysis conducted months earlier on the same topic also refuted claims that NSAIDs improved COVID-19 prognosis and showed that on the basis of 40 comparative studies consisting of 4,867,795 cases "the use of NSAIDs did not reduce mortality outcomes among people with COVID-19."[102] Another review, based on previous observational studies, systematic reviews and meta-analyses, concluded that NSAIDs did not worsen (or improve) disease outcomes in patients with COVID-19.[103] It was all hype for nothing!

In light of so much misinformation regarding COVID-19 treatments, it's crucial to dispel misconceptions surrounding certain touted remedies. One prime example is the widespread belief in the miraculous powers of chloroquine. Those absolutely convinced of its effectiveness have probably not read the results of a meta-analysis based on 28 randomized experimental studies concluding that treatment with hydroxychloroquine is associated with an increase, not a decrease, in mortality in COVID-19 patients.[104] Similarly, Ivermectin has also received particular attention as a potential treatment for COVID-19 disease on social media. However, a review of randomized experimental trials emphasized the limited and largely low-quality evidence supporting this treatment.[105] Another potential miracle cure that ended up at the center of heated media debates was the plasma of people who had recovered from COVID-19. Even in this case science debunked popular beliefs: a review of 13 studies concluded that plasma therapy did not confer any benefits for individuals severely or moderately affected by COVID-19.[106]

Unfortunately, there is limited availability of effective cures for COVID-19. A randomized trial published in *JAMA* indicated that immunomodulators, anti-platelet agents showed some efficacy in influencing survival post-COVID-19.[107] Treatment with a new oral antiviral drug named Paxlovid in the first five days of infection was shown to be effective in reducing progression to severe COVID-19 or mortality, regardless of vaccination status.[108] However, doctors and researchers highlighted some obstacles to the therapy's widespread use, including problems of "rebound" (a return of symptoms days after feeling better) and significant side effects.[109]

Inoculation against evidence-free opinions

In the quest to safeguard public health, the dissemination of accurate information is central. One of the essential ingredients for fighting a pandemic is effective communication and the development of messages capable of informing the public in a clear, simple and calm manner.[110] Establishing a communication strategy rooted in scientific principles and conveyed by trusted institutional figures can foster collaboration and cooperation among citizens, vital components in the collective effort to mitigate infections.[111] Correct information has the power to shape risk perception and motivate individuals to take protective measures. Numerous analyses suggest that effective communication can significantly reduce the virus's impact on mortality rates. A study highlighted that adequate knowledge, realistic risk perception and "healthy" individual attitudes toward COVID-19 showed a significant effect on promoting four life-saving behaviors: washing hands, correct habits during coughing, reducing the number of contacts and wearing a mask.[3] On the contrary, studies have shown that exposure to misinformation is linked with both risky behaviors and lower adherence to health regulations.[112]

Since the onset of the pandemic, a contentious issue has revolved around the role of experts in guiding interventions to mitigate the impact of COVID-19, both at the political and the behavioral level. This debate has been amplified by conflicting views and the issue of whether governments have been "following science's advice on managing COVID-19."[113] As analyzed in an article published in the *BMJ*, the success of certain countries in limiting the impact of SARS-CoV-2 could be evaluated by the degree to which policy leaders based their decisions upon the best available evidence. Notably, nations like the United Kingdom and the United States have become exemplars of governments seemingly choosing to disregard warnings from epidemiologists and public health scientists.[114] According to Richard Horton, editor of *The Lancet*, ignoring this advice caused what he called "the greatest failure of global science policy in a generation."[115]

Despite the undoubted importance of science in guiding policymaking, it remains to be seen who the "real" scientific experts to follow are. In the

Italian case, the communication of many renowned virologists was a complete disaster. The messages sent to the population were often incorrect, confused and contradictory. The bewilderment of citizens, at the mercy of television personalities and experts who spread unfounded truths throughout the course of the pandemic, has been one of the common threads of the COVID-19 strategy. Evidence-based facts have often been lost in the noise of erroneous opinions of experts with over-inflated egos, mainly driven by the need to seek publicity at all costs. Data survey results are merciless: a report published in April 2021 highlighted that only a small portion of Italians believed that communication during the health emergency was clear, high-quality and authoritative. Almost half of the population interviewed instead considered it confusing, and over a third classified it as anxiety-provoking and excessive.[116]

While numerous Western nations failed to meet the standards underlying effective communication during the pandemic, there are some positive examples. Countries like Taiwan, New Zealand and Vietnam have not only benefited from robust public health strategies, emphasizing prevention and community interventions, but also executed relatively successful communication campaigns. In Vietnam, the government responded swiftly to the crisis, implementing public health containment measures early on, coupled with a communication campaign characterized by timeliness and accuracy. The quality of information sources, clear and transparent content and reliable message transmission channels have been instrumental in promoting cognitive, emotional and behavioral changes that mitigated the risks of COVID-19 in the Eastern Asian nation.[117] Similarly, New Zealand's political measures against the pandemic were both effective and timely, focusing on promoting preventive behavior and empowering the community in infection containment. Prime Minister Jacinda Ardern's leadership stood out for its firm and clear communication style, which was simultaneously engaging and empathetic.[118] The approach to risk communication in New Zealand was founded on five key principles:

a   Reliance on scientific evidence,
b   Authoritative decision-making,
c   Collaboration with all stakeholders in crisis management,
d   Promotion of social solidarity,
e   Attention to citizen education.

An article that appeared in *JAMA* addressing the shortcomings in containing COVID-19 underscored the imperative for health science communities to enhance systematic efforts at science education.[119] One of the limits of several national strategies consisted of the difficulty of persuading sections of the population with little inclination toward scientific subjects to understand research findings. Researchers observed that there is a link between a low level of scientific education and susceptibility to COVID-19 conspiracy theories.[120] Interventions aimed at increasing citizens' scientific knowledge, especially within disadvantaged populations, are therefore imperative. Customized initiatives aimed at enhancing the comprehension of scientific information through clear, simple and transparent messages are also deemed essential.

Another critical step involves addressing scientists who make statements in the media. Many Italian experts who seized the spotlight during the pandemic, for example, expressed opinions without presenting data or evidence to substantiate their positions. Furthermore, they appeared uninformed about the best scientific literature on the topic during their television appearances. Shockingly, some of these individuals were subsequently rewarded with prestigious positions of power, indirectly conveying the misguided message that displaying hubris and disseminating misinformation are desirable traits in top positions within Italian healthcare institutions. Policy interventions are required to ensure that experts stay abreast of the latest scientific evidence in the literature before making public statements.

Equally vital is the need for top professionals to collaborate directly with policymakers, ensuring that policies are grounded in scientific evidence, rather than attempting to mold scientific evidence to fit policies. As highlighted by Taiwan's Vice President, Dr. Chen Chien-jen, "only facts should inform policies."[121] This echoed the words of Bertrand Russell when he said: "Never let yourself be diverted either by what you wish to believe, or by what you think would have beneficent social effects if it were believed. But look only and solely at what are the facts."[122]

Arguably the most disconcerting aspect of the COVID-19 communication failure in several nations has been the public sparring between "virologists" played out in newspapers, on TV and across social media platforms. Italy has probably provided a peculiar case study of how media sensationalism and disinformation can degenerate into chaos and popular confusion. During the pandemic, Italian media outlets have disseminated embarrassing insults even from well-known public figures, who attacked their opponents with epithets like "go back to the sewer,"[123] "I am fucking sick of it"[124] or "I do not talk about jackals and mosquitologists."[125] These personal attacks, devoid of any substantive argument, marked the lowest point of the pandemic communication. Italy, according to an analysis across a few European nations, stands out for a high percentage of insults and "toxic" comments on social media that include abuse, threats and hateful messages.[126] Witnessing renowned virologists exchanging insults was particularly disheartening. Scientific controversies constitute the essential basis for getting ever closer to an in-depth understanding of phenomena, including epidemics. A scientist should possess a flexible mindset that allows her or him to doubt ineluctably uncertain knowledge, prompting subsequent revisions in an iterative process that leads to greater certainty and a coherent accumulation of knowledge. Regrettably, the embarrassing arguments staged by many "virostars" represent the antithesis of the scientific process.

In the wake of recognized communication failures during the pandemic, one of the most pressing issues has been the imperative to combat false narratives that undermine science and public health. Addressing this challenge requires a structured approach to counter-disinformation actions capable of mitigating the impact of fake news. An article in *Nature Medicine* offered valuable suggestions on how to structure effective debunking messages.[127] According to the authors of the article, an effective debunking message should commence with presenting facts in a simple and memorable manner. The public should then be warned of the myths (but the myth should not be repeated more than once). Following this, the manipulation techniques used to mislead people should be identified and exposed. It is then crucial to reiterate the facts and emphasize the correct explanation. The authors explored some "prophylactic" approaches based on "inoculation against misinformation" consisting of two key components: first warning people that they may be misled by misinformation (to activate their psychological "immune system") and then preventing misinformation (tactic) by exposing them to a severely weakened dose of fake news combined with strong countermeasures and refutations (to generate cognitive "antibodies"). Once people have acquired "immunity," they can then indirectly spread the inoculation to others through offline and online interactions.

Recognizing the importance of combating the infodemia, or "too much information including false or misleading information in digital and physical environments during a disease outbreak,"[128] the WHO has developed recommendations to address news of false or dubious origin:[129]

1 Evaluate the reliability of the source.
2 Go beyond sensationalist headlines.
3 Identify the author of the information.
4 Check the publication dates of the news.
5 Examine the evidence supporting the thesis.
6 Check your prejudices.
7 Contact fact-checkers if in doubt.

In an insightful editorial featured in *Nature*, the key strategy to combat misinformation included inundating mass and social media with information that is accurate, easily digestible, engaging and shareable on mobile devices. The author of the editorial issued a call to action, urging scientists and informed individuals to leverage various platforms. As he put it: "Tweet. Write a comment for the press. Hold public lectures. Respond to journalists' requests. Share accurate information that you believe is valuable to the public. Correcting misrepresentations should be seen as a professional responsibility."[130] The sentiment echoes Noam Chomsky when he contends that intellectuals have the duty to "expose lies," even if it means challenging powerful figures or unsettling prevailing conventional wisdom.[131] Indeed, amidst the cacophony of opinions in TV debates and newspapers, a handful of scientist-activists have valiantly attempted to stem the tide of fake news and outlandish viewpoints. They have shared science, emphasizing the importance of not relying on anyone's opinion, however authoritative, but giving weight instead always to data, facts and evidence. Throughout the pandemic, the scientific information crucial for making lifesaving decisions has been readily available. As already noted, instead of hearing whoever's opinion, it was sufficient to look at the evidence including mortality statistics. These data often spoke for themselves. Sometimes they screamed.

References

1. Sule S, DaCosta MC, DeCou E, Gilson C, Wallace K, Goff SL. Communication of COVID-19 misinformation on social media by physicians in the US. *JAMA Network Open* 2023; **6**: e2328928.
2. Lee JJ, Kang K-A, Wang MP, *et al.* Associations between COVID-19 misinformation exposure and belief with COVID-19 knowledge and preventive behaviors: cross-sectional online study. *Journal of Medical Internet Research* 2020; **22**: e22205.
3. Xu H, Gan Y, Zheng D, *et al.* Relationship between COVID-19 infection and risk perception, knowledge, attitude, and four nonpharmaceutical interventions during the late period of the COVID-19 epidemic in China: online cross-sectional survey of 8158 adults. *Journal of Medical Internet Research* 2020; **22**: e21372.
4. Aghagoli G, Siff EJ, Tillman AC, Feller ER. COVID-19: misinformation can kill. *Rhode Island Medical Journal (2013)* 2020; **103**: 12–4.
5. Agamben G. L'invenzione di un'epidemia. Quodlibet. Published online on Feb 26, 2020. https://www.quodlibet.it/giorgio-agamben-l-invenzione-di-un-epidemia (accessed Jan 22, 2024).
6. Falcioni D. Italiani sempre più complottisti: per il 20% Covid creato in laboratorio, per il 5% non esiste. *Fanpage*. Published online Nov 24, 2020. https://www.fanpage.it/attualita/italiani-sempre-piu-complottisti-per-il-20-covid-creato-in-laboratorio-per-il-5-non-esiste/ (accessed Jan 22, 2024).
7. Ziniti A. Rapporto Censis, così la pandemia ha cambiato l'Italia: più negazionista, cospirazionista e fobica. *La Repubblica*. Published online Dec 3, 2021. https://www.repubblica.it/cronaca/2021/12/03/news/l_italia_irrazionale_che_esce_dalla_pandemia_negazionista_cospirazionista_credulona_e_fobica-328701909/ (accessed Jan 22, 2024).
8. Schaeffer K. Nearly three-in-ten Americans believe COVID-19 was made in a lab. Pew Research Center. Published online on Apr 8, 2020. https://www.pewresearch.org/short-reads/2020/04/08/nearly-three-in-ten-americans-believe-covid-19-was-made-in-a-lab/ (accessed Jan 22, 2024).
9. BBC. Coronavirus: Trump attacks 'China-centric' WHO over global pandemic. BBC News. Published online Apr 8, 2020. https://www.bbc.com/news/world-us-canada-52213439 (accessed Jan 22, 2024).

10. Bloom JD, Chan YA, Baric RS, *et al*. Investigate the origins of COVID-19. *Science* 2021; 372: 694.
11. Burns A. Trump: Obama born in Kenya. POLITICO. Published online May 25, 2012. https://www.politico.com/blogs/burns-haberman/2012/05/trump-obama-born-in-kenya-124569 (accessed Jan 22, 2024).
12. Wong E. Trump has called climate change a Chinese hoax. Beijing says it is anything but. *The New York Times*. Published online Nov 18, 2016. https://www.nytimes.com/2016/11/19/world/asia/china-trump-climate-change.html (accessed Jan 22, 2024).
13. Mark M. Trump just referred to one of his most infamous campaign comments: calling Mexicans 'rapists'. Business Insider. Published online on Apr 5, 2018. https://www.businessinsider.com/trump-mexicans-rapists-remark-reference-2018-4 (accessed Jan 22, 2024).
14. Kessler G, Rizzo S, Kelly M. Analysis | President Trump has made more than 20,000 false or misleading claims. Washington Post. Published online Feb 10, 2021. https://www.washingtonpost.com/politics/2020/07/13/president-trump-has-made-more-than-20000-false-or-misleading-claims/ (accessed Jan 22, 2024).
15. BBC News. False coronavirus claims by politicians debunked. Published online on Apr 16, 2020. https://www.bbc.com/news/av/52299689 (accessed Jan 22, 2024).
16. Marineau S. Russian disinformation in the time of Covid-19. The Conversation. Published online July 8, 2020. http://theconversation.com/russian-disinformation-in-the-time-of-covid-19-142309 (accessed Jan 22, 2024).
17. Brown L. China suggests Italy may be the birthplace of COVID-19 pandemic. *New York Post*. Published online Nov 20, 2020. https://nypost.com/2020/11/20/china-suggests-italy-may-be-the-birthplace-of-covid-19-pandemic/ (accessed Jan 22, 2024).
18. Il Sole 24 Ore. Coronavirus, lo sfogo della direttrice analisi del Sacco: «È una follia, uccide di più l'influenza». Burioni: «No a bugie» Published online on Feb 23, 2020. https://www.ilsole24ore.com/art/coronavirus-sfogo-direttrice-analisi-sacco-e-follia-uccide-piu-l-influenza-ACq3ISLB?refresh_ce=1
19. Virgilio G. Oramai è Burioni vs. Bassetti, il botta e risposta sul Coronavirus. Telefriuli. Published online Feb 15, 2020. https://www.telefriuli.it/cronaca/oramai-e-burioni-vs-bassetti-il-botta-e-risposta-sul-coronavirus/ (accessed Jan 22, 2024).
20. Il Tempo. Coronavirus in Italia: altro che rischio zero. Così i social massacrano Roberto Burioni e governo. Published online on Mar 29, 2020. https://www.iltempo.it/home-tv/2020/03/27/video/coronavirus-roberto-burioni-che-tempo-che-fa-2-febbraio-video-fabio-fazio-ministro-speranza-1303543/ (accessed Jan 22, 2024).
21. Rai. Roberto Burioni sul Coronavirus – Che tempo che farà 09/02/2020. Feb 9, 2020. https://www.youtube.com/watch?app=desktop&v=CaCRUFo3-Ig&ab_channel=Rai (accessed Jan 22, 2024).
22. Gandini S. Covid-19: rendere politica la rabbia – di Sara Gandini. Effimera. Published online on Mar 19, 2020. https://effimera.org/covid-19-rendere-politica-la-rabbia-di-sara-gandini/ (accessed Jan 22, 2024).
23. Rai. Coronavirus, la virologa Ilaria Capua: 'Questo virus è stato sopravvalutato'. Published online on Feb 24, 2020. https://www.la7.it/aggiornamenti-sul-coronavirus/video/coronavirus-la-virologa-ilaria-capua-questo-virus-e-stato-sopravvalutato-24-02-2020-309135 (accessed Jan 22, 2024).
24. Arnaldi V. Coronavirus, la virologa Ilaria Capua: "È una brutta influenza, meglio non andare in giro. Le Asl aiutino chi è in quarantena". Published online Feb 24, 2020. https://www.leggo.it/sanita/coronavirus_virologa_ilaria_capua_influenza_ultime_notizie_oggi-5070747.html (accessed Jan 22, 2024).

25. Ioannidis JPA. A fiasco in the making? As the coronavirus pandemic takes hold, we are making decisions without reliable data. STAT. Published online Mar 17, 2020. https://www.statnews.com/2020/03/17/a-fiasco-in-the-making-as-the-coronavirus-pandemic-takes-hold-we-are-making-decisions-without-reliable-data/ (accessed Jan 22, 2024).

26. Wang C, Horby PW, Hayden FG, Gao GF. A novel coronavirus outbreak of global health concern. *The Lancet* 2020; **395**: 470–3.

27. Rai Report. Era solo un influenza? Published online on Jan 25, 2021. https://www.raiplay.it/video/2021/01/Report-36ecb482-6064-4b6e-9e30-a0474334ff7f.html (accessed Jan 22, 2024).

28. Wu Z, McGoogan JM. Characteristics of and important lessons from the coronavirus disease 2019 (COVID-19) outbreak in China: summary of a report of 72 314 cases from the Chinese Center for Disease Control and Prevention. *JAMA* 2020; **323**: 1239–42.

29. Pipitone F. Covid, per il prof. Bernabei (CTS) non è un virus terribile: 'È una malattia normale'. Vesuvio Live. Published online Nov 7, 2020. https://www.vesuviolive.it/ultime-notizie/362978-bernabei-covid-malattia-normale/ (accessed Jan 22, 2024).

30. Gruppo Tv7. Intervista a Giorgio Palù (2 di 4). Primus Inter Pares. Published online on Oct 14, 2020. https://www.youtube.com/watch?v=jNAfIgGtOHw (accessed Jan 22, 2024).

31. Spadaro M. Covid, il dottor Baldanti del policlinico di Pavia: 'Omicron debole, si va verso "raffreddorizzazione" del virus'. StrettoWeb. Published online Jan 5, 2022. https://www.strettoweb.com/2022/01/covid-il-dottor-baldanti-omicron-debole-raffreddorizzazione-del-virus/1288955/ (accessed Jan 22, 2024).

32. Nidi A. 'Omicron non causa perdita gusto e olfatto'/Bassetti: 'Ha raffreddorizzato il Covid'. IlSussidiario.net. Published online Jan 3, 2022. https://www.ilsussidiario.net/news/omicron-non-causa-perdita-gusto-e-olfatto-bassetti-ha-raffreddorizzato-il-covid/2272351/ (accessed Jan 22, 2024).

33. Sablone L. La Gismondo smonta i catastrofisti: 'Omicron? Panico infondato'. Il Giornale. Published online Dec 2, 2021. https://www.ilgiornale.it/news/cronache/gismondo-smonta-i-catastrofisti-omicron-panico-infondato-1993295.html (accessed Jan 22, 2024).

34. Adnkronos. Variante Omicron, dati su sintomi e news: no allarme in Italia. Adnkronos. Published online Dec 10, 2021. https://www.adnkronos.com/Archivio/cronaca/variante-omicron-dati-su-sintomi-e-news-no-allarme-in-italia_DDHnZNIef2gPw68AqzP46 (accessed Jan 22, 2024).

35. Jones K. Dr. Marty Makary dismisses Christmas Omicron hysteria: 'No Need to Do Anything Different'. Mediaite. Published online Dec 16, 2021. https://www.mediaite.com/news/dr-marty-makary-dismisses-christmas-omicron-hysteria-no-need-to-do-anything-different/ (accessed Jan 29, 2024).

36. Perrero ME. Variante Omicron, cosa cambia? Il virologo Clementi: 'Sintomi lievi, no allarmismi'. La Gazzetta dello Sport. Published online Nov 30, 2021. https://www.gazzetta.it/salute/salute/30-11-2021/variante-omicron-cosa-cambia-il-virologo-clementi-sintomi-lievi-57455.shtml (accessed Jan 22, 2024).

37. Adnkronos. Covid, Zangrillo: 'Paranoia contagio creata dai media'. *Adnkronos*. Published online Dec 18, 2021. https://www.adnkronos.com/Archivio/cronaca/covid-zangrillo-paranoia-contagio-creata-dai-media_6RNcB3Ya1Bn JZUEB2RBOxC (accessed Jan 22, 2024).

38. Imperial College London: Report 49, Growth, population distribution and immune escape of Omicron in England. Published online on Dec 15, 2021. Scientific Advisory Group for Emergencies. https://www.gov.uk/government/publications/imperial-college-london-report-49-growth-population-distribution-and-immune-escape-of-omicron-in-england-15-december-2021 (accessed Jan 22, 2024).

39. Bhattacharyya RP, Hanage WP. Challenges in inferring intrinsic severity of the SARS-CoV-2 Omicron variant. *New England Journal of Medicine* 2022; **386**: e14.
40. Head E, van Elsland S. Omicron largely evades immunity from past infection or two vaccine doses | Imperial News | Imperial College London. Imperial News. Published online Dec 17, 2021. https://www.imperial.ac.uk/news/232698/modelling-suggests-rapid-spread-omicron-england/ (accessed Jan 22, 2024).
41. Sigal A, Milo R, Jassat W. Estimating disease severity of Omicron and Delta SARS-CoV-2 infections. *Nature Reviews Immunology* 2022; **22**: 267–9.
42. Nyberg T, Ferguson NM, Nash SG, *et al.* Comparative analysis of the risks of hospitalisation and death associated with SARS-CoV-2 Omicron (B.1.1.529) and Delta (B.1.617.2) variants in England: a cohort study. *The Lancet* 2022; **399**: 1303–12.
43. Faust JS, Du C, Liang C, *et al.* Excess mortality in Massachusetts during the Delta and Omicron waves of COVID-19. *JAMA* 2022; **328**: 74–6.
44. Li H, Yuan K, Sun Y-K, *et al.* Efficacy and practice of facemask use in general population: a systematic review and meta-analysis. *Transl Psychiatry* 2022; **12**: 1–15.
45. Ayers JW, Chu B, Zhu Z, *et al.* Spread of misinformation about face masks and COVID-19 by automated software on Facebook. *JAMA Internal Medicine* 2021; **181**: 1251–3.
46. 60 Minutes. March 2020: Dr. Anthony Fauci talks with Dr Jon LaPook about COVID-19. Published online on March 8, 2020. https://www.youtube.com/watch?v=PRa6t_e7dgI&ab_channel=60Minutes
47. Radio Popolare. Coronavirus, il virologo Pregliasco: 'I cittadini in Italia devono stare tranquilli'. Radio Popolare. Published online Jan 30, 2020. https://www.radiopopolare.it/coronavirus-virologo-pregliasco/ (accessed Jan 22, 2024).
48. La7. Coronavirus, Ricciardi (OMS): 'Le mascherine chirurgiche non servono, il virus penetra attraverso la garza'. Published online on March 10, 2020. https://www.la7.it/dimartedi/video/coronavirus-ricciardi-oms-le-mascherine-chirurgiche-non-servono-il-virus-penetra-attraverso-la-garza-10-03-2020-312511 (accessed Jan 22, 2024).
49. De Bac M. Covid ora meno contagioso? L'epidemiologo Greco: «In alcune Regioni mascherine inutili». Corriere della Sera. Published online June 24, 2020. https://www.corriere.it/cronache/20_giugno_24/coronavirus-l-epidemiologo-donato-greco-in-alcune-regioni-mascherine-non-servono-piu-9388c214-b647-11ea-9dea-5ac3c9ec7c08.shtml (accessed Jan 21, 2024).
50. Roberto De Vogli. Uso nelle mascherine nelle scuole, alcuni studi ne hanno messo in dubbio l'efficacia. *Il Fatto Quotidiano*. Published online Jan 17, 2022. https://www.ilfattoquotidiano.it/2022/01/17/uso-nelle-mascherine-nelle-scuole-alcuni-studi-ne-hanno-messo-in-dubbio-lefficacia/6454616/ (accessed Jan 22, 2024).
51. Shi DS. Hospitalizations of children aged 5–11 years with laboratory-confirmed COVID-19 – COVID-NET, 14 states, March 2020–February 2022. *Morbidity and Mortality Weekly Report* 2022; **71**. https://doi.org/10.15585/mmwr.mm7116e1.
52. Flaxman S, Whittaker C, Semenova E, *et al.* Assessment of COVID-19 as the underlying cause of death among children and young people aged 0 to 19 years in the US. *JAMA Network Open* 2023; **6**: e2253590.
53. MacIntyre CR, Chughtai AA. Facemasks for the prevention of infection in healthcare and community settings. *BMJ* 2015; **350**: h694.
54. BBC News. Coronavirus: some countries wear face masks and others don't. Published online Mar 26, 2020. https://www.bbc.com/news/world-52015486 (accessed Jan 22, 2024).
55. Li Y, Liang M, Gao L, *et al.* Face masks to prevent transmission of COVID-19: a systematic review and meta-analysis. *American Journal of Infection Control* 2021; **49**: 900–6.

56. Howard J, Huang A, Li Z, *et al*. An evidence review of face masks against COVID-19. *Proceedings of the National Academy of Sciences* 2021; **118**: e2014564118.

57. Wang Y, Deng Z, Shi D. How effective is a mask in preventing COVID-19 infection? *Medical Devices & Sensors* 2021; **4**: e10163.

58. Andrejko KL. Effectiveness of face mask or respirator use in indoor public settings for prevention of SARS-CoV-2 infection – California, February–December 2021. *Morbidity and Mortality Weekly Report* 2022; **71**. https://doi.org/10.15585/mmwr.mm7106e1.

59. Abaluck J, Kwong LH, Styczynski A, *et al*. Impact of community masking on COVID-19: a cluster-randomized trial in Bangladesh. *Science* 2022; **375**: eabi9069.

60. Romiti C. I talebani delle mascherine non mollano. L'Opinione delle Libertà. Published online June 25, 2022. https://opinione.it/editoriali/2022/06/24/claudio-romiti_talebani-mascherine-covid-virus-bizzarri-silvestri/ (accessed Jan 22, 2024).

61. Leonhardt D. Why masks work, but mandates haven't. The New York Times. Published online on Apr 31, 2022. https://www.nytimes.com/2022/05/31/briefing/masks-mandates-us-covid.html (accessed Jan 22, 2024).

62. Cowger TL, Murray EJ, Clarke J, *et al*. Lifting universal masking in schools – Covid-19 incidence among students and staff. *New England Journal of Medicine* 2022; **387**: 1935–46.

63. Roessler M, Tesch F, Batram M, *et al*. Post-COVID-19-associated morbidity in children, adolescents, and adults: a matched cohort study including more than 157,000 individuals with COVID-19 in Germany. *PLOS Medicine* 2022; **19**: e1004122.

64. Bowe B, Xie Y, Al-Aly Z. Acute and postacute sequelae associated with SARS-CoV-2 reinfection. *Nature Medicine* 2022; **28**: 2398–405.

65. Open. Coronavirus, il virologo Clementi: "Il 90% dei positivi è asintomatico e l'epidemia è sotto controllo". Published online on Aug 14, 2020. https://www.open.online/2020/08/14/coronavirus-virologo-clementi-90-positivi-asintomatico-epidemia-sotto-controllo/(accessed Jan 22, 2024).

66. AGI. 'Il 95% dei contagiati è asintomatico, basta con l'isteria' dice il virologo Palù. Published online Jan 22, 2024. https://www.agi.it/cronaca/news/2020-10-24/coronavirus-palu-asintomatici-basta-isterie-10055193/ (accessed Jan 22, 2024).

67. La7. Ranieri G. (OMS): 'Su 100 persone 80 non hanno sintomi e 15 sono paucisintomatici'. Published online on May 8, 2020. https://www.youtube.com/watch?v=3ahkvViJKd0 (accessed Jan 22, 2024).

68. Istituto Superiore di Sanità. Epidemia COVID-19. Epicentro. Published online on Oct 13, 2020. https://www.epicentro.iss.it/coronavirus/bollettino/Bollettino-sorveglianza-integrata-COVID-19_13-ottobre.pdf (accessed Jan 22, 2024).

69. Lavezzo E, Franchin E, Ciavarella C, *et al*. Suppression of a SARS-CoV-2 outbreak in the Italian municipality of Vo. *Nature* 2020; **584**: 425–9.

70. Buitrago-Garcia D, Egli-Gany D, Counotte MJ, *et al*. () Occurrence and transmission potential of asymptomatic and presymptomatic SARS-CoV-2 infections: A living systematic review and meta- analysis. *PLoS Medicine* 2020; **17**(9): e1003346

71. TG24 S. Covid, atti inchiesta Bergamo, Guerra: 'Tampone a tutti una scemenza'. Published online Mar 5, 2023. https://tg24.sky.it/cronaca/2023/03/05/bergamo-covid-inchiesta (accessed Jan 22, 2024).

72. World Health Organization. China Joint Mission on Covid 19. Final report. WHO. https://www.who.int/docs/default-source/coronaviruse/who-china-joint-mission-on-covid-19-final-report.pdf?fbclid=IwAR3IKi2bwW69O81xcSZuXecEmqvrMdSeejXXMQg5E7cO34YacliBFmBxiaY (accessed Jan 22, 2024).

73. Bai Y, Yao L, Wei T, *et al*. Presumed asymptomatic carrier transmission of COVID-19. *JAMA* 2020; **323**: 1406–7.
74. Wu JT, Leung K, Leung GM. Nowcasting and forecasting the potential domestic and international spread of the 2019-nCoV outbreak originating in Wuhan, China: a modelling study. *The Lancet* 2020; **395**: 689–97
75. Mandavilli A. In the W.H.O.'s coronavirus stumbles, some scientists see a pattern. *The New York Times*. Published online June 9, 2020. https://www.nytimes.com/2020/06/09/health/coronavirus-asymptomatic-world-health-organization.html (accessed Jan 22, 2024).
76. Michael E. Is asymptomatic spread common in COVID-19? *Healio*. Published online on Jun 12, 2020. https://www.healio.com/news/primary-care/20200612/is-asymptomatic-spread-common-in-covid19 (accessed Jan 22, 2024).
77. Li R, Pei S, Chen B, *et al*. Substantial undocumented infection facilitates the rapid dissemination of novel coronavirus (SARS-CoV-2). *Science* 2020; **368**: 489–93.
78. Tindale LC, Stockdale JE, Coombe M, *et al*. Evidence for transmission of COVID-19 prior to symptom onset. *Elife* 2020; **9**: e57149.
79. Furukawa NW, Brooks JT, Sobel J. Evidence supporting transmission of severe acute respiratory syndrome coronavirus 2 while presymptomatic or asymptomatic. *Emerging Infectious Diseases* 2020; **26**: e201595.
80. Fox M. Most coronavirus cases are spread by people without symptoms, CDC now says. CNN. Published online Nov 21, 2020. https://www.cnn.com/2020/11/20/health/cdc-coronavirus-spread-asymptomatic-website-wellness/index.html (accessed Jan 22, 2024).
81. Adnkronos. Covid, Tarro: 'Gli asintomatici non sono contagiosi'. Adnkronos. Published online Dec 12, 2020. https://www.adnkronos.com/Archivio/cronaca/covid-tarro-gli-asintomatici-non-sono-contagiosi_7klFZKBB60vMQi2xRGA3x5 (accessed Jan 22, 2024).
82. La Repubblica. Bassetti: 'Il caso Genoa è la Waterloo dei tamponi'. Published online Sept 29, 2020. https://genova.repubblica.it/cronaca/2020/09/29/news/bassetti_ii_caso_genoa_la_waterloloo_dei_tamponi_-268871034/ (accessed Jan 22, 2024).
83. Il report quotidiano diventa un caso, Bassetti: 'Non ha più senso, anche i dati dei deceduti sono falsati'. la Repubblica. Published online Jan 11, 2022. https://genova.repubblica.it/cronaca/2022/01/11/news/bassetti_basta_con_il_report_quotidiano_sui_contagi_non_ha_piu_senso_il_sottosegretario_alla_salute_costa_ha_ragione_-333431697/ (accessed Jan 19, 2024).
84. Huffington Post. Lopalco contro la 'dittatura del tampone': 'Il sistema rischia il tilt'. HuffPost Italia. Published online Sept 19, 2020. https://www.huffingtonpost.it/cronaca/2020/09/19/news/lopalco_contro_la_dittatura_del_tampone_il_sistema_rischia_il_tilt_-5299267/ (accessed Jan 22, 2024).
85. Askanews. Il governatore Vincenzo De Luca contro "la tamponite". Published online on Apr 10, 2020. https://askanews.it/old/op.php?file=/politica/2020/04/10/il-governatore-vincenzo-de-luca-contro-la-tamponite-top10_20200410_162451/ (accessed Jan 22, 2024).
86. Roberto De Vogli. Coronavirus, la credibilità dell'Oms è al minimo: troppi errori nella gestione della pandemia. Il Fatto Quotidiano. Published online June 12, 2020. https://www.ilfattoquotidiano.it/2020/06/12/coronavirus-la-credibilita-delloms-e-al-minimo-troppi-errori-nella-gestione-della-pandemia/5832622/ (accessed Jan 22, 2024).
87. Rodriguez G. Coronavirus. "Negli altri Paesi Ue il problema è stato sottostimato, non siamo gli 'untori' d'Europa. Ma in ogni caso per lasciarci alle spalle il pericolo dovremo aspettare maggio-giugno". Intervista a Walter Ricciardi. Quotidiano Sanità. Published online on Mar 2, 2020. https://www.quotidianosanita.it/scienza-e-farmaci/articolo.php?articolo_id=81950 (accessed Jan 22, 2024).

88. La Vecchia C. Covid, gli esperti: 'Gli asintomatici non dovrebbero fare i tamponi'. SondrioToday. Published online on Dec 29, 2021. https://www.sondriotoday.it/attualita/coronavirus/tamponi-covid-positivi-contatti-tracciamento.html (accessed Jan 22, 2024).
89. Sullivan CB, Schwalje AT, Jensen M, *et al.* Cerebrospinal fluid leak after nasal swab testing for coronavirus disease 2019. *JAMA Otolaryngology–Head & Neck Surgery* 2020; **146**: 1179–81.
90. Sethuraman N, Jeremiah SS, Ryo A. Interpreting diagnostic tests for SARS-CoV-2. *JAMA* 2020; **323**: 2249–51.
91. Giordano G, Blanchini F, Bruno R, *et al.* Modelling the COVID-19 epidemic and implementation of population-wide interventions in Italy. *Nature Medicine* 2020; **26**: 855–60.
92. Liang L-L, Tseng C-H, Ho HJ, Wu C-Y. Covid-19 mortality is negatively associated with test number and government effectiveness. *Scientific Reports* 2020; **10**: 12567.
93. Normiel D. Coronavirus cases have dropped sharply in South Korea. What's the secret to its success? *Science.* Published online on Mar 17, 2020. https://www.science.org/content/article/coronavirus-cases-have-dropped-sharply-south-korea-whats-secret-its-success (accessed Jan 23, 2024).
94. Wang CJ, Ng CY, Brook RH. Response to COVID-19 in Taiwan: big data analytics, new technology, and proactive testing. *JAMA* 2020; **323**: 1341–2.
95. Sheridan C. Fast, portable tests come online to curb coronavirus pandemic. *Nature Biotechnology* 2020; **38**: 515–8.
96. Sridhar D. Without mass testing, the coronavirus pandemic will keep spreading. Foreign Policy. Published online Jan 29, 2024. https://foreignpolicy.com/2020/03/23/coronavirus-pandemic-south-korea-italy-mass-testing-covid19-will-keep-spreading/ (accessed Jan 23, 2024).
97. Milazzo M. "Siamo centomila medici". Lettera al Ministro Della Salute. IS Media. Published online Apr 18, 2020. https://www.scinardo.it/appello-medici/ (accessed Jan 23, 2024).
98. McKay D, Heisler M, Mishori R, Catton H, Kloiber O. Attacks against healthcare personnel must stop, especially as the world fights COVID-19. *The Lancet* 2020; **395**: 1743–5.
99. Perico N, Cortinovis M, Suter F, Remuzzi G. Home as the new frontier for the treatment of COVID-19: the case for anti-inflammatory agents. *The Lancet Infectious Diseases* 2023; **23**: e22–33.
100. HuffPost Italia. Lancet: gli antinfiammatori bloccano l'infezione da Covid. Remuzzi: 'I vaccini un miracolo della medicina'. Published online Aug 29, 2022. https://www.huffingtonpost.it/covid/2022/08/29/news/gli_antinfiammatori_bloccano_linfezione_da_covid_sui_social_insulti_a_speranza-10104062/ (accessed Jan 23, 2024).
101. Roberto De Vogli. COVID, i fans riducono le ospedalizzazioni? Una lettura attenta dice che non è così. *Il Fatto Quotidiano.* Published online Aug, 2022, 2020. https://www.ilfattoquotidiano.it/2020/06/12/coronavirus-la-credibilita-delloms-e-al-minimo-troppi-errori-nella-gestione-della-pandemia/5832622/ (accessed Jan 22, 2024). https://www.ilfattoquotidiano.it/2022/08/30/covid-i-fans-riducono-le-ospedalizzazioni-una-lettura-attenta-dice-che-non-e-cosi/6784921/
102. Zhou Q, Zhao S, Gan L, *et al.* Use of non-steroidal anti-inflammatory drugs and adverse outcomes during the COVID-19 pandemic: a systematic review and meta-analysis. *EClinicalMedicine* 2022; **46**: 101373.
103. Laughey W, Lodhi I, Pennick G, *et al.* Ibuprofen, other NSAIDs and COVID-19: a narrative review. *Inflammopharmacol* 2023; **31**: 2147–59.

104. Axfors C, Schmitt AM, Janiaud P, *et al*. Mortality outcomes with hydroxychloroquine and chloroquine in COVID-19 from an international collaborative meta-analysis of randomized trials. *Nature Communications* 2021; **12**: 2349.
105. Cruciani M, Pati I, Masiello F, Malena M, Pupella S, De Angelis V. Ivermectin for prophylaxis and treatment of COVID-19: a systematic review and meta-analysis. *Diagnostics* 2021; **11**: 1645.
106. Iannizzi C, Chai KL, Piechotta *et al*. Convalescent plasma for people with COVID-19: a living systematic review. *Cochrane Database of Systematic Reviews* 2023(5): CD013600.
107. Writing Committee for the REMAP-CAP Investigators. Long-term (180-day) outcomes in critically ill patients with COVID-19 in the REMAP-CAP randomized clinical trial. *JAMA* 2023; **329**: 39–51.
108. Najjar-Debbiny R, Gronich N, Weber G, *et al*. Effectiveness of Paxlovid in reducing severe coronavirus disease 2019 and mortality in high-risk patients. *Clinical Infectious Diseases* 2023; **76**: e342–9.
109. Kozlov M. COVID drug Paxlovid was hailed as a game-changer. What happened? *Nature* 2023; **613**: 224–5.
110. Reddy BV, Gupta A. Importance of effective communication during COVID-19 infodemic. *Journal of Family Medicine and Primary Care* 2020; **9**: 3793–6.
111. Pian W, Chi J, Ma F. The causes, impacts and countermeasures of COVID-19 "infodemic": a systematic review using narrative synthesis. *Information Processing & Management* 2021; **58**: 102713.
112. Roozenbeek J, Schneider CR, Dryhurst S, *et al*. Susceptibility to misinformation about COVID-19 around the world. *Royal Society Open Science* 2020; **7**: 201199.
113. Are governments following the science on Covid-19? *The Economist*. Published online on Nov 11, 2020. https://www.economist.com/graphic-detail/2020/11/11/are-governments-following-the-science-on-covid-19 (accessed Jan 23, 2024).
114. Baker MG, Wilson N, Blakely T. Elimination could be the optimal response strategy for Covid-19 and other emerging pandemic diseases. *BMJ* 2020; **371**: m4907.
115. Horton R. 'It's the biggest science policy failure in a generation'. *Financial Times*. Published online on Apr 24, 2020. https://www.ft.com/content/8e54c36a-8311-11ea-b872-8db45d5f6714 (accessed Jan 23, 2024).
116. CENSIS. Disinformazione e fake news durante la pandemia: il ruolo delle agenzie di comunicazione. Published online Apr 19, 2021. https://www.censis.it/comunicazione/disinformazione-e-fake-news-durante-la-pandemia-il-ruolo-delle-agenzie-di (accessed Jan 23, 2024).
117. Tam LT, Ho HX, Nguyen DP, Elias A, Le ANH. Receptivity of governmental communication and its effectiveness during COVID-19 pandemic emergency in Vietnam: a qualitative study. *Global Journal of Flexible Systems Management* 2021; **22**: 45–64.
118. McGuire D, Cunningham JEA, Reynolds K, Matthews-Smith G. Beating the virus: an examination of the crisis communication approach taken by New Zealand Prime Minister Jacinda Ardern during the Covid-19 pandemic. *Human Resource Development International* 2020; **23**: 361–79.
119. Miller BL. Science denial and COVID conspiracy theories: potential neurological mechanisms and possible responses. *JAMA* 2020; **324**: 2255–6.
120. Wright L, Steptoe A, Fancourt D. Predictors of self-reported adherence to COVID-19 guidelines. A longitudinal observational study of 51,600 UK adults. *The Lancet Regional Health – Europe* 2021; **4**. https://doi.org/10.1016/j.lanepe.2021.100061.

121. The New York Times. Taiwan's weapon against coronavirus: an epidemiologist as vice president, Hernandez J and Horton C (authors). https://www.nytimes.com/2020/05/09/world/asia/taiwan-vice-president-coronavirus.html (accessed Jan 23, 2024).

122. Caulfield T. Pseudoscience and COVID-19 – we've had enough already. *Nature* 2020.

123. HuffPost Italia. Rissa social fra virologi sulla seconda ondata. 'Saccente'... 'Torna nelle fogne'.. Published online June 27, 2020. https://www.huffingtonpost.it/cronaca/2020/06/27/news/rissa_social_fra_virologi_sulla_seconda_ondata_saccente_torna_nelle_fogne_-5244389/ (accessed Jan 23, 2024).

124. Il Messaggero. Covid, Zangrillo sbotta in diretta tv: "Ho le palle piene, il Cts dica la verità agli italiani". Published online July 22, 2020. https://www.ilmessaggero.it/salute/medicina/covid_zangrillo_sbotta_in_onda_la7_inizio_ad_averne_le_palle_piene-5361315.html (accessed Jan 23, 2024).

125. Il Mattino. Coronavirus, il virologo Palù: "Crisanti? Non parlo di sciacalli zanzarologi". Published online July 5, 2020. https://www.ilmattino.it/primopiano/sanita/coronavirus_virologi_palu_crisanti_scontro-5328589.html (accessed Jan 23, 2024).

126. L'espresso. L'Italia è un Paese fondato sull'insulto: da noi il dibattito online più violento d'Europa. Published online May 29, 2018. https://lespresso.it/c/archivio/2018/5/29/litalia-e-un-paese-fondato-sullinsulto-da-noi-il-dibattito-online-piu-violento-deuropa/22128 (accessed Jan 23, 2024).

127. van der Linden S. Misinformation: susceptibility, spread, and interventions to immunize the public. *Nature Medicine* 2022; 28: 460–7.

128. Infodemic. World Health Organization. https://www.who.int/health-topics/infodemic (accessed Jan 23, 2024).

129. Let's flatten the infodemic curve. World Health Organization. https://www.who.int/news-room/spotlight/let-s-flatten-the-infodemic-curve (accessed Jan 23, 2024).

130. Chomsky N. The responsibility of intellectuals. New York, NY: The New Press, 2017.

131. Eye P. Lord Bertrand Russell was all over fake news, 60 years before it was fashionable. The Sydney Morning Herald. Published online Mar 28; 2017. https://www.smh.com.au/public-service/lord-bertrand-russell-was-all-over-fake-news-60-years-before-it-was-fashionable-20170328-gv8duk.html (accessed Jan 23, 2024).

3

MEDICALIZATION

Non chiamateci eroi
Eravamo qui per voi

Contagiati
Dimenticati
Caduti nella scia

Giurammo di guarire il mondo
Anche chi, in estate, faceva il girotondo

Tra gli insulti della gente
Come fosse niente

Salvando vite ancora
Incontrammo la nostra ora

***

Don't call us heroes
We were just here for your sake

Infected
Forgotten
Fallen in the wake

We swore to mend the world's pain
Even those who danced in the summer chain

Amidst the insults on our way
We kept saving lives anyway

In our final hour
Bring us a flower

DOI: 10.4324/9781003511977-5

Francesco Gasparini, having enjoyed just over two years of well-deserved retirement after a lifetime dedicated to medicine as a doctor and anesthesiologist, found himself compelled to return to the front lines in the face of the relentless pandemic. Even in his respite, he couldn't turn away from the call to help. Veneto, particularly overwhelmed by the second wave, needed his selfless service. Wearing his scrubs once again, Gasparini lent his expertise to various medical facilities, including the civil hospital in Venice, and the towns of Dolo and Mirano. His commitment extended to medical guards, emergencies and the relentless pace of the emergency rooms.[1] Tragically, on December 11, at the Angelo hospital in Mestre, he succumbed to the very threat he had valiantly fought against.[2] At 67 years old, he left behind not just a career but a reservoir of untapped wisdom, professionalism and humanity. Gasparini, having tested positive for COVID-19 a month prior, saw his condition deteriorate rapidly, ultimately leading to his admission to intensive care. Despite lacking pre-existing health issues, he became one of the poignant casualties of the pandemic. In the United States, a similar destiny affected James Mahoney, a pulmonary specialist at University Hospital in Brooklyn, who was supposed to retire but decided to keep working when the pandemic overwhelmed New York.[3]

These stories are not isolated. Many more doctors, nurses and healthcare workers made similar courageous choices. They deliberately risked their own lives to save others. Therefore, these losses are particularly painful and moving.

"Naked against the virus"

There are more heart-breaking stories of medical personnel succumbing to the relentless grip of the coronavirus. Its impact has been particularly severe on them. According to a report by the World Health Organization, between January 2020 and May 2021, an estimated 115,000 healthcare workers lost their lives to COVID-19.[4] Italy has borne a staggering loss of doctors and nurses, an unprecedented toll in recent memory.[5] General practitioners, the backbone of primary healthcare, have been particularly affected.[6] During the initial wave, a letter from the Novara Medical Association to the governor of Lombardy highlighted that they were "left to their own devices in managing the emergency."[7] Struggling against a virus that impacted many, they faced a health battle without adequate protection and training and often limited access to essential resources such as swabs. Some have paid dearly for the deficiencies of underfunded National Health Systems unprepared to face the health crisis. Others, filled with a deep sense of despair and grief, decided to take their own lives.[8]

In both the United States and the United Kingdom too, the toll on healthcare workers during the pandemic has been overwhelming. A study published in *JAMA* revealed that from March 2020 to December 2021, 4,511 medical doctors lost their lives in the United States. Alarmingly, approximately 622 of these deaths were deemed "in excess" compared to the average of previous years. Most of them were directly attributable to the impact of SARS-CoV-2 and the extreme stress endured during those harrowing months.[9] Similarly, the United Kingdom witnessed a devastating loss of healthcare professionals. The British Medical Association (BMA) asserted that the English government had failed in its duty to protect doctors from avoidable harm and suffering during the pandemic. Two reports published in May 2022, drawing on the experiences of thousands of doctors, brought to light the profound and lasting impact of the pandemic. The reports exposed repeated errors, lapses in judgment and failures in government policy as contributing factors to the tragedies. The Chair of the BMA Council emphasized the moral duty of the government to safeguard health workers, yet decried the stark reality that doctors were let down by the inadequate pandemic preparedness and flawed decision-making. Much like the situation in Italy and in the United States, a shortage of personal protective equipment (PPE) left many of them without adequate protection. Healthcare workers ended up being infected at a higher rate than the general population. On top of the hundreds of healthcare workers who lost their lives, many others faced burnout, overwork, distress, trauma and isolation. At the root of this disaster are not only lethal mistakes by the English government but also chronic under-investment in health services that has left the United Kingdom ill prepared to deal with the pandemic.[10] As the International Council of Nurses (ICN) noted, the unacceptable number of deaths among healthcare workers reflects the government's failure to protect their most precious workforce during the health crisis.[4]

In Italy, protests from medical associations were not in short supply, particularly during the first wave. Numerous initiatives were launched to address critical shortages, including the lack of essential PPE such as gloves, glasses, visors and masks. Concerns also extended to the insufficient use of swabs and virus containment procedures in clinics and hospitals. Moreover, the inadequacy of intensive care and the pressing need for assisted breathing machines tested the safety of hospitals and local health services. On March 16, the Italian Federation of General Practitioners issued a press release titled "Naked against the Virus," denouncing the shortage of PPE for family doctors.[11] A poignant interview with Giuseppe Marzulli, former Medical Director of the Alzano Hospital, in one of the hardest-hit areas during the initial phase of the pandemic, likened the medical facility to a "circle from Dante's Inferno." He portrayed healthcare workers as "heroes sent to the massacre," deserving recognition for their civil valor.[12] In mid-December, the General Secretary of the Italian Doctors' Union and a family doctor in Rome penned a letter to then Prime Minister Giuseppe Conte, expressing the hope that decisions to combat the pandemic would take into consideration their anguished pleas. These professionals, often "sent into the trenches" without protection, were desperately seeking acknowledgment of their challenges.[13] As 2020 ended, a silent protest unfolded at the entrance of a major hospital in Brescia for five consecutive Fridays. Hundreds of doctors participated, symbolically turning their backs toward the management office building while facing the patients. The protest, titled "We Are All Hippocrates," drew attention to the severe shortages of healthcare personnel and organizational gaps resulting from years of underfunding and systematic weakening of the National Health System (NHS).[14]

The pandemic must be fought in the communities

These resonating protests have undeniably struck a chord within national health systems, prompting reflection on the critical need to fortify protective measures, bolster the workforce, increase intensive care bed capacity and enhance safety in hospitals and treatment departments. While these measures would undoubtedly have saved numerous lives, they alone would not have halted the relentless advance of the virus. As a press release from an association of surgeons and dentists in the province of Bergamo emphasized, during the worst times of the health crisis, there was an urgent need for effective coordination of community health interventions to shield healthcare personnel from infection. The crisis highlighted a critical error made by those countries that have been overwhelmed by the virus – treating the pandemic as purely medical problem. This led to the misguided belief that it could be fought solely within the confines of hospitals and the healthcare system. But isn't the pandemic a medical problem after all? Only to a partial extent. The pandemic is a public health – or, more accurately, a global health – problem. The true battleground against the pandemic lies in comprehensive preventive strategies that need to be implemented at a population level. While hospitals play a crucial role in treating the infected, the broader fight unfolds within communities, demanding coordinated efforts, widespread health education and strategic interventions to curb the transmission of the virus. Recognizing the global nature of the challenge, addressing the social and behavioral determinants of health and implementing preventive measures on a community scale are indispensable.

As observed in an article appearing in the Italian magazine *Salute Internazionale*, "a public health emergency was mistaken for an intensive care emergency ... [during the first waves of the pandemic] epidemiological investigations were not carried out, patients were not swabbed, doctors went around without personal protection ... and above all they inadvertently spread the infection." The author of the editorial then underlined another key point: "when the pandemic exploded, a large part of the available resources went to strengthening the hospital and intensive care system, with the media spotlight occupied by virologists, vaccine and intensive care experts, while there would be a need to understand where we went wrong or what could be done" to stop the virus through effective prevention interventions.[15]

The term "medicalization" may sound unnecessarily complex, but its essence lies in the process by which behavioral, social and even economic determinants of health are viewed through a narrow biomedical lens. In simpler terms, it involves seeing health as nothing more than the absence of disease and the adoption of a reductionistic biomedical perspective on health. This approach leads to confusion, with terms such as "health" and "healthcare" being mistakenly used interchangeably. Research, however, reveals that health determinants are not solely confined to medical interventions. Moreover, social, behavioral, political and economic factors play a far more significant role in determining health and disease patterns at the population level. Despite the overwhelming empirical evidence in support of the importance of "non-medical determinants of health," the dominance of the biomedical perspective, fueled by power-driven forces in the healthcare industry, tends to overshadow the multifaceted nature of health.

The overwhelming dominance of a reductionistic view of health is not only ingrained in our institutions and university system but also reinforced by large healthcare commercial interests, including the pharmaceutical and health insurance sectors. The aftermath of the pandemic in Italy saw the Italian Society of General Medicine and Primary Care, along with the Italian Federation of General Practitioners, inviting Sanofi, a French pharmaceutical company, to oversee the training program of general practitioners in health prevention.[16] This raises a critical question: what kind of expertise in prevention can a pharmaceutical company offer?

Advances in biomedical science, pharmaceuticals and medical interventions have, without a doubt, generated positive impacts on population health. However, a notable failure in the response of Western governments, still inadequately recognized even today, was the scarce emphasis on prevention and the social determinants of health.[17] An approach overwhelmingly focused on healthcare, aligned with a reductionist, reactive vision of health – responding to diseases after their onset – needs to be integrated with a systemic, proactive perspective designed to prevent and promote health, rather than waiting for illness to manifest. As argued by Lantz in an analysis of the COVID-19 policy responses in the United States, both the Trump and the Biden administrations heavily emphasized healthcare solutions and vaccines yet allocated insufficient resources to crucial so-called "non-pharmaceutical" interventions. These included contact tracing, rapid testing, indoor ventilation, masking, protective measures for frontline service workers and paid leave for sick workers. These interventions proved to be life-saving and were the only options available before the introduction of vaccines.[18]

In the initial months of the pandemic, I had the privilege of being interviewed by two members of an Italian association of family members of COVID-19 victims called *Noi Denunceremo*. This group dedicated its energies to analyzing the main mistakes of the pandemic while fostering crucial participatory and informative initiatives. One of the association's aims regarded an examination of the institutional responsibilities underlying the lack of COVID-19 prevention and assistance interventions. The movement serves as an inspiring example of how engaged citizens can become positive agents of social change. Indeed, the paramount importance of the active participation of communities in the design, implementation and evaluation of health promotion and protection programs is underlined in most university manuals for planning public health interventions. The pursuit of "culprits" through court investigations may serve to punish those who have neglected their duties or committed illegalities. Yet, it is even more crucial to address the systemic causes of these shortcomings. The most serious causes for Italy's failure to manage the pandemic effectively extend beyond individuals. They are structural problems requiring economic and political changes.

Paradoxically, some of the strongest advocates for reinforcing local prevention, were the very doctors and nurses who were bravely "on the front line," exposed to the virus on a daily basis. Recognizing the imperative of preventing overcrowding in IC units, healthcare professionals have prioritized interventions at the community level to stem the influx of patients approaching medical facilities. In a poignant letter addressed to the Minister of Health, signed by over 100,000 doctors, a resounding plea echoed: "In addition to protective equipment and swabs, we ask to strengthen the territory, the real weak point of the National Health Service." During the most challenging months, while some televised voices criticized efforts of population testing, doctors in hospitals and clinics remained resolute about the pivotal role of prevention in curbing the pandemic's spread. As the letter observed: "patients must be treated as soon as possible in the community. The mapping of these patients, whether asymptomatic or pauci-symptomatic, and of all the family members of the confirmed cases is essential to avoid falling into a vicious circle, with waves of returning infections as soon as the lockdown ends."[19]

These healthcare professionals contended that merely bolstering medical technologies and healthcare infrastructure was insufficient. While increasing IC beds is crucial, preventing the virus from reaching hospitals is paramount.

Although some cross-national studies have highlighted an inverse association between hospital bed capacity and COVID-19 mortality,[20] using OECD databases, a colleague and I estimated the correlations between the number of beds per thousand inhabitants and the number of deaths and infections per million inhabitants.[20] Analyses showed non-significant associations. In a letter to the *New England Journal of Medicine (NEJM)*, a group of doctors who had grappled with the epicenter of the pandemic crisis in Italy advocated for a shift from patient-centered care to community-centered care. According to them, the key interventions for managing COVID-19 must regard the entire population, not just hospitals and clinics. Protecting healthcare facilities and workers, they argued, necessitates comprehensive action at the community level.[21]

The tragic irony is that, in those weeks, prevention and epidemiological surveillance were loudly invoked after having long been underfunded and weakened by budget cuts and decisions that penalized their support in favor of more expensive and hyper-specialized treatments. Anyone who supported or contributed to the marginalization of prevention and dismantling of public health functions could have at least spared the crocodile tears over the tragedy caused by these ill-made decisions. Perhaps, some of the healthcare workers showing the banner "We Are All Hippocrates" on the roof of the public hospital of Brescia wanted also to scream "They Are All Hypocrites."

Prevention at the margins

Throughout the pandemic, the term "virologist" has echoed through the mass media, referring to experts in virology, a medical branch dedicated to the study of viruses and the diseases they cause. Virologists play a crucial role in understanding clinical manifestations, microbiological structures and mutations and in developing vaccines and drugs to combat virus-induced diseases. Their expertise is invaluable in deciphering the intricacies of the virus and its effects on individuals. However, the planning, execution and assessment of national strategies against SARS-CoV-2 require skills that extend well beyond the biological and clinical focus. While virologists excel in studying viruses and their pathogenicity, their expertise does not inherently cover the distribution of the virus and its determinants at the population level. The effective management of a pandemic demands a broader perspective encompassing behavioral, social, political and global determinants of health. During the pandemic, most media spokespersons seemed not fully aware of this and kept interviewing virologists about the epidemiology of the virus and the effectiveness of public health interventions to contain it. Of course, by interviewing the "wrong" experts they often obtained the wrong answers. As a professor at Northwestern University, Alessandro Vespignani humorously put it, "asking a virologist about the future course of the COVID-19 epidemic is akin to consulting a mechanic adept with pistons and car control units to predict how much traffic there will be on a highway outside Milan."[22]

The ancillary, marginal role assigned to prevention activities became evident not just through the delayed and inadequate actions of governments but also in the choice of experts tasked with leading national strategies against the pandemic. Perhaps the most globally recognized figure in the fight against the pandemic is Prof. Anthony Fauci, an authoritative immunologist and expert in internal medicine. Amidst the preposterous political and personal attacks he had to endure, he remained a prominent voice during the health crisis. Yet, he has often erroneously been portrayed as a public health expert, which clearly he is not. While Prof. Fauci boasts an impressive scientific background and extensive experience in the study of specific viruses such as HIV, SARS-CoV-1, avian flu, swine flu, Zika and Ebola, he should not be confused with a prevention specialist. Public health and prevention utilize different theories and methodological tools than immunology and medicine, emphasizing a population and community approach over an individual and biomedical one.

In the United States, the repercussions of failures in prevention were starkly lethal. According to Eric Topol, Director of Scripps Research Translational Institute, a major mistake in managing the pandemic was "not taking a test for almost two months."[23] The absence of a national program of timely testing left the country blind to the spread of COVID-19, hindering the ability to monitor transmission and anticipate the disease. Of course, as already mentioned, an important part of the blame for the abysmal failure of the United States should be placed on the anti-science policies of the Trump administration. Just to put things in context, the White House COVID-19 Task Force, a team of extreme importance in steering the pandemic response, was led by Mike Pence, well known for his evangelical extremism and for having propagated anti-scientific hoaxes such as the unfounded claim that "smoking doesn't kill."[24] Yet, the Biden administration too has largely failed to emphasize prevention interventions that have been successful abroad. For example, the strategy on testing remained largely unadopted and calls by experts to require a negative test before returning to work were ignored. On masks, there has been no serious attempt to adopt a mandate as happened in the most "successful" nations.[25]

If in the United States the prospect of adopting rigorous public health interventions and appointing an expert in prevention and epidemiology to lead the COVID-19 strategy seemed beyond consideration, in Italy the situation took an even more disheartening turn. A letter published in *Nature* scrutinizing the performance of the technical team in charge of the national COVID-19 containment strategy, the already mentioned CTS, revealed repeated dismissals of proposals to bolster community and preventive activities against the virus.[26] Notably, the CTS exhibited a total reluctance to devise a comprehensive strategy for identifying outbreaks and engaging experts distinguished for their proficiency in prevention and epidemiology.[27] During the initial waves, Italy adopted a belated stop-and-go strategy that proved insufficient in constructing a robust barrier against the highly contagious virus. The shortcomings extended beyond a dearth of ideas to strengthen population-based diagnostic capabilities. There was also a failure to attempt adopting a serious contact tracing strategy, the absence of effective policies on supported isolation and no interest in fortifying the health information system. This would have effectively linked diagnostic activities with contact tracing, reinforcing the capacity to navigate and respond to the evolving dynamics of the pandemic.

The Italian CTS will likely be remembered for its daily presentations, at 6 pm on live TV, providing statistics on the number of daily deaths and infections. These presentations, though serving as a public update, often provided raw data without contextual information and comprehensive analyses of possible interventions. They did offer a platform for questions from journalists, many of whom lacked basic expertise in epidemiology and public health. It's important to acknowledge that the CTS faced an arduous task and became a focal point for criticism and political pressure from those who deemed any measure to contain the pandemic as a form of authoritarianism. During the intense first waves, the government and CTS, in charge of deciding whether or not to impose a national lockdown, encountered a "Catch-22" scenario reminiscent of Joseph Heller's novel. The dilemma was clear: "open everything" and the virus will overwhelm hospitals and claim many victims; "shut everything down" and it will cause profound social discomfort and disrupt productive activities. But, there was a third option: a robust community health response centered on a comprehensive outbreak surveillance program, employing swabs, timely tracing and supported isolation. Regrettably, the CTS never believed in proactive virus prevention. In August 2020, it dismissed a proposal to improve strategies for testing, tracing and epidemiological surveillance among Italian regions without even a reply.[28]

Why did the Italian CTS seem unwilling to implement containment measures that had been proven to save lives elsewhere? While many factors could be mentioned, one of them may regard the lack of prevention focus of its members. According to a journalist from *La Repubblica*, one of Italy's major newspapers, the CTS included the "top experts" in the field,[29] but examining the profiles of those appointed makes one ponder. Of all the members of the CTS, 18 out of 20 came from institutions based in Rome. Perhaps the Italian capital concentrated the best scientists in public health and health policy in the country? A close look reveals another story. Most appointments in the Italian healthcare system and universities are dominated by power politics, rather than meritocratic or content-based criteria. Most CTS members lacked expertise in epidemiological analysis, surveillance of infectious disease outbreaks, prevention interventions and health promotion communication. Moreover, the background of key figures raised eyebrows. The top figure, tasked with appointing and coordinating all the other members, had no specific training in public health but rather was trained in accounting. His major expertise in terms of previous work experience regards earthquake management. The "number two" in the CTS was a gynecologist with no specific skills in prevention and health policies. Both had no experience in planning, implementing and evaluating health prevention campaigns for infectious diseases.[30] Most CTS members were clinicians temporarily "loaned" to prevention. While some of their insights may have brought valuable expertise in their own clinical subjects (anesthesiology, aging, neurology, orthopedics, head sciences, pulmonology, pediatrics, pharmaceutical services, military healthcare), their lack of full-time engagement in global health and health promotion raised questions about their preparedness for managing a national prevention strategy for an entire country. Perhaps it should not be too surprising that some CTS members confused COVID-19 with a "normal disease."[31] Finally, key figures of the CTS often found themselves in dual roles, such as simultaneously leading a pediatric department in a major hospital in Rome and spearheading the national COVID-19 prevention strategy for a population of almost 59 million people.[32] How does one manage to fully commit skills and energies to both positions and still keep sleeping at night?

The marginalization of prevention and public health experts was also observed in the United Kingdom. The UK Scientific Advisory Group for Emergencies (SAGE) scientific committee comprised professionals of considerable scientific prestige, particularly in infectious disease modeling, but with limited expertise in planning and logistics for public health interventions and pandemic management. The chief scientific advisor to the government, for example, boasted an impressive scientific profile in clinical pharmacology, vascular biology and endothelial cell physiology. His curriculum was a real guarantee in favor of the adoption of policies based on the best scientific evidence; however, he did not seem to be particularly strong on population health policy. Furthermore, the fact that he had worked for GlaxoSmithKline, a pharmaceutical company producing vaccines, and owned £600,000 worth of shares in the company, raised some controversy about a potential conflict of interest during the vaccination campaigns.[33]

When the pandemic unfolded, the UK government continued to rely on the old 2011 flu pandemic plan, and the government response consistently downplayed the importance of prevention interventions based on swabs, tracing and isolation. A critical public health and prevention function, the NHS Test and Trace program, was not only privatized but also overseen by a politician lacking qualifications in prevention, public health and epidemiology.[34] The expensive program was later evaluated as a total failure.[35]

Prevention was certainly not the SAGE's "cup of tea." Numerous experts voiced their concerns, with a group of 37 renowned epidemiologists publishing a plea in *The Lancet* on April 20, 2020, urging the English government to test the entire population every week until new infections disappeared for several weeks.[36] The appeal was, of course, completely ignored.

Failures in pandemic management in countries such as Italy, the United States and the United Kingdom should have prompted deeper reflection on what went wrong in the war against the virus. Analyzing the best practices from countries where COVID-19 deaths were effectively contained could have provided extremely valuable insights. This idea, however, has been dismissed. This may be because experts from Western countries are used to lecturing on global health in other (developing) nations, rather than humbling themselves by taking lessons? This ethnocentric attitude is perhaps best epitomized by the words of a deputy chief medical officer in England who, in response to a WHO recommendation to strengthen population testing strategies, stated that the "test, test, test was intended [only] for developing countries."[37]

Treating prevention as an ancillary discipline and entrusting the management of a pandemic to professionals who lacked full-time experience in epidemiology and public health is perhaps one of the reasons some high-income nations failed to effectively contain COVID-19. The topic needs further investigation. A skilled clinician can treat the illnesses of individual patients, but it takes a prevention expert to save the lives of thousands. While it's true that a collaborative effort is needed during a pandemic, this doesn't justify assigning leadership roles in pandemic planning and management to experts in medicine and clinical subjects. Scientists and medical specialists can certainly contribute within their areas of expertise, but they should not be entrusted with the task of leading preventive strategies. Imagine if during an emergency requiring urgent surgery, a public health expert, instead of simply helping in the surgical suite, directed the operations in place of the surgeon.

Sentinels "on the front line" against COVID-19?

On April 20, 2020, the Italian National Federation of Surgeons and Dentists put forth a crucial call to mobilize 66,000 family doctors, 7,800 pediatricians and other general practitioners to fight the virus. The aim of the call was to transform these professionals into "sentinels" of the communities "on the front line against COVID-19."[38] This initiative underscored the pressing need to establish a robust community health system, an imperative identified alongside the necessity to enhance safety measures within hospitals. Medical doctor, activist and author Vittorio Agnoletto echoed this sentiment in his book *Breathless*, emphasizing the absence of a strong primary healthcare system and local medical capacities to buffer hospitals against the effects of the virus.[39]

The contribution of family doctors, pediatricians and other medical practitioners in implementing community prevention efforts against COVID-19 cannot be overestimated. However, it's equally important to avoid placing excessive expectations about their potential ability to prevent SARS-CoV-2. Effective virus containment necessitates a supplementary system safeguarding not only hospitals but also local medical services. While territorial medicine practitioners can contribute significantly by promptly identifying unusual patterns in disease incidence and offering qualitative insights on diseases prevalent among patients, they cannot alone serve as "frontline sentinels" in the battle against the virus. An upstream strategy against the virus is essential. This can be carried out by a task force comprising epidemiologists, health policy analysts, data analysis experts and community health specialists free of clinical duties. Through well-coordinated efforts supported by robust epidemiological surveillance resources and technologies, these professionals can play a pivotal role in early outbreak detection and organize tailored preventive interventions at the community level.

Western governments have often made decisions regarding preventive interventions without precise information on the pandemic and used specific dates as references. However, as highlighted by Independent SAGE experts, effective decision-making for implementing preventive measures requires reliable "data, not dates." Epidemiological information is crucial for monitoring infection trends in various contexts such as schools, workplaces and communities. The collection of such data plays a fundamental role in governing diagnostic activities involving swabs and contact tracing measures. The challenge extends beyond the creation of tracking apps; it involves the establishment of technologically advanced surveillance systems. As a study published in *Science* emphasized, effective COVID-19 strategies require an early warning system capable of integrating various indicators to identify pandemic outbreaks. This integration of health and behavioral data enables continuous epidemiological monitoring, allowing for the prompt detection of any changes that warrant intervention. For instance, research indicates that activities such as doctors' searches, fever data and Google searches related to COVID-19 can often predict changes in the distribution of infections several weeks in advance. By amalgamating multiple epidemiological indicators, a real-time informational "thermostat" can be created, guiding the intermittent activation, intensification or relaxation of public health interventions. This dynamic approach ensures adaptability as the pandemic evolves and transforms over time.[40] As highlighted in an OECD report entitled "Big Data: A New Dawn for Public Health?" if governments really want to improve the management of new epidemic outbreaks, they need to invest in data collection and public health surveillance systems.[41]

For months, Italian epidemiologists have tried in vain to make their voices heard about the critical need for an effective epidemiological system to prevent and manage emerging pandemics like COVID-19. In an article published in *Epidemiology & Prevention*, professor of environmental epidemiology at Imperial College London Paolo Vineis and colleagues advocated for the strengthening of diagnostic capabilities and the activation of robust epidemiological surveillance systems. Their emphasis was on early identification of outbreaks, efficient tracing and the implementation of isolation and quarantine activities.[42] Numerous contributions in the literature have highlighted key sentinel indicators capable of promptly signaling changes in the pandemic.[43] In an open letter addressed to the Minister of Health, the Italian Association of Epidemiology (AIE) explicitly called for the creation of a surveillance system based on indicators capable of monitoring changes in COVID-19 incidence in detailed geographical areas.[44] The AIE stressed the significance of data georeferencing as a fundamental tool for generating maps and conducting frequent data processing, allowing for the effective monitoring of potential COVID-19 outbreaks and visualizing real-time changes in the pandemic over time. These data could not only aid in a better understanding of the pandemic but also be pivotal in evaluating the effectiveness of preventive measures. Despite requiring substantial economic investment, these tools, when combined with effective test and tracing systems, represent a relatively small cost compared to the economic repercussions caused by the pandemic and subsequent lockdowns.[45]

Italy is not a country for public health experts

In 2001–2003, I worked as a researcher at the Regional Epidemiological Service (SER) of the Veneto region. This period took place while I pursued my PhD in global health at the University of California, Los Angeles (UCLA). Although I was in the middle of my doctoral studies, I decided to take a break and return to Italy to have a "real world" experience in health promotion in the region where I had spent a significant portion of my life and where my closest connections reside. Thanks to the intuition of a colleague, I devoted my first professional efforts to creating the first surveillance system for monitoring the lifestyles and social determinants of health in Italy named the "Health Determinants Surveillance System (SSDS)."[46,47] Remarkably, this project that started in 2002 anticipated a very similar system created by the Italian Ministry of Health titled "Progress of Health Companies for Health" in Italy (PASSI), launched a few years later. Although there are no notes, citations in bibliographic references or acknowledgments of the work done in the context of the SDSS project in any document of the Italian Ministry of Health, they were productive months that I remember dearly. My ambition to make a difference to the public health of my region was clear, even though sometimes my friends told me: "I still haven't fully understood exactly what your job is."

After the completion of the first data collection of the SDSS project, a change in leadership occurred at the SER. The newly appointed director, a medical doctor, argued that my skills in public health and social epidemiology were seemingly mismatched with the institution's mission and activities, which had to focus primarily on public health and epidemiology. The argument was very curious precisely because only a few researchers in Italy, even today, have formal qualifications in social epidemiology. But perhaps even the director of the Center hadn't yet fully understood what my job was? Nevertheless, a few months later, I decided to leave and announced my resignation. I returned to Los Angeles to finish my PhD. I have no idea what then happened to the SER and how it contributed to prevention activities in Veneto. What I do know is that both the president of the Veneto region and the secretary in charge of strategic healthcare decisions affecting the activities of many centers including the SER ended up in prison on charges of corruption.[48,49]

This personal episode may seem inconsequential, yet it sheds light on the workings (or lack thereof) of public health institutions not just in Veneto but throughout Italy. The involvement of experts in social sciences applied to public health should be essential in institutions responsible for health protection and health promotion at the population level. Effective public health systems tackle health risk factors through a multidisciplinary and population-based approach – a concept seemingly absent in Italy. Could this deficiency be a key factor in our country's unpreparedness and struggles in handling the pandemic? Within the Italian university system, topics such as social epidemiology and health policy evaluation, for example, lack recognition as distinct disciplines. Epidemiology finds itself relegated to a university subsector in the field of medicine called "Hygiene and Preventive Medicine." Astonishingly, before the outbreak of the pandemic, there was almost a complete absence of university training in global health in Italy. For instance, at the University of Padova, where I work, there are no global health courses except for one that I teach to my community psychology students.

Students frequently approach me after my classes, at times brimming with enthusiasm about specializing in global health. Regrettably, I find myself grappling with embarrassment and a sense of defeat, compelled to advise them to seek advanced education abroad. Many had hoped that the pandemic would serve as a catalyst for change, particularly in the realm of education. Those familiar with the subject understand that effectively managing a pandemic requires a set of cross-cutting and multidisciplinary skills encompassing at least three disciplines unrelated to the qualifications of a doctor or virologist: epidemiology, public health and health policy. In addition to these technical-scientific expertise, "soft skills" such as leadership, teamwork, problem-solving, decision-making and human resources management are necessary. In an article co-authored with two of my colleagues, we investigated the critical areas that warrant intervention to enhance future

COVID-19 containment strategies in Italy. Among the recommendations, we mentioned the imperative to invest in public health, epidemiology and health policy, emphasizing a trans-disciplinary and international approach. Yet, even in the aftermath of a pandemic that incurred a staggering loss of lives and significant economic impact, prevention and public health have not yet assumed the pivotal roles they deserve within the National Health Service and Italian universities. An editorial by Rodolfo Saracci, former Director of the Analytical Epidemiology Unit of the International Agency for Research on Cancer, underscored this oversight in the Italian National Recovery and Resilience Plan. Saracci pointed out that prevention was practically absent from the plan. As he observed, "the 7 billion in investments is all designated for local assistance while for prevention, there is not even a minimal budget line."[50] Echoing this sentiment, an article by two experts from the Institute Mario Negri based in Milan adopted a similar critical tone: "five semesters have passed since the start of the pandemic, much has been done, and much has been learned about the defensive behaviors of both the virus and the population, yet the public health response remains similar to the pre-pandemic approach."[51]

The ancillary role given to prevention and public health and the overwhelming influence of the clinical and biomedical model in health are results of hierarchical dynamics guiding decision-making processes in Italian healthcare institutions and universities. The negligible contribution of experts in epidemiology and global health in the COVID-19 containment interventions reflects a chronic-degenerative disease of power that has obscured the nation's vision during the crisis. As emphasized by a former professor from the University of Padova, Schools of Public Health have not been developed because "they were never wanted." The appeals for trans-disciplinarity abound, yet when it comes to securing funding, recruiting personnel and advancing careers, the safeguarding of the narrow interests of some sectors prevails. The practice of "disciplinary territorial pissing" at the expense of the common good, however, stems from collective behavioral practices socialized in institutions dominated by rigid hierarchies and non-meritocratic relationships. In Italian healthcare institutions and universities, one of the most important social norms that contribute to career success is not merit and the capability to advance knowledge or outcomes in one's field but an attitude of unquestioning obedience. As noted by Andrea Crisanti, who worked most of his career abroad and joined the University of Padova for a couple of years, the country is plagued by a culture that suffocates transparency, merit and independence.[52] This deficiency stems from what Edward Banfield, in his classic work *The Moral Basis of a Backward Society*, termed "amoral familism" – a culture antithetical to community spirit, prioritizing personal gain and the maximization of individual advantages over civic meaning and the common good.[53] Of course, it is important not to generalize. In Italy, there are also exceptions that can spark a glimmer of hope for the future.

The United States' and United Kingdom's paradox

If the lack of expertise in public health may have harmed the pandemic response in Italy, a paradox emerged when evaluating the effectiveness of preventive interventions in the United States and the United Kingdom. The mere presence of the most prestigious public health universities in the world did not shield these nations from an abysmal public health failure. This begs the question: why have countries boasting the finest public health experts in the world faltered in implementing effective public health policies?

A former colleague at the University of Michigan, professor of global public health Scott Greer and other researchers, in their book titled *Coronavirus Politics: The Comparative Politics and Policies on COVID-19*,[54] have attempted an answer. After scrutinizing COVID-19 management policies globally, they concluded that the professional and political institutionalization of public health has exerted only limited influence on politics. While some are staunchly convinced that "science has failed" and indeed there are peculiar cases of renowned American and British experts spreading misinformation and negatively influencing public health policies and strategies,[55] two crucial aspects are overlooked. First, as stated before, the pandemic starkly revealed the self-congratulatory arrogance of politicians who, instead of consulting the foremost experts in the field, chose to disregard scientific recommendations. Second, the motto "follow the science" did not specify which science is required to combat a pandemic. Like journalists, many politicians too failed to base their decisions on the best scientific evidence because they often confused professionals proficient in virology and medical fields with experts in prevention and public health.

Amid the clamor, a few steadfast, clear and reliable voices emerged during the pandemic, exemplified by the English Independent SAGE. This group of experts established an independent technical committee alternative to the official SAGE, which had discredited itself on many grounds including aligning with the positions of experts advocating the herd immunity strategy. The Independent SAGE extended beyond creating a more diverse group of experts in terms of gender and ethnicity; it sought to include experts from disciplines extending well beyond those included in the reductionist and biomedical approach, such as health policies, health inequalities, global health and behavioral sciences. During the pandemic, this group of scientists effectively engaged the public and policy leaders with useful information, data, presentations and analyses of the pandemic, releasing hundreds of videos and dozens of documents. They will be remembered for having provided solid analyses and knowledge that was like a ray of light in a cacophony of errors and imprecisions.

References

1. Fortunati C. Medico anestesista in pensione, rientra in reparto e muore di Covid. Aveva risposto alla "chiamata alle armi" dell'Usl 3 riprendendo servizio. Sindacato Italiano Veterinari Medicina Pubblica Veneto. Published online Dec 11, 2020. https://www.sivempveneto.it/medico-anestesista-in-pensione-rientra-in-reparto-e-muore-di-covid-aveva-risposto-alla-chiamata-alle-armi-dellusl-3-rientrando-in-servizio/ (accessed Jan 23, 2024).
2. La Piazza Web. Mirano: il saluto al dottor Francesco Gasparini. Published online on Dec 12, 2020. https://www.lapiazzaweb.it/2020/12/mirano-il-saluto-al-dottor-francesco-gasparini/ (accessed Jan 23, 2024).
3. Naftulin J. A New York ICU doctor who postponed his retirement to treat coronavirus patients has died from COVID-19. Business Insider. Published online on May 19, 2020. https://www.businessinsider.com/nyc-icu-doctor-came-out-of-retirement-died-covid-19-2020-5 (accessed Jan 30, 2024).
4. World Health Organization. The impact of COVID-19 on health and care workers: a closer look at deaths. https://www.who.int/publications-detail-redirect/WHO-HWF-WorkingPaper-2021.1, Sep 2021. (accessed Jan 23, 2024).
5. Blasio ND. Salvare gli operatori sanitari. Salute Internazionale. Published online Mar 12, 2020. https://www.saluteinternazionale.info/2020/03/salvare-gli-operatori-sanitari/ (accessed Jan 23, 2024).
6. Federazione Nazionale degli Ordini dei Medici Chirurghi. Elenco dei Medici caduti nel corso dell'epidemia di Covid-19. Fnomceo. Published online Jan 19, 2024. https://portale.fnomceo.it/elenco-dei-medici-caduti-nel-corso-dellepidemia-di-covid-19/ (accessed Jan 23, 2024).
7. La Stampa. "I medici di famiglia isolati e abbandonati a se stessi nel gestire l'emergenza". Published online Mar 14, 2020. https://www.lastampa.it/novara/2020/03/14/news/i-medici-di-famiglia-isolati-e-abbandonati-a-se-stessi-nel-gestire-l-emergenza-1.38592944/ (accessed Jan 23, 2024).
8. Knoll C, Watkins A, Rothfeld M. 'I couldn't do anything': the virus and an E.R. doctor's suicide. *The New York Times*. Published online July 11, 2020. https://www.nytimes.com/2020/07/11/nyregion/lorna-breen-suicide-coronavirus.html (accessed Jan 30, 2024).
9. Kiang MV, Carlasare LE, Thadaney Israni S, Norcini JJ, Zaman JAB, Bibbins-Domingo K. Excess mortality among US physicians during the COVID-19 pandemic. *JAMA Internal Medicine* 2023; **183**: 374–6.
10. Iacobucci G. Covid-19: government failed to protect doctors during pandemic, BMA inquiry finds. *BMJ* 2022; 377: o1235.
11. Federazione Italiana Medici di Medicina Generale. Nudi contro il virus. Published online on Mar 16, 2020. https://www.fimmg.org/index.php?action=pages&m=view&p=43&art=3863 (accessed Jan 23, 2024).
12. Rai Presa Diretta. Giuseppe Marzulli racconta il disastro della prima ondata. Feb 1, 2021. https://www.youtube.com/watch?v=zci_vPbRQ40 (accessed Jan 23, 2024).
13. Adnkronos. Covid, in Italia record di medici morti: 'Una catastrofe'. Published online Jan 8, 2021. https://www.adnkronos.com/Archivio/salute/sanita/covid-in-italia-record-di-medici-morti-una-catastrofe_35bgYIkYhxVssh8pR9JLxE (accessed Jan 23, 2024).

14. Conca M. Coronavirus e operatori sanitari: flash mob di "Siamo Tutti Ippocrate". Prima Brescia. Published online Dec 4, 2020. https://primabrescia.it/cronaca/coronavirus-e-operatori-sanitari-flash-mob-di-siamo-tutti-ippocrate/ (accessed Jan 23, 2024).

15. Blasio ND. C'era una volta il Piano pandemico. SaluteInternazionale. Published online Apr 15, 2020. https://www.saluteinternazionale.info/2020/04/cera-una-volta-il-piano-pandemico/ (accessed Jan 23, 2024).

16. Quotidiano Sanità. Medicina generale. Sanofi sigla accordo con Fimmg e Simg per formare i medici del future. Published online on Apr 23, 2020. https://www.quotidianosanita.it/lavoro-e-professioni/articolo.php?articolo_id=84420 (accessed Jan 23, 2024).

17. Lantz PM. The medicalization of population health: who will stay upstream? *The Milbank Quarterly* 2019; **97**: 36.

18. Lantz PM, Goldberg DS, Gollust SE. The perils of medicalization for population health and health equity. *The Milbank Quarterly* 2023; **101**: 61–82.

19. Quotidiano Sanità. Coronavirus. L'appello di 100 mila medici a Governo e Regioni: "Pazienti vanno trattati il più presto possibile sul territorio". Published online on Apr 18, 2020. https://www.quotidianosanita.it/lavoro-e-professioni/articolo.php?articolo_id=84198 (accessed Jan 23, 2024).

20. De Vogli R, Buio MD, De Falco R. Effects of the COVID-19 pandemic on health inequalities and mental health: effective public policies. *Epidemiologia e Prevenzione* 2021; **45**: 588–97.

21. Nacoti M, Ciocca A, Giupponi A, *et al.* At the epicenter of the Covid-19 pandemic and humanitarian crises in Italy: changing perspectives on preparation and mitigation. *NEJM Catalyst Innovations in Care Delivery* 2020. https://catalyst.nejm.org/doi/pdf/10.1056/CAT.20.0080.

22. Telese L. Vespignani a TPI: "I virologi italiani non hanno capito nulla, per sconfiggere il virus servono le 3T". The Post Internazionale. Published online May 3, 2020. https://www.tpi.it/cronaca/vespignani-coronavirus-intervista-virologi-italiani-e-3t-20200503595940/ (accessed Jan 23, 2024).

23. Bajaj S. Six lessons we've learned from Covid that will help us fight the next pandemic. *Smithsonian Magazine*. Published online on Dec 30, 2022. https://www.smithsonianmag.com/science-nature/six-lessons-weve-learned-from-covid-that-will-help-us-fight-the-next-pandemic-180981371/ (accessed Jan 23, 2024).

24. Silverstein J. Mike Pence said smoking 'doesn't kill' and faced criticism for his response to HIV. Now he's leading the coronavirus response. CBS News. Published online Feb 29, 2020. https://www.cbsnews.com/news/coronavirus-mike-pence-health-science-smoking-hiv/ (accessed Jan 23, 2024).

25. Simmons-Duffin S, Huang P. A year in, experts assess Biden's hits and misses on handling the pandemic. NPR. Published online Jan 18, 2022. https://www.npr.org/sections/health-shots/2022/01/18/1073292913/a-year-in-experts-assess-bidens-hits-and-misses-on-handling-the-pandemic (accessed Feb 4, 2024).

26. Pistoi S. Examining the role of the Italian COVID-19 scientific committee. *Nature Italy* 2021. https://www.nature.com/articles/d43978-021-00015-8.

27. Day M. Covid-19: identifying and isolating asymptomatic people helped eliminate virus in Italian village. *BMJ* 2020; **368**: m1165.

28. Quotidiano Sanità. Tamponi. Ecco il piano "Crisanti" al vaglio del Governo: 300 mila tamponi al giorno. Published online on Sep 1, 2020. https://www.quotidianosanita.it/governo-e-parlamento/articolo.php?articolo_id=87541 (accessed Jan 23, 2024).

29. Menichini R. Covid 19, oltre mille al comando tra task force, comitati, istituzioni. Ma non ci sono le donne. la Repubblica. Published online Apr 30, 2020. https://www.repubblica.it/politica/2020/04/30/news/donne_task_force_catena_di_comando_covid19-255273362/ (accessed Jan 23, 2024).

30. Berizzi P. Figli di potenti assunti senza concorso. Ecco la Parentopoli di Bertolaso. *la Repubblica*. Published online Mar 27, 2010. https://www.repubblica.it/cronaca/2010/03/27/news/parentopoli_bertolaso-2932413/ (accessed Jan 23, 2024).

31. Pipitone F. Covid, per il prof. Bernabei (CTS) non è un virus terribile: 'È una malattia normale'. Vesuvio Live. Published online Nov 7, 2020. https://www.vesuviolive.it/ultime-notizie/362978-bernabei-covid-malattia-normale/ (accessed Jan 22, 2024).

32. Magani N. Locatelli, 'retromarcia' Cts: "quasi tutti asintomatici"/"No panico, scuole aperte". IlSussidiario.net. Published online Oct 18, 2020. https://www.ilsussidiario.net/news/locatelli-retromarcia-cts-quasi-tutti-asintomatici-no-panico-scuole-aperte/2082699/ (accessed Jan 23, 2024).

33. Roach A. Hancock: No conflict of interest in Vallance holding vaccine shares. Evening Standard. Published online Sept 24, 2020. https://www.standard.co.uk/news/uk/patrick-vallance-vaccine-shares-denies-conflict-interest-a4555141.html (accessed Jan 23, 2024).

34. Cooper H, Szreter S. After the virus: lessons from the past for a better future. Cambridge, UK: Cambridge University Press, 2021.

35. COVID-19: Test, track and trace (part 1) – Committees. UK Parliament. Published online Mar 10, 2021. https://committees.parliament.uk/work/906/covid19-test-track-and-trace-part-1/publications/ (accessed Jan 23, 2024).

36. Peto J, Alwan NA, Godfrey KM, *et al*. Universal weekly testing as the UK COVID-19 lockdown exit strategy. *The Lancet* 2020; **395**: 1420–1.

37. Shridar D. Britain, 'herd immunity' and 'following the science'. In: Preventable: how a pandemic changed the world and how to stop the next one. Penguin Books, 2022.

38. Quotidiano Sanità. Coronavirus. "Un nuovo modello di gestione è possibile. Coinvolgere i medici di famiglia per la Fase 2". Ecco la proposta della Fnomceo. Quotidiano Sanità. Published online on Apr 21, 2020. https://www.quotidianosanita.it/lavoro-e-professioni/articolo.php?articolo_id=84349 (accessed Jan 23, 2024).

39. Agnoletto V. Senza respiro. Un'inchiesta indipendente sulla pandemia Coronavirus, in Lombardia, Italia, Europa. Come ripensare un modello di sanità pubblica. Altreconomia, 2020.

40. Kogan NE, Clemente L, Liautaud P, *et al*. An early warning approach to monitor COVID-19 activity with multiple digital traces in near real time. *Science Advances* 2021; **7**: eabd6989.

41. Organization Economic Cooperation and Development (OECD). Big data: a new dawn for public health? OECD, 2019. https://doi.org/10.1787/f24cb567-en.

42. Vineis P, Bisceglia L, Forastiere F, Salmaso S, Scondotto, S. Covid-19: arrivare preparati all'autunno. *Epiemiologia & Prevenzione* **44**(4): 202–204. (accessed Jan 23, 2024).

43. Saracci R. Covid. Mortalità non può essere il dato di riferimento per le scelte. Quotidiano Sanità. Published online on Feb 2, 2021. https://www.quotidianosanita.it/lettere-al-direttore/articolo.php?articolo_id=92086 (accessed Jan 23, 2024).

44. Associazione Italiana Epidemiologia. Lettera aperta della Associazione Italiana di Epidemiologia per le azioni di contrasto alla pandemia di COVID-19. Epidemiologia.it. Published online Oct 28, 2020. https://www.epidemiologia.it/6566 (accessed Jan 23, 2024).

45. Organization Economic Cooperation and Development (OECD). Testing for COVID-19: a way to lift confinement restrictions. Published online on May 4, 2020. https://www.oecd.org/coronavirus/policy-responses/testing-for-covid-19-a-way-to-lift-confinement-restrictions-89756248/ (accessed Jan 23, 2024).

46. De Vogli R. Socioeconomic determinants of health behaviours: does psychosocial stress matter? PhD dissertation, University of California Los Angeles. 2003; 1–213.

47. De Vogli R, Santinello M. Unemployment and smoking: does psychosocial stress matter? *Tobacco Control* 2005; **14**: 389–95.

48. Pietrobelli G. Galan torna libero dopo due anni e mezzo: 'In 15 anni di presidenza mai un'azione in cambio di qualcosa'. *Il Fatto Quotidiano*. Published online Jan 6, 2017. http://www.ilfattoquotidiano.it/2017/01/06/galan-torna-libero-dopo-due-anni-e-mezzo-in-15-anni-di-presidenza-mai-unazione-in-cambio-di-qualcosa/3299465/ (accessed Jan 23, 2024).

49. Sindacato Italiano Veterinari Medicina Pubblica Veneto. Sanità e mazzette, a processo politici e manager cliniche private. Published online May 5, 2011. https://www.sivempveneto.it/sanita-e-mazzette-a-processo-politici-e-manager-di-cliniche-private/ (accessed Jan 23, 2024).

50. Saracci R, Forastiere F, Vineis P. Dov'è la prevenzione nel Piano Nazionale di Ripresa e Resilienza? Scienza in rete. Published online May 12, 2021. https://www.scienzainrete.it/articolo/dov-prevenzione-nel-piano-nazionale-di-ripresa-e-resilienza/rodolfo-saracci-francesco (accessed Jan 23, 2024).

51. Clavenna A, Bonati M. Strategie per contrastare la pandemia, aspettiamo l'autunno? Scienza in rete. Published online July 1, 2022. https://www.scienzainrete.it/articolo/strategie-contrastare-pandemia-aspettiamo-lautunno/antonio-clavenna-maurizio-bonati/2022-07 (accessed Jan 23, 2024).

52. Ditta A. Polemica Zaia-Crisanti, lo sfogo del professore: 'In Italia non ci sono cultura del merito e indipendenza'. The Post Internazionale. Published online May 26, 2020. https://www.tpi.it/cronaca/polemica-zaia-crisanti-italia-cultura-merito-indipendenza-20200526608925/ (accessed Jan 23, 2024).

53. Banfield EC, Banfield LF. The moral basis of a backward society, 1. New York: The Free Press, 1967.

54. Greer SL, King EJ, da Fonseca EM, Peralta-Santos A, editors. Coronavirus politics: the comparative politics and policy of COVID-19. Ann Arbor: University of Michigan Press, 2021.

55. Howard J. We want them infected: how the failed quest for herd immunity led doctors to embrace the anti-vaccine movement and blinded Americans to the threat of COVID. Hickory, NC: Redhawk Publications, 2023.

4

"LAISSEZ-FAIRE THE VIRUS"

"No heroes, no cowards!! Staff in a state of agitation." These words adorned a banner unfurled on the roof of San Carlo hospital in Milan, bearing the sentiment of a nurse who decided to voice his protest publicly. Originating from a letter by emergency doctors and resuscitators, the missive highlighted the dire situation in hospitals that were so overwhelmed that healthcare workers found themselves compelled to make choices that were "neither clinically nor ethically tolerable."[1] What does it mean? The indelible images of emergency services besieged, patients laid out on stretchers in makeshift examination rooms, still linger in our memories. Faced with such healthcare shortages, how were the overstretched workers expected to cope? A sentence from the new, updated Italian pandemic plan explicitly acknowledged an uncomfortable truth known among healthcare personnel and administrators: in times of scarce resources, prioritizing care for certain patients becomes a necessity. The words used could not be clearer: "the imbalance between needs and available resources may make it necessary to adopt triage criteria in accessing therapies." However, the text adds, "when scarcity makes resources insufficient compared to need, ethical principles can allow scarce resources to be allocated so as to provide necessary treatments preferentially to those patients who are most likely to benefit from them."[2]

While this may seem like a radical departure from the Hippocratic oath or a surrender of the ideal of providing care without distinctions, it is crucial to recognize the complex web of causes leading to such decisions. Doctors and nurses found themselves in the agonizing position of choosing whom to save because they had no choice. When hospitals were inundated beyond capacity, with limited intensive care beds available, someone inevitably faced

DOI: 10.4324/9781003511977-6

delayed treatment and, in essence, became a "sacrifice." Yet, the true culprits behind these "ethically and morally intolerable choices" are not the health-care workers.

Human sacrifices on the altar of the economy

"From an economic point of view, COVID-19 could also be slightly advantageous in the long term, disproportionately eliminating dependent elderly people" are the words expressed in an article that appeared in the *Telegraph*, a widely read English newspaper.[3] Also in the United Kingdom, the ex–chief scientific adviser to the government noted (referring to the Prime Minister): "He says his party 'thinks the whole thing is pathetic and Covid is just Nature's way of dealing with old people' – and I am not entirely sure I disagree with them."[4] Another consultant to the English government appears to have said, "…protect the economy, and if that means some pensioners die, too bad."[5] A similar expression was given by the president of the General Confederation of Industry of Macerata in Italy, who, in reference to social distancing measures, observed: "people are tired; never mind if someone dies."[6] The former governor of Liguria, later arrested on corruption charges, noted that the victims of the virus were mostly very elderly patients "not essential to the country's productive effort."[7] In the United States, there was no shortage of similar "contributions." A lieutenant governor of Texas noted that many would rather die than see the economy ruined by public health measures.[8] In Brazil, the former president Bolsonaro remarked: "I'm sorry for the deaths, but it's the fate of all of us."[9]

While these statements show a lack of empathy consistent with a potential psychopathic personality disorder, they offer direct insight into an approach that deems sacrificing human lives to protect the economy acceptable. Throughout the pandemic, influential economic and political groups exerted pressure on governments to avoid restrictions, public health interventions and prevention measures. Often, these forms of political influence remained implicit and distant from public scrutiny. At times, however, they came to the fore. An article published in *Internazionale* titled "How Much Is the Life of Human Beings Worth?" tackled the analyses of two economists who decided to calculate the value of human life in relation to the costs of prevention strategies.[10] The first is the director of the Toulouse School of Economics who argued that the economic losses from COVID-19 deaths were a lesser evil than the costs of a lockdown, estimating a lifetime value of 3 million euros per person.[11] To reach this conclusion, the economist compared the losses resulting from the death of 30,000 people with the cost resulting from a fall in GDP equal to 20%, concluding that these deaths were preferable to the costs of a lockdown. The second is an English economist, the author of a cost-benefit analysis for the Institute of Economic Affairs, a conservative think tank inspired by free market principles, who seemed to imply that 400,000 premature deaths could be an acceptable "cost" to protect the economy.[12]

This calculated indifference toward the value of some lives aligns well with the philosophical aberrations of modern society. Notably, there is a parallelism between laissez-faire economic principles and social Darwinism, a philosophical doctrine celebrating the "evolutionary success" of individuals possessing traits desirable for survival.[13] Upon reflection, the concept of "nature" as the primary arbiter of the "struggle for life" seamlessly fits the vision of the market as the principal arbiter between winners and losers in society. For laissez-faire economists, markets are akin to what the laws of nature are to social Darwinists. Social Darwinism and laissez-faire economics share the assumption that competition, whether for life or for profit, must not be curtailed or limited. The market, like nature, should be left free to reward productive actors with wealth and penalize inefficient ones with failure, just as the laws of nature reward adaptive individuals with survival and punish those who fail with extinction. In both philosophical doctrines, there is no compassion for the sick, the weak, the inefficient, the poor and all those who are "behind" in economic or evolutionary terms. Both theories view any interference capable of impeding market affairs, such as social welfare policies or redistributive taxation, as a kind of "curse in disguise" or an obstacle to progress.

There are also important differences between these two philosophies though: while for the laissez-faire economist, social protection policies represent obstacles to economic prosperity, for the social Darwinist, they promote the "survival of the most incapable." Despite this nuance, both schools of thought find acceptable the idea of sacrificing some human lives on the altar of evolutionary or economic "progress." It may be coincidental that from 1848 to 1853 the founder of social Darwinism, Herbert Spencer, served as the editor of the London-based magazine *The Economist*. During the period when Spencer worked for the magazine, editors expressed their objections to the passage of laws such as the Public Health Act, pointing out that "suffering and evil are nature's warnings; they cannot be eliminated; and the impatient attempts of benevolence to banish them from the world by law ... have always produced more harm than good."[14] According to the social Darwinian philosophy, even war, death, and famine are necessary for advancing human progress and "biological purification." A (un)memorable passage in Spencer's most important book, entitled *Social Statics*, reads: "under the natural order of things, society is constantly expelling its unwholesome, imbecilic, slow, wavering, and unfaithful members." And although "it seems difficult that widows and orphans should be left to struggle for life and death ... yet, when considered not separately, but in connection with the interest of universal humanity, these harsh fatalities are full of benefits." The conclusion is brutal, honest and repugnant: "imperfect beings are failures of nature ... If they are complete enough to live, they live, and it is good that they live. If they are not complete enough to live, they die and it is better for them to die."[15]

Herd immunity or social murder?

Former British Prime Minister Boris Johnson left an indelible memory in the collective imagination of the pandemic. After assuring that the coronavirus would not prevent him from shaking hands with people and boasting of having done so with infected patients in a hospital, he tested positive a few weeks later.[16] He ended up in intensive care and survived. Previously, he had supported, more or less explicitly, the desire to adopt a policy inspired by principles of "herd immunity,"[17] publicly announcing that "many families will lose their loved ones" due to the virus.[18] But what did BoJo actually mean by "herd immunity"? During an interview on a BBC program called *Newsnight*, Graham Medley, one of the government's scientific advisors, explained what it is. The term, well-known among epidemiologists and public health experts, has been primarily used in scientific discussions regarding vaccination coverage for a pathogen. It refers to that level of immunity in a population considered sufficient to allow even unvaccinated people to be safe.[19] Herd immunity has been history's way of ending pandemics, thanks to vaccines. At the time of Johnson's statements, vaccines against SARS-CoV-2 were not yet available, but according to some experts herd immunity could be achieved even without them. As one of the supporters of this approach pointed out, "the virus must spread. The more it spreads the better, because the more people will develop immunity."[20] Rather than "herd immunity," it needed to be more appropriately called "mass infection."[21]

British government advisors were not the only ones to entertain the idea of adopting this strategy. Even overseas, some had high hopes of achieving herd immunity through mass infections. The world was particularly shocked by the adoption of this approach in the United States, where over a million people died due to COVID-19. In an article in the *British Medical Journal*, Drew Altman called the American strategy a "deplorable" performance, the product of a policy failure based largely on the idea of letting the virus spread at the price of an "acceptable" number of coronavirus deaths.[22] The political pressure to "let the virus run its course" in the United States produced a manifesto called the Great Barrington Declaration (GBD), signed at the American Institute for Economics Research, a conservative, free-market, libertarian foundation based in Great Barrington, Massachusetts. Although the foundation claims to be independent, it receives funding from multinational corporations such as Exxon Mobil and organizations such as the Charles Koch Foundation, both of which have been known to spread and support climate change denial.[23,24] In this sense, it is a "corporate-libertarian" foundation, for the type of freedom it promotes concerns powerful private enterprises, not the general public. As highlighted in an article that appeared on the *BMJ* blog, GBD has significantly influenced the policies of some countries by underlining the benefits of the herd immunity approach and opposing any form of preventive intervention.[25] The targets of its political pressure included not only governments but also public health organizations such as the WHO and the Centers for Disease Control and Prevention (CDC). The latter found itself under attack especially on social media outlets where concerted smear campaigns were waged on the basis of false information. As revealed by a CDC official, the organization seemed to be often on the defensive and at one point even even maintained a guilty silence about the risks to the public posed by COVID-19.[26]

Another country that has somewhat flirted with the idea of herd immunity, only to be overwhelmed by waves of COVID-19 deaths, is Brazil. The failure of the Brazilian COVID-19 strategy resulted in more than 700,000 deaths, many of them preventable. In the first months of the pandemic, an area of Brazil called Manaus came to the attention of public health scientists for being an extreme case of how not to act against the virus.[27] As explained in an editorial appearing in the *BMJ*, Manaus was revealed to be "the final nail in the coffin of the natural herd immunity hypothesis."[28] In an additional analysis that appeared in *Science*, it is explained how this unfortunate city has become a prototype of the damage that can occur if the virus is allowed to run its course without any intervention.[29] If the Bolsonaro government's strategy amplified the lethal effects of the virus among Brazilians, it also seems to have caused damage to the international community by creating conditions for the origin of new variants. In another article that appeared in *Nature*, Brazil is described not only as a pandemic "disaster" but also as a country that acted as a "super spreader" of the variant Gamma (which first emerged within its borders), to the detriment of other Latin American countries.[30]

In Sweden too the idea of herd immunity through mass infection was considered a plausible and achievable national goal. The Swedish strategy stood out for not having adopted quarantines for those returning after a trip abroad and for not having imposed or recommended the use of masks even for visitors to retirement homes. The epidemiologist in charge of the national strategy, Anders Tegnell, ended up at the center of numerous controversies for advising the Swedish government not to take preventive measures and to let the virus run wild. At the end of April 2020, he explained that in his opinion Stockholm could have reached herd immunity within a few weeks.[31] In reference to a possible second wave, he explained that Sweden had a "high level of immunity" and was anticipating a low number of cases.[32] Of course, such a prediction was wrong. The international scientific community and public health experts criticized Sweden's approach in an editorial in *Nature* accusing the government of "not having followed the scientific method." As observed in the article, "Sweden was well equipped to prevent the COVID-19 pandemic from becoming serious" but decided to let the virus spread. Indeed, Sweden enjoys an extremely advantageous position compared to other nations in terms of COVID-19 risk: low population density, relatively fair socioeconomic conditions, high education and a high level of trust in authorities and institutions. Despite this, during 2020, Sweden recorded mortality rates from COVID-19 ten times higher than those of neighboring Norway and paid dearly in terms of human lives for the strategy of failing to protect the elderly in retirement homes, in extreme cases leaving them to suffocate to death without treatment. "Many elderly people were given morphine instead of oxygen despite available supplies, ending their lives" explained the authors of the same editorial.[33] As analyzed by an empirical analysis published in *Nature Human Behavior*, the combination of non-pharmaceutical public health interventions, very advantageous social, economic and political conditions compared to the European average and timely vaccination campaigns has allowed Denmark, Finland and Norway to remain at pre-pandemic life expectancy levels throughout 2020 and 2021. This was not the case for Sweden, however, where the mirage of achieving herd immunity caused "substantial ... non-recoverable damage," despite improvements in the following years.[34] Although Anders Tegnell assured everyone that the Swedish strategy was "sustainable," the evidence incontrovertibly showed that the country, especially in 2020, failed to protect its weakest citizens from the pandemic, generating what the King of Sweden acknowledged as a "total fiasco."[35]

Italy has never followed a herd immunity strategy, yet the idea of promoting mass infection found some support and a number of researchers even signed the GBD.[36] An epidemiologist, interviewed several times in the Italian mass media, explained that "the virus must spread so that more people develop immunity" and make it possible "to cure the infection also with the plasma of recovered patients."[37] Of course, as already stated, evidence had amply demonstrated that using the plasma of those who have recovered is ineffective.

The disastrous results of the herd immunity strategy were widely predicted by epidemiologists and analytical models. Governments had been warned: without a rapid response aimed at suppressing the coming outbreaks, millions of bodies would have to be buried.[38] As put in an article published in *Nature*, herd immunity was nothing more than a "false promise" that "could lead to untold death and suffering."[39,40] And this is exactly what happened. In another article published in *The Lancet* signed by over 30 experts in the field of global health, the herd immunity strategy was depicted as a "dangerous fallacy not supported by scientific evidence."[41] Prof. Anthony Fauci also criticized it as "ridiculous."[42]

Fortunately, despite the public outbursts, no country has gone "all the way" in adopting this strategy. Some governments have instead embraced stop-and-go interventions and applied some public health programs in a delayed, confusing and fragmented manner. However, Kamran Abbasi in the *BMJ* came down hard on them: "when politicians and experts say they are willing to allow tens of thousands of premature deaths for the sake of herd immunity or in the hope of supporting the economy, isn't this premeditated and reckless indifference towards human life? When politicians intentionally ignore scientific advice, international and historical experience, and their own alarming statistics and models because taking action goes against their political strategy or ideology, is it legal?" According to Abbasi, it is not; letting COVID-19 spread without doing anything to protect people from its impact could be classified as "social murder."[43]

Children as human shields

As described by Jonathan Howard in his brilliant exposé titled *We Want Them Infected*,[44] one of the arguments raised by proponents of the herd immunity strategy included the notion of letting children become infected early by the virus in order to protect adults. As an epidemiologist and official in the US Department of Health and Human Services explained: "infants, kids, teens, young people, young adults, middle aged with no conditions, etc. have zero to little risk … so we use them to develop herd … we want them infected."[45] A neuroradiologist and senior fellow in healthcare policy at the Hoover Institution, a conservative think tank, echoed the same view: "Children have virtually zero risk of getting a serious complication, virtually a zero risk of dying … Children only rarely transmit the disease."[46] A professor of medicine at Harvard Medical School too made a similar argument: "The weakness of the virus is the near inability to kill young people," and he added: "whether schools are open or not, children are less at risk from COVID-19 than from influenza."[47] According to two American epidemiologists, this "strategy" would not only protect adults and old people but also benefit children too. In an essay entitled "Should We Let Children Catch Omicron," these authors argued that "a more laissez-faire approach to kids and Covid makes public health sense, too," and then added, "Shielding kids from exposure only increases their future risk … Serious complications from the disease are rare among children, and the circulating virus allows adults to be naturally boosted … By rebuilding population immunity among the least at-risk, moreover, we help buffer risk for those most vulnerable."[48]

Across the pond, there were similar enthusiastic proposals about "using children as human shields." A sociologist at Nottingham Trent University made the argument that school closures were "depriving children of the opportunity to acquire immunity to the infection"[49] and critically questioned the idea of "prevent[ing] every death regardless of the cost." As he explained: "death is a normal part of life … we should acknowledge that many frail old people might see COVID-19 infection as a relatively peaceful end compared with, say, several years of dementia or some cancers."[50] Another academic, a professor of computational biology at University College London, further clarified these points, saying: "I'm not sure how to convey this message in a half-acceptable way. But if the objective were to send SARS-CoV-2 into endemicity, then healthy kids have to be exposed to the virus, ideally earlier than later. This is not 'eugenism'; it is bog-standard infectious disease epidemiology."[51] Maybe, but it sounds like a type of epidemiology that could be very popular in ancient Sparta, not in societies committed to protecting the right to health of their most vulnerable citizens.

In Italy, the idea of letting the virus infect children became popular among a few experts. An epidemiologist observed in the first months of 2022: "if masks actually avoid contact with the virus, [a] perplexity arises: the immune system of children at this age is in formation and needs to be 'trained' in order to make them become healthier adults and less susceptible to infections."[52] Of course, data on pediatric hospitalizations showed that "training" children by exposing them to COVID-19 was unhealthy at best, lethal at worst.[53] Although scientific evidence indicates that children are at lower risk of dying or getting hospitalized due to COVID-19 than adults and old people, the idea that they are invulnerable to the disease is another egregious example of disinformation. There are obstacles in identifying the actual number of COVID-19 deaths among children, including difficulties in terms of assigning the most adequate diagnosis on death certificates. Moreover, there is a scarcity of studies on this topic. Yet, the Centers for Disease Control and Prevention's COVID Data Tracker, on December 31, 2023, reported a total of 1,757 children aged 0–17 years who had died because of the virus in the United States alone. The same dataset showed that there were 7,059 deaths among young people aged 18–29 years old.[54] A study published in *JAMA* showed that between August 1, 2021, and July 31, 2022, COVID-19 was a leading cause of death in children and young people aged 0 to 19 years in the United States.[55] Moreover, estimates by UNICEF that included data from 95 countries indicate that on January 29, 2024, the total number of child deaths due to COVID-19 was 5,507 for ages 0–4, 2,797 for ages 5–9, 3,372 for ages 10–14 and 5,815 for ages 15–19, for a total of 17,491 fatalities.[56]

Death is the most tragic tip of the iceberg when it comes to the health impact of COVID-19 on children. A paper published in *JAMA Pediatrics* showed that in England alone, from February 1, 2020, to January 31, 2022, there were 10,540 hospitalizations among children and adolescents due to COVID-19.[57] Also, some children have developed multisystem inflammatory syndrome, a severe condition that involves multiple organs, requiring hospitalization. This disease was originally described as a Kawasaki disease-like illness due to its symptomatology; however, further research showed that, unlike Kawasaki disease, which rarely necessitates intensive care, the multisystem inflammatory syndrome causes significant rates of critical illnesses. In the United States, from April 2020 to May 2022, there were 4,868 pediatric hospitalizations for multisystem inflammatory syndrome and 2,387 hospitalizations for Kawasaki disease.[58] A meta-analysis and systematic review published in the *Journal of Infection and Public Health* showed that nearly one-quarter of pediatric patients hit by the disease ended up with long-term COVID symptoms, which widely involved multi-organ systems. Symptoms including dyspnea, fatigue and headache occurred most frequently. Other symptoms were myocarditis, splenomegaly, appendicitis, developmental regression, memory impairment and cognitive difficulties.[59] Less risky than influenza?

Health for sale

The normalization of sacrificing human for some "higher" economic purpose is consistent with political positions that have undermined the pandemic response in additional ways. The idea of not caring for "unproductive" members of society to protect the economy is often associated with long-standing support for neoliberal policies aimed at gradually weakening the role of the state to allow the market to operate "freely." Advocates of the "laissez-faire the virus" approach have usually strongly opposed preventive measures against SARS-CoV-2, dismissing them as ineffective and even harmful. This has often not only undermined public health recommendations but also fueled skepticism and non-compliance among the general public. Of population health measures implemented to contain the virus, lockdowns have been a subject of considerable debate among experts, with opinions varying on their effectiveness and impact. While some considered this intervention useless, it's essential to examine the science of its effectiveness while acknowledging its limitations and social and psychological costs. The COVID-19 crisis has disproportionately affected certain economic sectors, exacerbating inequalities[60] and socioeconomic stress, particularly among less affluent segments of the population. Lockdowns have added to the misery of the most disenfranchised sections of society. These measures had to be avoided, but at what cost? In spite of the loud reactions and controversies they generated, a significant portion of studies questioning the effectiveness of lockdowns showed to be insufficiently rigorous.[61] One study, published in *Scientific Reports* by a Brazilian doctor in March 2021, claimed that spending more time at home did not necessarily correlate with lower COVID-19 deaths. However, the research faced methodological issues and was retracted.[62] Additional research efforts have raised legitimate doubts about the actual impact of lockdowns on reducing COVID-19 mortality.[63] Yet, epidemiologists and public health experts, as well as numerous other scientific contributors, have argued the exact opposite, supporting the idea that lockdowns prevented more severe mortality scenarios.[50, 64–66]

A curious case regards a project called the Santa Clara study, whose results suggested that COVID-19 was no more lethal than the seasonal flu[67] and was co-authored by a prominent epidemiologist and professor from Stanford University. The study made headlines and was used by libertarian and right-wing activists to claim that the lockdown was an unjustified overreaction.[68,69] This research effort was also found to be flawed and ended up estimating a grossly inaccurate COVID-19 fatality rate. As Andrew Gelman, Director of the Center for Applied Statistics at Columbia University, noted, "I think the authors of the article cited above [the Santa Clara study] owe us all an apology."[70] The Stanford University professor, a prophet of scientific rigor, famous for having previously published an article arguing that "most published research results are false," had published some false results himself. As noted in another editorial, the expert "exposed the weaknesses of medical science," but then "medical science returned the favor."[71] Moreover, the study has been criticized because of an important conflict of interest: it was partly financed by an airline company,[72] that could obtain obvious benefits from research demonstrating that COVID-19 was not dangerous.[73]

Instances of studies attacking prevention measures based on inaccurate data, funded by stakeholders with vested interests in discrediting prevention interventions, raise strong suspicions. Neoliberal values and the ideology that preaches a minimal role for government interventions seem to be at the root of a particularly distorted view of public health. Herd immunity advocates have promoted an individual-centric approach to the pandemic, downplaying the significance of collective efforts for public health. This perspective, espoused by various figures, including authors, politicians, economists, major corporations and members of the global financial elite, seems to embody Margaret Thatcher's ideological stance, encapsulated in the famous phrase "There's no such thing as society. There are individual men and women and there are families."[74] This emphasis has probably contributed to weak, fragmented public health responses and hindered the unity needed to combat a global health crisis effectively.

Measures aimed at safeguarding public health have often been perceived, especially in the West, as unwarranted intrusions into personal freedom. The disdain for state interventions, seen as interference with the free market, became evident as proponents of neoliberal approaches argued that prevention measures equated to authoritarianism, suggesting a trade-off between pandemic control and democratic freedoms. However, the scientific evidence has shown that effective COVID-19 management is associated with good governance, not authoritarianism. While countries successful in managing COVID-19 such as Vietnam have resorted to some rigid measures, democracies such as South Korea, Australia, Japan and New Zealand have demonstrated successful pandemic management without heavily sacrificing democratic principles.

The influence of laissez-faire economics has significantly hampered the pandemic response in the realm of healthcare as well. This approach, driven by a narrow focus on economic interests, has undermined national health systems making nations ill prepared to handle the demands of a pandemic. Rooted in neoliberal economic theories, this ideology contends that state interventions are inherently inefficient and incapable of adequately addressing citizens' health needs. In the decades preceding the pandemic, many countries witnessed transformations consisting of a gradual shift toward privatization and budget cuts for healthcare.[75] Furthermore, the progressive defunding of public health and prevention programs, exacerbated by economic austerity following the 2008 crisis, has had profound effects. Privatization has led to a fragmentation of healthcare services, diminishing the ability to coordinate public health strategies with local community medicine. These policies have also resulted in a reduction in healthcare facilities, personnel and the number of intensive care unit beds. A *Lancet* study highlighted the consequences of outsourcing services in the United Kingdom following the 2012 healthcare reform, revealing a significant increase in mortality.[76] Instead of enhancing efficiency, the involvement of private providers in the national healthcare system seems to generate negative effects as the profit motive of private investors often instigates counterproductive reductions in healthcare personnel, detrimentally affecting healthcare provision. A parallel study involving Italy produced similar findings, demonstrating an association between decreases in public health spending and increases in avoidable mortality.[77] Italy's disinvestment in public healthcare manifested in substantial reductions in the number of hospitals and healthcare personnel, coupled with significant cuts in community healthcare investments. In the years leading up to the pandemic, Italy witnessed a one-third reduction in intensive care beds, despite falling below the European average for this critical indicator.[78]

Cost containment policies and privatizations have not spared specialist outpatient care and residential community care structures.[79] However, it is crucial to note that the first expenses often slashed during times of crisis are those related to prevention. Following the onset of the pandemic, urgent investments were needed not only in hospitals and intensive care but also in epidemiological prevention and surveillance. Unfortunately, these resources had already been depleted due to what is euphemistically termed "healthcare spending optimization." Despite Italy dedicating a higher percentage of health spending to prevention than the OECD average, the country's lag in terms of epidemiological intelligence and public health interventions. The closure of the National Center of Epidemiology a few years before the pandemic stands as a glaring example of political short-sightedness that perceives prevention as an unnecessary cost.

As articulated by Carlo Montaperto, the medical director of the Milan polyclinics, and Mirco Nacoti, an anesthetist at the Papa Giovanni XIII hospital, "prevention does not bring profits" economically and "does not make noise" politically.[80] In increasingly market-influenced and private-sector-oriented national health systems, community health interventions are deemed less "profitable" than lucrative sectors like high surgery, cardiology and social-assistance residences. Nacoti pointed out that this economic disparity resulted in an imbalance of power between prevention and healthcare, even at a political level, as economic power often translates into political influence. In this paradoxical system of incentives, if prevention is highly effective and leads to fewer hospitalizations, it could ironically mean lower revenues for healthcare companies and less political influence.[80]

The glaring influence of economic and political stakeholders on public health has become so apparent that seemingly unjustified decisions are now considered normal. The selection of an economist like Mario Monti for the WHO super commission on health policies serves as a clear symptom of the shadow cast by neoliberal ideology and economics over global health. Don't get me wrong: Monti is a serious, sober and capable professional and politician. In spite of his capability as an economist and his political integrity, his appointment raised questions about his expertise in global health. Moreover, Monti's tenure as the head of the Italian government from November 2011 to April 2013 is often remembered for healthcare cuts and a concerning rise in "out of pocket" healthcare spending, even though these trends began a year before his leadership and were in part caused by the effects of the 2008 global financial downturn.[81,82] Regardless, the decision to entrust Monti with the leadership of the WHO super commission on health policies suggests that actual experience in global health is not a prerequisite for such a role. Instead, it appears that having considerable influence and power in the economic and political spheres is of greater importance. Yet, Monti deserves some credit for having candidly revealed, during a TV interview, a doubt shared by many: "I also wondered what I had to do with the WHO when they called me."[83]

Economy or health is a false dichotomy

"A generation is leaving, the one that saw the war, smelled it and felt its privations, between fleeing to an air raid shelter and the anxious search for something to feed themselves. Gone are hands hardened by calluses, faces marked by deep wrinkles, memories of days spent under the scorching sun or the biting cold. Hands that have moved rubble, mixed cement, bent iron, in a vest and newspaper hat. Those of the Lambretta, the Fiat 500 or 600, the first refrigerators, and the black and white television are gone. They leave us, wrapped in a sheet, like Christ in the shroud, those of the economic boom who with their sweat rebuilt this nation of ours, giving us that well-being which we have taken advantage of with impunity. Experience, understanding, patience, resilience, respect, qualities now forgotten, are gone. They leave without a caress, without anyone shaking their hand, without even a last kiss."[84] These touching words from Fulvio Marcellitti, a police inspector, were shared in a social media message during the pandemic. The rhymes talk about thousands of elderly people who have passed away silently, depriving society of their wisdom, experience and memories. Was their death really a "fair" price to pay to "save" the economy and allow everyone the much-desired "normality"? No, it was not fair at all and did not even save the economy.

The idea of safeguarding the economy by allowing the virus to spread, although widely endorsed in some political circles, has been proven to be an illusion. The most effective way to safeguard production activities was not to permit the uncontrolled spread of the virus but rather to combat it through preventive measures. Countries that have effectively managed the pandemic, prioritizing prevention and implementing robust virus containment policies, have not only minimized the worst health effects but also mitigated its economic impact. A study featured in *The Lancet* conducted an empirical analysis, comparing GDP growth and the stringency of lockdown measures during the initial 12 months of the pandemic for Organization for Economic Co-operation and Development (OECD) countries. The project focused on those countries that pursued either virus elimination or virus mitigation strategies. Results revealed that the "elimination-oriented approach" outperformed the "mitigation-oriented approach" in terms of GDP growth across various time periods. Countries opting for elimination witnessed a return to pre-pandemic levels of GDP growth by early 2021, while those employing less vigorous strategies experienced lingering negative growth. Moreover, the study highlighted that nations choosing swift action to eliminate SARS-CoV-2 not only protected their economies but also avoided the worst restrictions on civil liberties.[85] This seems counterintuitive, but some countries adopting effective prevention interventions have not even resorted to a lockdown. A compelling example is Taiwan, which experienced minimal movement restrictions yet successfully saved thousands of lives and curtailed economic damage.

Those who have long attacked prevention measures as useless and harmful have also failed to recognize another essential point: it was not so much public health measures that contributed to the COVID-19 economic crisis and social disruption. The most important cause of the crisis was the virus itself. Some research efforts provide support for this hypothesis. A study using cell phone log data from customer visits to more than 2.25 million businesses across 110 different industries in the United States highlighted that legal shutdown orders represented only a modest part of the massive changes to consumer behavior. While overall consumer traffic fell by 60%, legal restrictions accounted for only 7% of this reduction. The choice to stay at home and protect oneself from the virus, regardless of preventive measures, played a far more important role than lockdowns in causing the economic effects of the pandemic.[86] As an IMF report explained, the contraction of the economy occurs even without public health interventions precisely because many activities are affected by the voluntary choices and behaviors of the population.[87] Sadly, the idea of letting the virus spread to save the economy resulted in excess avoidable deaths and did not help nations earn a cent. On the contrary, as Nassim Taleb explained in April 2020, governments "didn't want to spend pennies in January [2020], now they're spending trillions."[88]

What did a country like Sweden gain by snubbing territorial prevention activities to limit the virus? The numbers on the decline in GDP in 2020 of the Scandinavian countries speak for themselves: Denmark, Sweden, Norway and Finland suffered contractions of 8.5%, 8.3%, 5.3% and 5.2%, respectively. Unlike the growth of GDP, however, the loss of human lives cannot be amendable. An analysis in *Nature Human Behavior* explains: Sweden, "unlike its Scandinavian neighbors, suffered a substantial loss in life expectancy in 2020. Although in 2021 Swedish life expectancy then recovered quickly to return to near 'normal' levels, the years of life lost during the period of high mortality [COVID-19] cannot be recovered."[34]

The decision to abandon preventive measures to protect productive activities has been a monumental failure, showing that the idea of choosing between health and the economy is a false dilemma.[89] As emphasized in an article in *Nature*, governments such as those of the United Kingdom and Sweden erred in assuming the inevitability of the respiratory pathogen's spread. Instead, they should have made "all reasonable efforts to delay the spread of a virus until medical interventions would be available."[90] Moreover, as the authors of an article in *The Lancet* explain, the "laissez-faire" virus strategy has created the conditions for the spread of new variants of concern. Countries adopting a "live with the virus" stance have inadvertently become potential sources of global threats, creating conditions for the spread of new and worrisome mutations. This has not only endangered the health of populations worldwide but also undermined the effectiveness of preventive strategies employed by countries adopting a more proactive approach.

The collapse of the Great Wall

"China dangerously resembles a pressure cooker: a country with its borders closed for two and a half years. The economy is doing badly. What they manage to save from the Chinese economic miracle is at the price of frightening sacrifices," explained a well-known journalist from an important Italian newspaper at the end of summer 2022.[91] In the same days, the news arrived that China had overtaken the United States in terms of average life expectancy at birth (Figure 4.1). It was a historic result, to say the least, but one that went unnoticed in the Western media. In 1960, the United States had a lead of more than 25 years of life expectancy over China, but this gap has been vaporized by over 60 years of failed health policies and increased mortality, especially among middle-aged US males, combined with rapid transformations in the determinants of health in the Asian powerhouse. The definitive overtaking, however, is attributable to the diverse management of the pandemic in the two countries.

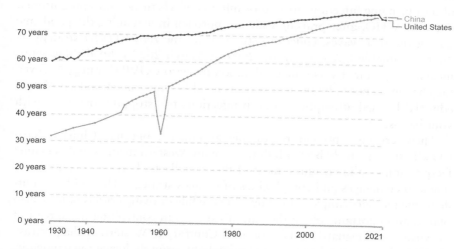

FIGURE 4.1 The surpassing: life expectancy at birth in China and in the United States (1930–2021)

Note: Period life expectancy is a metric that summarizes death rates across all age groups in one particular year. For a given year, it represents the average lifespan for a hypothetical group of people if they experienced the same age-specific death rates throughout their lives as the age-specific death rates seen in that particular year.

Sources: From Our World in Data, "Life expectancy at birth – period tables – Various sources" [dataset], with data from "Human Mortality Database," 2023; United Nations, "World Population Prospects," 2022; Zijdeman et al., "Life Expectancy at Birth 2," 2015; James C. Riley, "Estimates of Regional and Global Life Expectancy, 1800–2001," 2005. Retrieved February 14, 2024 from https://ourworldindata.org/grapher/life-expectancy?time=1930.latest&facet=none& showSelectionOnlyInTable=1&country=USA~CHN

The Chinese strategy, sometimes called the "zero COVID" approach (although in reality it has always been an aspiration rather than a real goal), which contemplated very rigid and burdensome measures for people, has been the target of numerous attacks by the Western media. The newspaper *The Observer*, for example, carried the headline "China insists on Zero COVID strategy that doesn't work."[92] An article in Bloomberg asserted that China's "Zero COVID strategy has become Xi's Nemesis. The result is an economic mess."[93] The *New York Times* too joined the chorus with catchy headlines such as "China's Zero COVID Mess Proves Autocracy is Bad for Everyone."[94]

Some criticisms of China's Zero COVID strategy are legitimate, especially concerning the impact of some draconian interventions on people's freedom. Furthermore, there have been valid concerns about the sustainability of maintaining strict prevention measures in response to the emergence of highly transmissible new variants." As underlined in a couple of editorials in *The Time*[95] and the *Financial Times*,[96] with the arrival of Omicron the idea of bringing infections to zero or minimal levels turned into pure utopia. Even the WHO, after praising China's approach in managing the pandemic during the first waves, ended up stigmatizing the zero COVID strategy as "not sustainable." A letter in the *BMJ* in March 2022 echoed these sentiments, suggesting it was time to abandon the zero COVID strategy.[97] Given the challenges posed by the highly transmissible Omicron variants, a *Nature* editorial likened attempting to curb infections to "stopping the wind with your hands."[98]

These critiques present reasonable arguments, but has China's Zero-COVID strategy truly been a failure, as many Western media pundits claim? Despite some valid critiques, most of these intellectual attacks overlook the nuanced challenges and complexities of China's strategy. The rigid and burdensome measures implemented by China, while drawing criticism, have also played an important role in the nation's success in controlling the spread of the virus and safeguarding the economy. Contrary to Western media portrayals, China's economy demonstrated remarkable growth during the pandemic, outpacing those of Western nations and other emerging countries. In 2021, China's GDP surged by an impressive 8.1%, a noteworthy achievement for a country having a "bad economy." One factor contributing to China's economic success during the early stages of the pandemic was the targeted and localized nature of its strict interventions. While certain sectors experienced significant impacts, highly targeted, localized measures enabled a swift return to pre-pandemic economic levels. This contrasts with the experience of many Western countries, which saw dramatic GDP declines while implementing less rigorous and less punctual stop-and-go strategies.

Chinese health policies have not only had significant impacts on the economy but have also proven to be effective at the public health level. Shortly

after the first COVID-19 deaths were reported, China demonstrated remarkable efficiency by swiftly implementing stringent measures – which would
be unthinkable for a Western nation. For example, during the first dramatic
waves of the pandemic, Chinese health authorities conducted mass testing on
all 9 million inhabitants of Wuhan within a remarkably short timeframe.[75]
The stringent lockdown imposed in Wuhan, criticized globally, proved to be
briefer than those adopted in European countries such as Italy. Moreover,
China's strategy in 2021 and 2022 involved the prompt identification of new
outbreaks, followed by rigid but highly targeted and localized lockdowns.[99]
Remarkably, this proactive approach allowed China to restore relative normalcy to both its society and its economy more swiftly than anticipated.[100]
The zero COVID strategy, relying on preventive measures such as testing,
tracing and isolating, proved successful until the emergence of the Omicron
variants, which posed new challenges and rendered the idea of virus elimination unattainable. While many Western commentators have labeled the
zero COVID strategy a failure, COVID-19 death figures from the first two
years of the pandemic offer a totally different perspective. An article in *The
Lancet*, published during the early months of the pandemic, emphasized the
incredible speed with which China organized national interventions, citing it
as the crucial factor behind their success. As highlighted in a *Science* article,
"China's aggressive zero COVID strategy has worked very well" up until the
Omicron variants arrived, with China reporting only a few thousand deaths –
a fraction of the figures seen in countries like the United States.[101] Also, in
an article published in *The Lancet Respiratory Medicine*, it is stressed that
"Chinese policy has been enormously successful."[102] Even in Western media,
there have been some acknowledgments of the positive impact of China's
zero COVID approach. An editorial in *The Guardian*, for example, recognized that despite facing "bad press,"[103] the Chinese policy of elimination,
employing mass testing, specific lockdowns and case surveillance with rigorous quarantines and isolations prevented a humanitarian catastrophe. The
fog raised over the evaluation of the Chinese strategy by Western media can
be cleared by comparing China's COVID-19 death figures against those of
the United States. At the end of 2022, the United States had recorded over 1.2
million deaths; if China had had the same indicator of COVID-19 deaths per
million inhabitants, with a population four times larger, it would have had to
bury over 4 million corpses. Consider also India, a country with a very large
population such as is found in China. According to WHO estimates, much
disputed by the New Delhi government, India had an excess mortality caused
by the pandemic of around 4.7 million deaths in 2020 and 2021.[104]

Despite significant actions in terms of prevention, the advent of the
Omicron variants marked the collapse of China's defences against the virus. By mid-2022, the laissez-faire approach to the virus had gone global,
on by statements from US President Joe Biden and the WHO declaring

the "end" of the pandemic. It was at this juncture that maintaining the zero COVID strategy became impossible. The new SARS-CoV-2 variants introduced a level of elusiveness and contagiousness that had profound repercussions for China's preventive measures. While the zero COVID strategy had proven effective in saving lives nationally and even globally (by averting new variants),[101] these new mutations posed an insurmountable challenge. Scientists understood that abruptly abandoning the zero COVID policy before achieving effective vaccination could have resulted in a public health disaster. Suddenly deciding to "live with the virus," as expected, caused significant problems for the healthcare system. According to various scientific contributions in the literature, the sudden abolition of zero COVID policies in China would have caused a "tsunami" of infections and nearly 2 million deaths.[105,106]

These predictions were probably exaggerated, but China has indeed been overwhelmed by Omicron. To adapt its approach, the Asian nation has resorted to what is referred to as the "dynamic zero COVID strategy."[102] This approach was designed to provide a window of opportunity for the country to prepare and improve mass vaccinations, particularly among the elderly and those with underlying conditions.[107] Nonetheless, it was found to be inadequate. In late November 2022, widespread protests erupted against the perceived rigidity of China's preventive measures, leading Western media to label the country as a "health dictatorship." A month later, responding to mounting pressure, Chinese authorities made a decisive shift by abandoning most of the restrictive controls. Patients with mild symptoms were no longer encouraged to get tested, let alone asymptomatic ones. People who tested positive at home were no longer asked to report their test results.[108] Travel in public was no longer restricted by electronic health cards, and lockdowns were now even more localized and targeted and no longer required for entire municipal areas or cities. From January 8, 2023, onward, people started to travel abroad again. The die was cast.

The sudden relaxation of policies inevitably caused a rapid increase in infections. Overwhelmed by a struggling healthcare system and hundreds of thousands of elderly people dying, Chinese authorities decided to adopt new criteria for counting COVID-19 fatalities, excluding most deaths from reporting thanks to a narrower definition of mortality. Afterwards, Chinese authorities decided to effectively stop counting cases and deaths, abandoning mass testing almost completely. In a notable shift, Wang Guiqiang, an infectious disease expert working for the Chinese government, declared at a State Council press conference on December 20 that "the main cause of death from Omicron infection is the underlying diseases." This echoed the contentious Hamlet-like debate about "deaths with or by COVID-19" that characterized so much public discussion in the West in the early phases of the pandemic.

Now it has found resonance and popularity in the Far East.[109] It marked a stark departure from China's earlier approach, which had distinguished itself not only for the effectiveness of its prevention strategies but also for rigorous population-wide testing in repeated waves of the virus.

The main reasons behind the Chinese health crisis caused by Omicron are to be found not only in the rapid abandonment of prevention measures but also in an insufficient vaccination rate, especially among the elderly. In contrast to other countries that pursued the zero COVID approach but then achieved high immunization rates, especially in vulnerable groups, such as Australia and New Zealand, China faced unique challenges. As of the end of November 2022, only 40% of individuals aged over 80 had received a complete course of two vaccinations and a booster shot. These vaccinations were based on Chinese-licensed vaccines that were not specifically designed to target the Omicron variants. This left a vulnerable segment of the population at heightened risk. The crisis unfolded in China at a time when the rest of the world was experiencing a general relaxation of virus-related measures. However, the impact of Omicron was not limited to China alone. Other nations that had either relaxed or abandoned zero COVID policies without implementing robust vaccination campaigns faced similar challenges.[110]

There were two major lessons learned from the Chinese challenge faced in the context of the arrival of Omicron variants. First, it showed the importance of a comprehensive and well-executed vaccination strategy, especially targeting high-risk groups like the elderly, in preventing a sharp increase in mortality caused by the relaxation of major prevention strategies. Second, despite the declaration of the "end of the pandemic" and a revision in the nomenclature of major variants – originally identified through Greek alphabet letters like Alpha and Delta, different strains of Omicron were now named BA.4, BA.5 or BQ.1.1 or XBB.1.5 affecting the perception of their threat[111] – as Martin Hibberd, professor of emerging infectious diseases at the London School of Hygiene & Tropical Medicine, pointed out, "Omicron has a reputation for being milder, but that's only if you're vaccinated." If you're not, the expert explained, as in countries like Hong Kong, or if you're poorly vaccinated, as is the case in China, "it can [still] be deadly."[102]

Western pundits, once quick to condemn China's stringent measures, then blamed the Asian nation for easing restrictions, conveniently forgetting that these were the very same measures adopted in Europe and in the United States in early 2020. The irony lies in the fact that, during the earlier waves of the pandemic, rich countries had implemented some of the strictest and most extensive lockdowns worldwide and those who criticized such measures were often dismissed as supporters of unfounded conspiracy theories. As already stated, the uncontrolled spread of Omicron made strict prevention measures unrealistic and unsustainable. However, before criticizing nations that have limited large-scale COVID-19 infections and deaths, commentators from Europe, the United Kingdom and the United States should look in the mirror and reflect on the millions of dead buried due to their failed governments' strategies.

References

1. Mackinson T. Milano, il grido dei medici del San Paolo e del San Carlo costretti a decidere chi salvare: "Le carenze erano ben note, ora ci troviamo a fare intollerabili scelte sull'accesso alle cure". *Fatto Quotidiano*. Nov 19, 2020. https://www.ilfattoquotidiano.it/2020/11/19/milano-il-grido-dei-medici-del-san-paolo-e-del-san-carlo-costretti-a-decidere-chi-salvare-le-carenze-erano-ben-note-ora-ci-troviamo-a-fare-intollerabili-scelte-sullaccesso-alle-cure/6008132/?fbclid=IwAR1jwbVd4H-GXUqNWwivQ0c3nl9cICfN_K5-gRVFNYD8Irvoyt kuJlXM_pE
2. Fassari L. Pronto il nuovo Piano Pandemico 2021–2023. "Se risorse sono scarse privilegiare pazienti che possono trarne maggior beneficio". Ecco le misure: formazione, scorte Dpi e farmaci e organizzazione dei servizi. Quotidiano Sanità. Jan 11, 2021. https://www.quotidianosanita.it/governo-e-parlamento/articolo.php?articolo_id=91385 (accessed Jan 23, 2024).
3. Roberts J. Telegraph journalist says coronavirus 'cull' of elderly could benefit economy. Metro. Published online Mar 11, 2020. https://metro.co.uk/2020/03/11/telegraph-journalist-says-coronavirus-cull-elderly-benefit-economy-12383907/ (accessed Jan 23, 2024).
4. Weaver M. 'Nature's way of dealing with old people': the damning messages revealed to Covid inquiry. *The Guardian*. Published online Oct 31, 2023. https://www.theguardian.com/uk-news/2023/oct/31/natures-way-of-dealing-with-old-people-the-damning-messages-revealed-to-covid-inquiry (accessed Jan 27, 2024).
5. Walker P. No 10 denies claim Dominic Cummings argued to 'let old people die'. The Guardian. Published online Mar 22, 2020. https://www.theguardian.com/politics/2020/mar/22/no-10-denies-claim-dominic-cummings-argued-to-let-old-people-die (accessed Jan 23, 2024).
6. Rai News. Covid, Guzzini: 'La gente è stanca, pazienza se qualcuno muore'. Poi si scusa. rainews. Published online Dec 15, 2020. https://www.rainews.it/dl/rainews/articoli/covid-guzzini-gente-stanca-pazienza-se-qualcuno-muore-c986eef1-07f0-4eef-86fe-5cb8ab1ed013.html (accessed Jan 23, 2024).
7. La Stampa. "Anziani non indispensabili allo sforzo produttivo del Paese", è bufera sul tweet del governatore Toti. Published online Nov 1, 2020. https://www.lastampa.it/savona/2020/11/01/news/anziani-non-indispensabili-allo-sforzo-produttivo-del-paese-e-bufera-sul-tweet-del-governatore-toti-1.39488593/ (accessed Jan 23, 2024).
8. Beckett L. Older people would rather die than let Covid-19 harm US economy – Texas official. *The Guardian*. Published online Mar 24, 2020. https://www.theguardian.com/world/2020/mar/24/older-people-would-rather-die-than-let-covid-19-lockdown-harm-us-economy-texas-official-dan-patrick (accessed Jan 23, 2024).
9. Sturloni G. Le peggiori sparate sul coronavirus sentite nel 2020. Wired Italia. Published online on Dec 22, 2020. https://www.wired.it/attualita/politica/2020/12/22/peggiori-sparate-scienziati-politici-coronavirus/ (accessed Jan 23, 2024).

10. Coin F. Quanto vale una vita? Internazionale. Published online Jan 5, 2021. https://www.internazionale.it/opinione/francesca-coin/2021/01/05/quanto-vale-una-vita (accessed Jan 23, 2024).

11. Gollier C. Covid-19: 'Confiner les personnes vulnérables, plutôt que les jeunes et les actifs'. *Le Monde*. Published online Nov 4, 2020. https://www.lemonde.fr/idees/article/2020/11/04/confiner-les-personnes-vulnerables-plutot-que-les-jeunes-et-les-actifs_6058401_3232.html (accessed Jan 23, 2024).

12. Jessop J. The UK lockdown and the economic value of human life. *Economic Affairs* 2020; **40**: 138–47.

13. Gray TS. Spencer, Herbert (1820–1903). In: Routledge encyclopedia of philosophy, 1st edn. London: Routledge, 2016. https://doi.org/10.4324/9780415249126-DC076-1.

14. Russell B. Freedom versus organization: the pattern of political changes in the 19th century European history. New York: W.W. Norton & Co., 1934.

15. Spencer H. Social statics: the conditions essential to human happiness specified, and the first of them developed. New York: Robert Schalkenbach Foundation, 1995.

16. Reuters. "Johnson – Coronavirus will not stop me shaking hands." Published online March 3, 2020. https://www.reuters.com/article/idUSKBN20Q1K2/ (accessed Jan 23, 2024).

17. The Independent. No 10 fails to deny reports Boris Johnson told Italian PM he wanted 'herd immunity'. Published online June 4, 2020. https://www.independent.co.uk/news/uk/politics/coronavirus-no-10-boris-johnson-italian-pm-herd-immunity-pierpaolo-sileri-a9548786.html (accessed Jan 23, 2024).

18. The Guardian. Coronavirus: Johnson warns 'many more families are going to lose loved ones' – video. Published online Mar 12, 2020. http://www.theguardian.com/politics/video/2020/mar/12/coronavirus-johnson-warns-many-more-families-are-going-to-lose-loved-ones-video (accessed Jan 23, 2024).

19. Omer SB, Yildirim I, Forman HP. Herd immunity and implications for SARS-CoV-2 control. *JAMA* 2020; **324**: 2095–6.

20. Science. "Critics slam letter in prestigious journal that downplayed COVID-19 risks to Swedish schoolchildren." Published October 6, 2020. https://www.science.org/content/article/critics-slam-letter-prestigious-journal-downplayed-covid-19-risks-swedish (accessed Jan 21, 2024).

21. Gurdasani D, Drury J, Greenhalgh T, *et al*. Mass infection is not an option: we must do more to protect our young. *Lancet* 2021; **398**: 297–8.

22. Altman D. Understanding the US failure on coronavirus – an essay by Drew Altman. *BMJ* 2020; **370**: m3417.

23. Greenhalgh T, McKee M, Kelly-Irving M. The pursuit of herd immunity is a folly – so who's funding this bad science? *The Guardian*. Published online Oct 18, 2020. https://www.theguardian.com/commentisfree/2020/oct/18/covid-herd-immunity-funding-bad-science-anti-lockdown (accessed Jan 23, 2024).

24. Ahmed N. Koch-funded PR agency aided Great Barrington declaration sponsor. *Byline Times*. Published online Oct 13, 2020. https://bylinetimes.com/2020/10/13/koch-funded-pr-agency-aided-great-barrington-declaration-sponsor/ (accessed Jan 23, 2024).

25. Yamey, G., & Gorski, D. "Covid-19 and the new merchants of doubt." BMJ. Published online September 13, 2021. https://blogs.bmj.com/bmj/2021/09/13/covid-19-and-the-new-merchants-of-doubt/ (accessed January 23, 2024).

26. Mandavilli A. 'We were helpless': despair at the CDC as the Covid pandemic erupted. *The New York Times*. Published online March 21, 2023. https://www.nytimes.com/2023/03/21/health/covid-cdc.html (accessed Jan 23, 2024).

27. BBC. Why are so many babies dying of Covid-19 in Brazil? BBC News. Published online Apr 14, 2021. https://www.bbc.com/news/world-latin-america-56696907 (accessed Jan 23, 2024).

28. Taylor L. Covid-19: is Manaus the final nail in the coffin for natural herd immunity? *BMJ* 2021; 372: n394.

29. Buss LF, Prete CA, Abrahim CMM, *et al.* Three-quarters attack rate of SARS-CoV-2 in the Brazilian Amazon during a largely unmitigated epidemic. *Science* 2021; 371: 288–92.

30. Rodrigues M. Will Brazil's COVID disaster sway its presidential election? *Nature* Published online Sept 22, 2022. https://doi.org/10.1038/d41586-022-03015-w.

31. Friedman TL. Friedman: is Sweden getting it right with its COVID-19 approach? *The Mercury News*. Published online Apr 30, 2020. https://www.mercurynews.com/2020/04/30/friedman-is-sweden-getting-it-right-with-its-covid-19-approach/ (accessed Jan 23, 2024).

32. Bjorklund K. The inside story of how Sweden botched its coronavirus response. Foreign Policy. Published online Jan 29, 2024. https://foreignpolicy.com/2020/12/22/sweden-coronavirus-covid-response/ (accessed Jan 23, 2024).

33. Brusselaers N, Steadson D, Bjorklund K, *et al.* Evaluation of science advice during the COVID-19 pandemic in Sweden. *Humanities & Social Sciences Communications* 2022; 9: 1–17.

34. Schöley J, Aburto JM, Kashnitsky I, *et al.* Life expectancy changes since COVID-19. *Nature Human Behaviour* 2022; 6: 1649–59.

35. Henley J. King of Sweden blasts country's 'failed' coronavirus response. The Guardian. Published online Dec 17, 2020. https://www.theguardian.com/world/2020/dec/17/king-sweden-failed-covid-strategy-rare-royal-rebuke-lockdown-hospitals-cases (accessed Jan 23, 2024).

36. Valigia Blu. Il prof. Silvestri di Pillole di Ottimismo chiede chiarimenti a Valigia Blu per un articolo. Ecco la nostra risposta. Valigia Blu. Published online Oct 17, 2020. https://www.valigiablu.it/scambio-silvestri-valigia-blu/ (accessed Jan 23, 2024).

37. Ganding S, Capria MM. Cos'ha lasciato in ombra il Covid-19. Epidemiologia e insensatezze dell'emergenza coronavirus. Giap. Published online May 17, 2020. https://web.archive.org/web/20200517080558/https://www.wumingfoundation.com/giap/2020/05/ombra-covid19/ (accessed Jan 23, 2024).

38. COVID-19 | The myth of herd immunity. Institute for Health Metrics and Evaluation as author. Published on October 1, 2020. https://www.healthdata.org/news-events/newsroom/videos/covid-19-myth-herd-immunity (accessed Jan 23, 2024).

39. Aschwanden C. The false promise of herd immunity for COVID-19. *Nature* 2020; 587: 26–8.

40. Aschwanden C. Nature Magazine. COVID-19 herd immunity strategies could bring 'untold death and suffering'. *Scientific American*. https://www.scientificamerican.com/article/covid-19-herd-immunity-strategies-could-bring-untold-death-and-suffering/ (accessed Jan 23, 2024).

41. Alwan NA, Burgess RA, Ashworth S, *et al.* Scientific consensus on the COVID-19 pandemic: we need to act now. *The Lancet* 2020; 396: e71–2.

42. Coronavirus updates: Fauci calls 'herd immunity' declaration embraced by White House 'ridiculous'. ABC News. Published online October 15, 2020. https://abcnews.go.com/Health/live-updates/coronavirus/?id=73623859 (accessed Jan 23, 2024).

43. Abbasi K. Covid-19: social murder, they wrote – elected, unaccountable, and unrepentant. *BMJ* 2021; 372: n314.

44. Howard J. We want them infected: how the failed quest for herd immunity led doctors to embrace the anti-vaccine movement and blinded Americans to the threat of COVID. Hickory NC: Redhawk Publications, 2023.

45. Diamond, D. "'We want them infected': Trump appointee demanded 'herd imm unity' strategy, emails reveal." Politico. Published online December 16, 2020. https://www.politico.com/news/2020/12/16/trump-appointee-demanded-herd-immunity-strategy-446408 (accessed Jan 27, 2024).

46. Howard J. 'Infants, kids, teens, young people, young adults, middle aged with no conditions etc. have zero to little risk ... so we use them to develop herd ... we want them infected ...' In: *We want them infected: how the failed quest for herd immunity led doctors to embrace the anti-vaccine movement and blinded Americans to the threat of COVID.* Hickory, NC: Redhawk Publications, 2023: 173.

47. Kulldorff M. Herd immunity is still key in the fight against Covid-19. *The Spectator.* Published online Aug 8, 2020. https://www.spectator.co.uk/article/herd-immunity-is-still-key-in-the-fight-against-covid-19/ (accessed Jan 29, 2024).

48. Krug A. Should we let children catch Omicron? UnHerd. Published online Feb 2, 2022. https://unherd.com/2022/02/should-we-let-children-catch-omicron/ (accessed Jan 29, 2024).

49. Dingwall R. Coronavirus UK – why closing schools is (generally) a bad idea. Social Science Space. Published online Mar 18, 2020. https://www.socialsciencespace.com/2020/03/coronavirus-uk-why-closing-schools-is-generally-a-bad-idea/ (accessed Jan 29, 2024).

50. Science Media Centre. "Expert reaction to a preprint looking at the impact of lockdowns, as posted on the Johns Hopkins Krieger School of Arts and Sciences website." Published online February 2, 2022. https://www.sciencemediacentre.org/expert-reaction-to-a-preprint-looking-at-the-impact-of-lockdowns-as-posted-on-the-john-hopkins-krieger-school-of-arts-and-sciences-website/ (accessed Jan 23, 2024).

51. Science-Based Medicine. "Should an infectious disease epidemiologist comment on child vaccination?" Published online February 11, 2022. https://sciencebasedmedicine.org/unkind-largely-unqualified-and-highly-judgmental/ (accessed January 29, 2024).

52. De Vogli R. Uso nelle mascherine nelle scuole, alcuni studi ne hanno messo in dubbio l'efficacia. Il Fatto Quotidiano. Published online Jan 17, 2022. https://www.ilfattoquotidiano.it/2022/01/17/uso-nelle-mascherine-nelle-scuole-alcuni-studi-ne-hanno-messo-in-dubbio-lefficacia/6454616/ (accessed Jan 22, 2024).

53. Shi DS. Hospitalizations of children aged 5–11 years with laboratory-confirmed COVID-19 – COVID-NET, 14 states, March 2020–February 2022. *MMWR Morbidity and Mortality Weekly Report* 2022; **71**. https://doi.org/10.15585/mmwr.mm7116e1.

54. CDC. COVID Data Tracker. Centers for Disease Control and Prevention. Published online Mar 28, 2020. https://covid.cdc.gov/covid-data-tracker (accessed Jan 29, 2024).

55. Flaxman S, Whittaker C, Semenova E, *et al.* Assessment of COVID-19 as the underlying cause of death among children and young people aged 0 to 19 years in the US. *JAMA Network Open* 2023; **6**: e2253590.

56. Arora A. COVID-19 confirmed cases and deaths. UNICEF. Published online May 17, 2021. https://data.unicef.org/resources/covid-19-confirmed-cases-and-deaths-dashboard/ (accessed Jan 29, 2024).

57. Ward JL, Harwood R, Kenny S, *et al.* Pediatric hospitalizations and ICU admissions due to COVID-19 and pediatric inflammatory multisystem syndrome temporally associated with SARS-CoV-2 in England. *JAMA Pediatrics* 2023; **177**: 947–55.

58. Molloy MJ, Auger KA, Hall M, *et al.* Epidemiology and severity of illness of MIS-C and Kawasaki disease during the COVID-19 pandemic. *Pediatrics* 2023; **152**: e2023062101.

59. Zheng Y-B, Zeng N, Yuan K, *et al.* Prevalence and risk factor for long COVID in children and adolescents: a meta-analysis and systematic review. *Journal of Infection and Public Health* 2023; **16**: 660–72.
60. Reducing inequality benefits everyone – so why isn't it happening? *Nature* 2023; **620**: 468–468.
61. Lewis D. What scientists have learnt from COVID lockdowns. *Nature* 2022; **609**: 236–9.
62. Savaris RF, Pumi G, Dalzochio J, Kunst R. Retracted article: stay-at-home policy is a case of exception fallacy: an internet-based ecological study. *Scientific Reports* 2021; **11**: 5313.
63. Herby, J., Jonung, L., & Hanke, S. H. "A systematic literature review and meta-analysis of the effects of lockdowns on COVID-19 mortality II." medRxiv. Published online August 30, 2023. https://www.medrxiv.org/content/10.1101/2023.08.30.23294845v1 (accessed January 23, 2024).
64. Flaxman S, Mishra S, Gandy A, *et al.* Estimating the effects of non-pharmaceutical interventions on COVID-19 in Europe. *Nature* 2020; **584**: 257–61.
65. Soltesz, K., Gustafsson, F., Timpka, T., Jaldén, J., Jidling, C., Heimerson, A., ... & Bernhardsson, B. "Inferring the effectiveness of government interventions against COVID-19." Science. Published online December 15, 2020. https://www.science.org/doi/10.1126/science.abd9338 (accessed January 23, 2024).
66. Chernozhukov V, Kasahara H, Schrimpf P. Causal impact of masks, policies, behavior on early Covid-19 pandemic in the U.S. *Journal of Econometrics* 2021; **220**: 23–62.
67. Bendavid E, Mulaney B, Sood N, *et al.* COVID-19 antibody seroprevalence in Santa Clara County, California. *International Journal of Epidemiology* 2020; **50**(2): 410–9.
68. Ioannidis JPA. A fiasco in the making? As the coronavirus pandemic takes hold, we are making decisions without reliable data. STAT. Published online Mar 17, 2020. https://www.statnews.com/2020/03/17/a-fiasco-in-the-making-as-the-coronavirus-pandemic-takes-hold-we-are-making-decisions-without-reliable-data/ (accessed Jan 22, 2024).
69. The New York Times. "Opinion | A study said Covid wasn't that deadly. The right seized it." Published online May 14, 2020. https://www.nytimes.com/2020/05/14/opinion/coronavirus-research-misinformation.html (accessed January 23, 2024).
70. McCormick E. Why experts are questioning two hyped antibody studies in coronavirus hotspots. *The Guardian.* Published online Apr 23, 2020. https://www.theguardian.com/world/2020/apr/23/coronavirus-antibody-studies-california-stanford (accessed Jan 23, 2024).
71. Wired. "A prophet of scientific rigor - and a Covid contrarian." Published online October 12, 2020. https://www.wired.com/story/prophet-of-scientific-rigor-and-a-covid-contrarian/?fbclid=IwAR0QefSGHMUkSgY9mwK6ZCbJek1iyxkErfM4i27IqKOBccu0fLyzBChjk1U (accessed January 23, 2024).
72. Lee SM. JetBlue's founder helped fund a Stanford study that said the coronavirus wasn't that deadly. BuzzFeed News. Published online May 15, 2020. https://www.buzzfeednews.com/article/stephaniemlee/stanford-coronavirus-neeleman-ioannidis-whistleblower (accessed Jan 23, 2024).
73. Landsverk G. A controversial study on coronavirus was partly funded by an airline founder who's criticized lockdowns, according to a new investigation from BuzzFeed News. Business Insider. https://www.businessinsider.com/buzzfeed-stanford-coronavirus-study-funded-by-jetblue-founder-2020-5 (accessed Jan 23, 2024).
74. The Guardian. "Margaret Thatcher: a life in quotes." Published online April 8, 2013. https://www.theguardian.com/politics/2013/apr/08/margaret-thatcher-quotes (accessed January 26, 2024).

75. Burki T. China's successful control of COVID-19. *The Lancet Infectious Diseases* 2020; **20**: 1240–1.
76. Goodair B, Reeves A. Outsourcing health-care services to the private sector and treatable mortality rates in England, 2013–20: an observational study of NHS privatisation. *The Lancet Public Health* 2022; **7**: e638–46.
77. Quercioli C, Messina G, Basu S, McKee M, Nante N, Stuckler D. The effect of healthcare delivery privatisation on avoidable mortality: longitudinal cross-regional results from Italy, 1993–2003. *Journal of Epidemiology and Community Health* 2013; **67**: 132–8.
78. Organisation for Economic Co-operation and Development Italy: Fewer Hospital Beds, Less Time Spent in Hospitals. Published online November 7, 2019. https://www.oecd.org/italy/italy-fewer-hospital-beds-less-time-spent-in-hospitals.htm (accessed January 23, 2024).
79. In 10 anni chiusi 173 ospedali, personale ridotto di 46 mila unità, scarsi progressi sull'assistenza territoriale e sempre più spazio al privato. Ecco com'è arrivato il Ssn di fronte al Covid. Quotidiano Sanità. Published online July 7, 2021. https://www.quotidianosanita.it/studi-e-analisi/articolo.php?articolo_id=96379 (accessed Jan 23, 2024).
80. Radiotelevisione Italiana (RAI) Presa Diretta 2020/21 – C'era una volta la sanità pubblica - Video. RaiPlay. Published online February 1, 2021. https://www.raiplay.it/video/2021/02/Presa-diretta—Cera-una-volta-la-sanita-pubblica-0b7d6ab0-bb1e-4abf-a1a9-ced2de43d5d2.html (accessed Jan 23, 2024).
81. Paterlini M. Italy's health system reforms on hold. *The Lancet* 2013; **381**: 1085–6.
82. World Bank open data. World Bank. https://data.worldbank.org (accessed Jan 23, 2024).
83. La Repubblica Monti: Servizio sanitario nazionale a rischio. *la Repubblica*. Published online Nov 27, 2012. https://www.repubblica.it/politica/2012/11/27/news/monti_servizio_sanitario-47544859/ (accessed Jan 23, 2024).
84. Biagioli F. 'Se ne vanno', la poesia da brividi che rende omaggio all'intera generazione di nonni strappata via senza neanche una carezza. greenMe. Published online Apr 21, 2020. https://www.greenme.it/lifestyle/arte-e-cultura/poesia-omaggio-nonni-morti-coronavirus/ (accessed Feb 7, 2024).
85. Oliu-Barton M, Pradelski BSR, Aghion P, *et al*. SARS-CoV-2 elimination, not mitigation, creates best outcomes for health, the economy, and civil liberties. *The Lancet* 2021; **397**: 2234–6.
86. Goolsbee A, Syverson C. Fear, lockdown, and diversion: comparing drivers of pandemic economic decline 2020. *Journal of Public Economics* 2021; **193**: 104311.
87. International Monetary Fund Research Dept. Chapter 2 the at lockdown: dissecting the economic effects. In: World economic outlook. Oct 2020. International Monetary Fund. https://www.elibrary.imf.org/display/book/9781513556055/ch02.xml (accessed Jan 23, 2024).
88. Avishai B. The pandemic isn't a black swan but a portent of a more fragile global system. *The New Yorker*. Published online Apr 21, 2020. https://www.newyorker.com/news/daily-comment/the-pandemic-isnt-a-black-swan-but-a-portent-of-a-more-fragile-global-system (accessed Jan 21, 2024).
89. Dorn F, Khailaie S, Stoeckli M, *et al*. The common interests of health protection and the economy: evidence from scenario calculations of COVID-19 containment policies. *The European Journal of Health Economics* 2023; **24**: 67–74.
90. Sridhar D. Five ways to prepare for the next pandemic. *Nature* 2022; **610**: S50.
91. Piazzapulita, Federico Rampini: 'La Cina? Una pentola a pressione'. *Libero Quotidiano*. https://www.liberoquotidiano.it/news/spettacoli/televisione/33001897/piazzapulita-federico-rampini-cina-pentola-a-pressione.html (accessed Jan 23, 2024).

92. Observer. "China is insisting on a zero-Covid approach that isn't working." https://observer.com/2022/04/china-zero-covid-policy-analysis/ (accessed January 23, 2024).

93. Bloomberg. "China's 'zero Covid' has become Xi's nemesis." Published online April 17, 2022. https://www.bloomberg.com/opinion/articles/2022-04-17/china-corona-virus-outbreak-xi-jinping-s-covid-zero-is-failing(accessed January 23, 2024).

94. The New York Times. "China's 'zero Covid' mess proves autocracy hurts every-one." Published online April 13, 2022. https://www.nytimes.com/2022/04/13/busi-ness/china-covid-zero-shanghai.html (accessed January 23, 2024).

95. Time. "Asia has kept COVID-19 at bay for 2 years. Omicron could change that." Published online January 18, 2022. https://time.com/6139851/asia-omicron-covid-surge/ (accessed January 23, 2024).

96. Financial Times. "China's zero-Covid goal is no longer sustainable." https://www.ft.com/content/a34a67aa-f4ea-4f6b-b162-568919007e57 (accessed January 23, 2024).

97. BMJ. "Is it time to end China's 'zero Covid' policy?" Published online January 23, 2024. https://www.bmj.com/content/376/bmj.o707/rr (accessed January 23, 2024).

98. Mallapaty S. China's zero-COVID strategy: what happens next? *Nature* 2022; **602**: 15–6.

99. Myers SL. Facing new outbreaks, China places over 22 million on lockdown. *The New York Times*. Published online Jan 13, 2021. https://www.nytimes.com/2021/01/13/world/asia/china-covid-lockdown.html (accessed Jan 23, 2024).

100. Chen S, Zhang Z, Yang J, *et al*. Fangcang shelter hospitals: a novel concept for responding to public health emergencies. *The Lancet* 2020; **395**: 1305–14.

101. Normile D. China quietly plans a pivot from 'zero COVID'. Science. https://www.science.org/content/article/china-quietly-plans-pivot-zero-covid (accessed Jan 23, 2024).

102. Burki T. Dynamic zero COVID policy in the fight against COVID. *The Lancet Respiratory Medicine*. 2022; **10**: e58–9.

103. Spinney L. The 'zero-Covid' approach got bad press, but it worked – and it could work again. *The Guardian*. Published online Mar 28, 2022. https://www.theguardian.com/commentisfree/2022/mar/28/no-covid-approach-bad-press-but-worked (accessed Jan 23, 2024).

104. Taylor L. Covid-19: true global death toll from pandemic is almost 15 million, says WHO. *BMJ* 2022; **377**: o1144.

105. Cai J, Deng X, Yang J, *et al*. Modeling transmission of SARS-CoV-2 Omicron in China. *Nature Medicine* 2022; **28**: 1468–75.

106. Xiao H, Wang Z, Liu F, Unger JM. Excess all-cause mortality in China after ending the zero COVID policy. *JAMA Network Open* 2023; **6**: e2330877.

107. Times G. Tedros' remarks on China's zero-COVID 'irresponsible'. Global Times. https://www.globaltimes.cn/page/202205/1265409.shtml (accessed Jan 23, 2024).

108. Normile D. China is flying blind as pandemic rages. Science. https://www.science.org/content/article/china-flying-blind-pandemic-rages (accessed Jan 23, 2024).

109. Dyer O. Covid-19: China stops counting cases as models predict a million or more deaths. *BMJ* 2023; **380**: 2.

110. Financial Times. "Hong Kong Omicron deaths expose limits of fraying zero-Covid policy." https://www.ft.com/content/6e610cac-400b-4843-a07b-7d870e8635a3 (accessed January 23, 2024).

111. Prater E. Meet the biology professor who named the surging 'Kraken' COVID variant. He has more to help make sense of Omicron's 'alphabet soup'. Fortune Well. Published online January 5, 2023. https://fortune.com/well/2023/01/05/kraken-variant-omicron-covid-name-ryan-gregory-biology-professor/ (accessed Jan 23, 2024).

5

INEQUITY

"He had lost all certainty, he had gone haywire," lamented the brother of Laurent, a bartender who, in the waning days of 2020, tragically chose to end his life by throwing himself onto the train tracks. Once employed at a club, he worked the shift from five in the afternoon until midnight. However, the stringent restrictions imposed by the Italian government to contain the COVID-19 pandemic not only cost him his job but also compelled him to return to live with his father. His brother reflected, "He was completely closed in on himself."[1] In a parallel tragedy during the same period, a 59-year-old entrepreneur from Gricignano d'Aversa, in southern Italy, was found lifeless by his son in the warehouse of his family's shoe factory. He had taken his own life with a noose around his neck. The family business, which had thrived for three generations, succumbed to the crisis precipitated by the coronavirus pandemic. Deprived of orders for an extended period, the once thriving enterprise became an insurmountable burden, an unbearable weight on the shoulders of its dedicated owner.[2] Similarly, in December 2020, a 53-year-old man tragically threw himself into the Tiber River in Rome from a height of 15 metres, an event witnessed by a friend who bravely attempted to save him, risking succumbing to the river's currents. He never recovered from the economic fallout of the coronavirus and the associated lockdown measures. His advertising agency, specializing in organizing disco events, suffered profound setbacks due to the restrictive measures, and the weight of the crisis proved too much for him to bear.[3]

The announced suicide crisis that did not happen

These are only a few of the heart-wrenching stories underscoring the profound human toll exacted by the economic repercussions of the pandemic.

DOI: 10.4324/9781003511977-7

Many others have been affected by the crisis. The COVID-19 pandemic has not only unleashed a public health calamity but also reverberated as a profound socioeconomic shock. According to the World Bank's Global Economic Prospects, the year 2020 witnessed a staggering 4.3% contraction in global GDP, [4] coupled with estimates from the International Labor Office (ILO) indicating a loss of 225 million jobs worldwide.[5] The United States and Japan experienced respective GDP declines of 3.6% and 5.3%, while Europe bore the brunt of the pandemic with a striking 7.4% drop.[6] In Italy, the economic fallout was even more severe, with a GDP decrease of 8.9% in 2020, leading to a loss of nearly 1 million employed individuals between February 2020 and 2021.[7] Hundreds of thousands of businesses succumbed to the crisis, closing their doors permanently.[8]

Given these alarming statistics, it was widely expected that the pandemic would inflict a severe toll on mental health. Individuals grappling with job loss and economic instability are particularly susceptible to a spectrum of problems including anxiety, panic attacks, sleep disorders, stress and, notably, depression.[9] Moreover, economic downturns have historically been linked to self-destructive behaviors, as evidenced by the aftermath of the Great Recession of 2008.[10]

Some experts who opposed COVID-19 prevention interventions were absolutely convinced that lockdowns would lead to a surge in suicides.[11] However, despite these dire predictions, the anticipated surge of suicides never occurred. While the socioeconomic impacts were undoubtedly severe, surprisingly, quantitative analyses published in the scientific literature indicate that in 2020, there were no increases in suicide rates compared to previous years. In fact, some regions witnessed decreasing trends.[12] An analysis of the main causes of death from 2015 to 2020 in the United States, one of the countries hit hardest by the health emergency, shows a significant reduction in suicides, which fell from 47,511 in 2019 to 44,834 in 2020. A similar scenario unfolded in Canada.[13,14] In Sweden, suicide rates in January–June 2020 showed a slight decrease compared to the corresponding rates in January–June 2019.[15] Peru too experienced a decrease in suicides, homicides and road accidents.[16] The pandemic appears to have had no negative effects on suicides in England, as underlined by an article appearing in the *British Medical Journal*.[17] In Australia, a study that analyzed the early effects of the COVID-19 pandemic found no significant changes in the rate of suspected suicide in the year 2020 compared to average rates for the years 2015–2019.[18] Similarly, a study in Norway showed stable levels of suicidal ideation and suicide deaths during the first six months of the COVID-19 pandemic compared to pre-pandemic levels.[19] In Germany, suicide rates remained in line with those for previous years.[20] In Italy, a report analyzing deaths recorded between March 1 and April 30, 2020, revealed a 19% decrease in suicides among men and a 27% decrease among women compared to the five-year average from 2015 to 2019.[21] A systematic review of the literature encompassing 18 countries showed an increase in suicides and suicide attempts in six countries and a decrease in four.[22] Another analysis involving data from 33 countries concluded that there is no evidence supporting the hypothesis of a higher-than-expected number of suicides during the pandemic years.[23]

These data contradict the worrying dire predictions. Yet, the literature would seem to indicate that some populations have been disproportionately affected by the pandemic, including children and adolescents. A rapid systematic review of the effects of past pandemics highlighted their significant effects on psychosocial stress, severe worry, feelings of helplessness, suicides and behavioral problems such as substance abuse.[24] In 2020, in Japan, a nation that did not even implement a national lockdown, suicide rates among women and adolescents increased for the first time in 11 years.[25,26] Research conducted in Texas showed that rates of suicidal ideation and suicide attempts among 11- to 21-year-olds were higher during some months of 2020 than in 2019.[27] In spite of these results, a systematic review and meta-analysis of 47 observational studies on adolescents and young people showed that, during the pandemic, temporal suicidal trends showed increases that were not statistically significant.[28] Another review observed an upward trend in suicidal ideation and suicide attempts, while confirming a stable historical trend in suicide rates.[29]

While the observed reduction in suicides in 2020 may offer an optimistic outlook, caution must guide our interpretation.[30] Historically, crises, whether wars or pandemics, have elicited varied social responses. On one front, such adversities can amplify isolation, prejudice, latent racism and xenophobia.[31,32] Conversely, they may paradoxically foster reciprocity, solidarity and a less stressful lifestyle in certain population segments. Could it be that, on an aggregate level, the shock of the pandemic's impact on suicide risk for some was counteracted by protective factors like interpersonal support, enhanced belonging and a collective commitment to health? The answer remains elusive. It's crucial to acknowledge that even if this counterbalance theory holds true, it offers little solace to those grappling with the loss of a loved one to suicide. At a population level, the anticipated suicide crisis did not materialize, defying expectations, including my own. However, rather than serving as a reason to relax our vigilance, these findings should be a catalyst for reinforcing support and equity measures that proved to save lives in times of hardship. Governments should redouble efforts to avert social conditions that can drive particularly sensitive individuals like Laurent to "lose all certainty."

Psychodemia

In the wake of concerns expressed by professionals about the potential capacity of the COVID-19 pandemic to generate a mental health crisis,[33] there has been a proliferation of investigations into psychological health, including online analyses with more or less reliable samples.[34] Indeed, the phenomenon of suicide may be only the tip of the iceberg of a larger psychosocial condition. Some studies carried out in the United Kingdom,[35,36] in the United States[37] and in the Czech Republic[38] have highlighted worrying increases in psychological stress during the first months of the pandemic compared to previous years. Furthermore, according to the Health at a Glance 2021 report, an increase in anxiety and depression has been observed in almost all OECD countries.[39] However, the findings are not unequivocal. A Dutch study found no increase in the prevalence of anxiety and depressive symptoms in March 2020 compared to 12 months earlier.[40] A Danish investigation even showed a reduction in depressive symptoms in adults living at home with their children during a lockdown.[41]

Unlike suicides, and despite conflicting results, the international literature seems unanimous in concluding that the pandemic has generated deleterious effects on mental health. There are multiple mechanisms capable of explaining why. First, it is important to highlight the mental health effects of long COVID.[42] A study, published in the early stages of the pandemic, showed that many hospitalized and discharged patients returned to hospitals and more than one in ten died.[39] The deterioration in physical health caused by long COVID has certainly had a notable impact on psychological well-being. A study in *The Lancet* showed that in the months following diagnosis, a significant proportion of survivors of the COVID-19 disease are victims of various psychological conditions, psychiatric problems[40] and neurological diseases. A study by Kim and colleagues showed that some neuropsychiatric conditions persist for up to two years after acute infection, with significant implications for quality of life.[43]

Another poignant impact of the pandemic on mental health has been the trauma associated with losing close relatives, with the bereavement of children who lost their parents. According to estimates from a study published in *The Lancet*, more than 5 million children have lost a parent or caregiver due to COVID-19.[44] In the United States alone, it is reported that between April 1, 2020, and June 30, 2021, over 140,000 children had to grapple with the traumatic loss of a parent or grandparent who cared for them. Significantly, the risk of such loss was disproportionately higher among children facing greater socioeconomic disadvantage or belonging to ethnic minorities.[45] The sudden and often unexpected nature of bereavement, compounded by the inability to participate in funeral rites, can give rise to prolonged psychological stress, anxiety, depression and even suicidal ideation among the affected children.[46] Among the consequences of the pandemic, it is also important to underline the trauma and sense of guilt of those who have involuntarily infected their family members, inadvertently causing their death. The drama is in some ways even more painful in cases of people who did not believe in the dangers of the virus or were completely unaware that they had contracted the virus.[38]

Another way the pandemic has caused mental health effects involves social distancing measures. In Italy and other countries, the rapid spread of the coronavirus prompted governments to introduce rigid SARS-CoV-2 control measures. The main objective of these interventions was to reduce the speed of the spread of the virus to limit mortality and overcrowding in intensive care units. However, isolation and quarantine are experiences that can be unpleasant, as they can cause, for example, separation from loved ones and loss of freedom.[47] Lockdowns especially appear to have contributed to mental health issues, causing increases in psychosocial problems such as anxiety, depression and social isolation.[48] Lockdowns have particularly affected people living in overcrowded homes without access to a garden or a balcony and in disadvantaged areas of large cities.

The pandemic has also generated negative effects on quality of life and interpersonal relationships.[49] Lockdowns may also have increased the risk of exposure to domestic violence, especially against women and children.[50] For many vulnerable groups and frail elderly people, lockdowns have increased loneliness and the feeling of being a burden on their family and society in general. The scientific evidence is quite unanimous in underlining that (positive) social relationships are an important protective factors for health, being inversely correlated with mortality.[46] A longitudinal study using data provided by the University College London Covid-19 Social Study, conducted during the first wave of the pandemic, showed a clear socioeconomic gradient not only with respect to coronavirus-related adversity (COVID-19 diagnosis) but also with respect to socio-relational effects, with particular reference to the hospitalization or death of a loved one. To some, this may appear insignificant in terms of health. Yet, a review and meta-analysis that included 90 studies with more than 2 million participants suggested that loneliness is as deadly as smoking cigarettes.[51]

The unjust virus: it affects everyone, but it is not democratic

When two well-known figures from the Italian economic and political world, Flavio Briatore and Silvio Berlusconi, ended up in the hospital in the summer of 2020, many believed SARS-CoV-2 to be an "egalitarian" virus that did not discriminate. Before them, political figures such as Donald Trump, Boris Johnson and Jared Bolsonaro had also been hospitalized after publicly mocking and denying the danger of the viurs. Briatore and Berlusconi were admitted to the San Raffaele Hospital in Milan a few weeks apart, under the care of the same doctor, "famous" for having stated in the summer of 2020 that the virus was "clinically dead." The virus, however, was more alive than ever. It struck then, as it struck later, without "leaving behind" even some of the most powerful men in the world. Iran's Deputy Health Minister Iraj Arirchi, after being infected, described SARS-CoV-2 as "a democratic virus, [which] does not distinguish between poor and rich or between statesmen and ordinary citizens."[52] The philosopher Slavoj Zizek, in his book *Virus*, agreed: "He was profoundly right about this – we are all in the same boat."[53]

Data do not support the idea of a democratic virus. SARS-CoV-2 does not only affect the elderly, the sick, individuals with previous pathologies and the immunosuppressed; the virus hits much harder precisely those who are in social and economic difficulties. The scientific evidence is unequivocal: the most disadvantaged social classes have higher COVID-19 infection, hospitalization and mortality rates than the general population.[54] In the United States, areas characterized by higher socioeconomic deprivation showed a higher prevalence of SARS-CoV-2 infection.[55] A study examining COVID-19 mortality in nursing home residents in England reported that virus-related deaths were more common in lowerincome groups.[56] A systematic literature review that included over 50 studies observed that African American and Hispanic populations had disproportionately higher rates of infection, hospitalization risk and mortality related to SARS-CoV-2 than whites.[57] Another contribution showed that the decrease in life expectancy in Hispanic and non-Hispanic blacks was two to three times greater than in the non-Hispanic white population, reversing years of progress in reducing racial and ethnic disparities. The life expectancy of African American male citizens living in the United States is now 67.7 years – a low level of longevity not seen since 1998.[58] Socioeconomic inequalities are also associated with a higher risk of long COVID.[20] Moreover, a study based on 12 longitudinal surveys of the UK adult population noted that the pandemic may have exacerbated existing mental health inequalities.[59]

The scientific evidence in favor of the hypothesis that COVID-19 "targets" the most vulnerable is overwhelming. In an editorial published in *The Lancet*, Richard Horton stated, perhaps a little provocatively, that "COVID-19 is not a pandemic," but a syndemic.[9] A syndemic, or synergistic epidemic, refers to the aggregation of two or more simultaneous or sequential epidemics or clusters of diseases that exacerbate the prognosis and health burden of a population. The term was developed by anthropologist Merrill Singer in the mid-1990s to challenge a biomedical approach to diseases, which studies individual pathologies as separate entities from other diseases, regardless of the social contexts that determine them. According to Singer, syndemics are caused by poverty, stress or structural violence and must be studied in light of the social, economic and political determinants that influence them.[10] Indeed, regarding the COVID-19 pandemic, at least two categories of diseases appear to have interacted with one another: the SARS-CoV-2 infection and non-communicable or chronic diseases that worsen its prognosis. These conditions, however, share a common third category of determinants: socioeconomic factors.[60] The main chronic diseases increasing the risk of COVID-19 mortality, such as hypertension, diabetes, cardiovascular diseases and obstructive pulmonary disease, are in fact more prevalent among the less well-off populations.[61] Major behavioral risk factors (e.g., obesity and cigarette smoking) that influence pathologies associated with COVID-19 deaths (e.g., type 2 diabetes and respiratory diseases) are also socially stratified.[62]

There are various reasons that explain why people living in disadvantaged socioeconomic conditions are more exposed to COVID-19 infection, hospitalization and death. First, scientific evidence shows that some occupations are more exposed to risk factors for mental and physical health, including ergonomic risks, repetitive work, long hours, shift work and low wages. These characteristics lead to increased exposure to respiratory diseases, some types of cancer and hypertension, all conditions associated with a greater risk of mortality from COVID-19. At the same time, some types of employment, in which certain vulnerable socioeconomic categories are over-represented, such as jobs in the fields of sanitation, social and health care and door-to-door delivery, are at greater risk of contagion.[26] Among the professional categories at higher risk of being exposed to SARS-CoV-2 contagion, there are also workers in the meat and poultry processing industry.[26, 29] The most vulnerable socioeconomic groups in society also have less job security, less flexibility and less ability to stay at home during a lockdown,[28] as well as fewer opportunities for social distancing and less access to protective equipment.[29]

Another mechanism capable of explaining the relationship between socioeconomic conditions and severe COVID-19 outcomes is inequalities in access to healthcare, which before and during the pandemic contributed significantly to differences in the prevalence of chronic diseases in social groups with heterogeneous levels of income, education and employment.[27] Barriers to access to healthcare facilities aggravate the prevention, treatment and care of COVID-19 disease in materially deprived or socially marginalized groups. Furthermore, individuals suffering from chronic diseases (such as cancer or cardiovascular diseases), which affect the less well-off social classes much more frequently, are less likely to receive assistance during the spread of the virus since health services, during the most critical phases, are overwhelmed by too many infections.[26, 63]

Inequalities in housing conditions also create a greater risk of contracting COVID-19 in the less well-off classes. Homelessness and exposure to poor-quality housing are associated with worse health outcomes: for example, humid environments increase the risk of respiratory diseases such as asthma, while overcrowding can lead to higher infection rates. Socially disadvantaged neighborhoods are more likely to contain smaller homes with a lack of outdoor space, as well as having higher population densities,[64] being more exposed to pollution and having fewer green spaces for exercise. The combination of these factors increases the risk of contracting the COVID-19 disease.[26] Furthermore, in crowded neighborhoods it is more complicated to apply social distancing rules. Finally, the most vulnerable people are more likely to live in neighborhoods classified as food deserts, which hinder access to healthy foods, a protective factor against severe COVID-19 outcomes.

A final mechanism capable of explaining why poor, less educated and socially disadvantaged people have been particularly affected by the pandemic is chronic stress and the cumulative impact of adverse events over the course of life. Many years ago, psychologists described the emblem of the stressed person as a man who is too busy, with a hectic lifestyle, and who perhaps works in the world of business or high finance. But scientific evidence shows that chronic stress is much more prevalent among less well-off social strata. Research has highlighted that allostatic load, an indicator of stress capable of influencing the speed with which individuals age biologically, is a much more widespread phenomenon among poorer and less educated individuals. If COVID-19 risk is positively related to age, individuals with higher biological age may also be more susceptible to the adverse effects of the pandemic.[36]

Vaccine apartheid

When the former governor of the Lombardy region stated that the distribution of vaccines had to be prioritized "on the basis of GDP,"[65] implying that the richest Italian regions had to be covered first, there was great public dismay. The expression must be appreciated for its candid nature, for it is rare to learn directly from the words of members of the elite how much they care about principles of equity. In addition to being an important dimension in understanding who is most affected by death and disease, equity is also an essential component of any analysis and strategy of global health issues. The missteps in pandemic management were not just limited to overlooking social disparities within nations but also extended to neglecting the glaring inequalities on the international stage. To contain the spread of the virus, joint international actions coordinated by organizations such as the WHO, UN agencies and national governments were necessary to avoid inequitable distribution of vaccines.[66] Unfortunately, such collaborative mechanisms were lacking. Instead of triggering virtuous cycles of international solidarity, the availability of new vaccines has generated a selfish, frenetic competition for doses, with the richest, most powerful countries dominating the scene. The "vaccinationalism" of wealthier countries generated what could be called a "vaccination apartheid," where poorer nations were left without access to vaccines during the worst years of the pandemic. In November 2020, European Union countries, the United Kingdom and the United States had already secured 80% of the doses of Pfizer/BioNTech vaccines, while low-income nations in sub-Saharan Africa were unable to cover even a small fraction of their population."[67]

Anthony Costello, professor emeritus at University College London and a member of the Independent SAGE, did not mince words when addressing countries that, in his view, indirectly contributed to the creation of "vaccine apartheid." In December 2021, he delivered a stark assessment, arguing that millions would succumb to COVID-19 because of a lack of vaccination coverage in the most impoverished countries. Highlighting the glaring disparity, he pointed out that the rates of fully vaccinated individuals in high-income and low-income countries at the time were 69% and 3.5%, respectively. Costello accused the UK, Canada, Germany and other EU states of endorsing a policy that deliberately obstructed access to vaccines. He contended that these nations were defending an immoral economic system that prioritizes the interests of big pharmaceutical patents over the lives of millions. In light of this, he raised a provocative question: whether states facilitating this obstruction could be held accountable and prosecuted before the International Criminal Court for crimes against humanity.[68] Amidst this criticism, some countries have garnered praise for their efforts to promote equity in vaccination. Notably, China has received commendation for its commitment to supplying vaccines to numerous developing countries from the World Economic Forum.[69] Yet, by time the pandemic was declared "over," disparities in vaccine access left most poor countries largely uncovered (Figure 5.1).

The self-centeredness exhibited by countries contributing to "vaccination apartheid" has proven to be an epidemiological boomerang. The virus, indifferent to geographical borders, has exploited the gaps in global health strategies that neglected social inequalities between nations and provided the coronavirus with ample opportunities to proliferate. Human rights theories and principles, often criticized as abstract slogans, showed their tangible impact on people's lives. The health crisis vividly demonstrated that safeguarding everyone's right to health was not only a moral imperative but also a pragmatic approach. A global commitment toward equitable vaccine distribution was, in fact, a practical necessity. In the initial stages of vaccination campaigns, the WHO took a step toward addressing this issue by introducing the Covid-19 Vaccine Global Access (COVAX) Facility. The primary objective of COVAX was ambitious: to vaccinate at least 60% of the world's population by July 2022. This global allocation mechanism sought not only to ensure affordable prices but also to provide all countries with access to a diverse portfolio of vaccines, particularly benefiting low- and middle-income nations through significantly reduced prices.

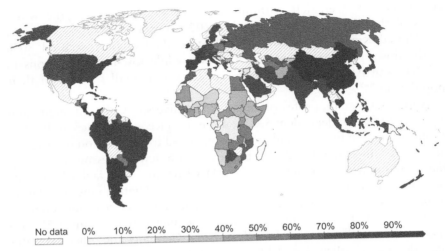

FIGURE 5.1 Vaccine apartheid at the "end of the pandemic": share of people who had received at least one dose of COVID-19 vaccine on May 3, 2023

Note: Total number who had received at least one vaccine dose, divided by the population of the country

Source: Official data collated by Our World in Data – Last updated 14 February 2024 – processed by Our World in Data. "people_vaccinated_per_hundred" [dataset]. Official data collated by Our World in Data – Retrieved 14 February 2024 from https://ourworldindata.org/grapher/share-people-vaccinated-covid?tab=map&time=2023-05-03

However, the success of COVAX hinged on substantial funding to procure the required vaccines. Despite commitments from governments and private partners, the allocated funds fell woefully short of the magnitude of the challenge. Calls for a collaborative approach to vaccine allocation and distribution, based on values of equity and solidarity, were widespread. Yet, the neglect of a comprehensive strategy for vaccine allocation by both governments and the private sector resulted in the initiative's failure. In an article published in *Nature Medicine*, a mathematical model sought to assess the potential impact of wealthy nations' relinquishing a portion of their vaccines for equitable distribution to less affluent countries. The study drew the conclusion that adopting a more equitable strategy, with affluent nations sharing their vaccines with the less privileged, could have saved at least 1 million lives in 2021 alone.[70]

When the right to profit of a few wins over the right to health of all

When Jonas Salk was asked who should own the patent on his polio virus vaccine, he replied: "People, I would say. There is no patent. Can the sun be patented?"[71] The development and authorization of COVID-19 vaccines less than a year after the outbreak of the pandemic was one of the most remarkable achievements in the history of immunization. The speed with which the world mobilized was exceptional and unprecedented. However, the approval of effective vaccines was just the first step; their widespread and affordable distribution globally became paramount. In addition to robust aid measures and international collaboration, as an editorial in *Nature* argued, there was a need for "a waiver of the patent on COVID vaccines" to ensure broader access, especially in economically challenged countries. According to the author of the editorial, this intervention was "fair and reasonable."[72] Shobita Parthasarathy, professor of public policy at the University of Michigan, proposed to escalate the production of generic drugs throughout the world, especially in developing countries. This might have been possible if the World Trade Organization (WTO) had approved the proposal submitted by India and South Africa to temporarily give up intellectual property rights on COVID-19 vaccines and other technologies, including some patents and trade secrets. Hundreds of WTO member countries had given their support to the proposal, but the United States, the United Kingdom and the European Union, under pressure from large pharmaceutical multinationals, blocked its passage.[73] Even during a pandemic that has killed millions, the private profit of a few has been placed before the right to life of all. Appeals from scientists and public health experts to ensure that vaccine-producing countries help developing countries both by suspending intellectual property rights on vaccines and by transferring technological and logistical aid to ensure greater vaccination coverage worldwide were repeated.[74] Without success.

A report titled "The Double Dose of Inequalities," released by Amnesty International during the initial phases of the vaccination campaign, underscored how major pharmaceutical companies contributed to perpetuating inequities in vaccine access worldwide.[75] The report highlighted how "vaccine manufacturers have played a decisive role in limiting global vaccine production and hindering equitable access to a life-saving product." Despite benefiting from billions of dollars in government funding and advance orders that mitigated the financial risks associated with drug development, these companies maintained a monopoly on intellectual property, obstructed technology transfers and vehemently opposed measures and public policies aimed at expanding global vaccine production. Companies like Pfizer, BioNTech and Moderna have disproportionately supplied vaccines to affluent nations, prioritizing profit over global health accessibility. Despite their corporate missions projecting their philanthropic image, such as Pfizer's commitment to "fair and equitable distribution," BioNTech's aim to "make vaccines available around the world as quickly as possible" and Moderna's self-portrayal as dedicated to "delivering effective, affordable vaccines and therapies to all populations," their actions tell a different story. These pharmaceutical giants actively contributed to "vaccine apartheid" and undermined initiatives by the

WHO regarding vaccination coverage in Africa. An editorial in *BMJ* exposed the interference of the kENUP Foundation, a consultancy firm hired by Bi-oNTech, opposing a new WHO-sponsored technology transfer hub in Cape Town, South Africa. The hub was intended to empower African researchers and entrepreneurs to produce patent-free versions of mRNA vaccines. Ellen't Hoen, a lawyer and global health activist, criticized such interference, stating, "if you run a nonprofit foundation and you go around trying to stop people from developing life-saving vaccines, I don't know what your agenda is, but it really has a bad smell."[76]

Yet, pointing fingers solely at Big Pharma for the "vaccine apartheid" is akin to addressing a symptom rather than its underlying problem. In an increasingly globalized market where companies compete more and more aggressively against one another, their professed social responsibility often proves to be more illusion than substance. Companies are happy to contribute to social causes only to the extent that their profits remain unaffected and their public image is enhanced. It is the responsibility of governments to enact laws and regulations capable of addressing these idiosyncrasies. An article in *Nature* argued that the COVID-19 pandemic has exposed misconceptions surrounding vaccine intellectual property policies and demonstrated how alternative policies could have ensured universal access. The article examined two myths: "the myth of the need for patents" and "the myth of unimpeded access by patents." The first suggests that without patent protection, critical molecular technologies necessary for rapid vaccine development might not have been developed. The second claims that patents are not hindering access to COVID-19 vaccines and treatments. Facts, assured the author of the article, led instead to the opposite conclusion. In addition to limiting access to patents and know-how needed to produce vaccines and antivirals, big pharmaceutical companies like Pfizer have resisted efforts by low- and middle-income countries to adapt effective COVID-19 treatments like Paxlovid to local health needs."[77]

Some argue that Pfizer, Moderna and other patent holders have made large investments in vaccine development and "deserve" to profit from their monopoly power. But doesn't the same principle also apply to governments, and therefore taxpayers, who have provided billions of dollars in research grants and advance purchase agreements, especially during the early stages of the pandemic?[78] Furthermore, companies like Pfizer unilaterally decided to increase the price of COVID-19 vaccines many months after the agreements and state aid were obtained. Will they return part of the profits obtained from this price increase to governments? No, they won't.

Mariana Mazzucato, a professor at University College London, astutely exposed the prevailing ideology in Western societies that falsely claims the private sector to be the primary source of technological innovations. The reality, however, is quite different. Many technologies that have enriched major companies, such as Apple and Microsoft, owe their development to state aid and basic research funded by government institutions.[79] Historically, breakthrough innovations like fiber optics, computers, airplanes and radar are deeply rooted in scientific research funded by government institutions, particularly in military research by organizations like the Pentagon. An article in the *Proceedings of National Academies of Sciences* demonstrated how public funding from the National Institutes of Health contributed significantly to the publications associated with new drugs approved by the Food and Drug Administration between 2010 and 2016.[80] While patent liberalization might not automatically ensure universal access to COVID-19 vaccines in poorer countries, the complexity of vaccine production know-how and the need for supportive industrial processes could be addressed through international cooperation and development aid. The development of vaccines in record time demonstrates that when there is political will and real interest in solving a problem that affects everyone, the wealthiest countries can act effectively and efficiently through forms of public-private cooperation. But, the humanitarian ethos has been overwhelmed by the logic of profit. Moreover, as an illustrative example of the application of double standards, affluent countries, despite decades of advocating for free markets and trade, have embraced a significant degree of protectionism to safeguard the interests of private oligopolies that receive public subsidies. At times, the geopolitics of Western nations seems to be based on hypocrisy, rather than democracy.

Bill Gates and how the ultra-rich can save the world?

The ethical lapses in international cooperation are starkly exemplified by the actions of one of the most prominent figures in global health, Bill Gates. Despite being a charismatic public figure who has purportedly contributed to global health policies through extensive financing of programs and interventions in developing countries, as well as authoring a book entitled *How to Prevent the Next Pandemic*, Gates has staunchly opposed the temporary liberalization of intellectual property rights on COVID-19 vaccines.[68] During a global security conference in Munich in 2022, when asked about the WHO's goal of vaccinating at least 70% of the world's population by July 2022, Gates dismissively remarked, "it's too late for that."[81] In an article appearing in *The Lancet*, which analyzed the effectiveness of COVID-19 vaccines in saving millions of lives and was funded by the Bill & Melinda Gates Foundation, stressed that "inadequate access to vaccines in countries with low income has limited the impact of vaccines, reinforcing the need for equity and global vaccine coverage."[82] The authors, of course, did not dare to criticize those who helped fund their article, but the inconsistency is unmissable. Bill Gates was not alone in his resistance to COVID-19 vaccine patent liberalization. Other leaders of private organizations that have generously funded interventions against SARS-CoV-2, such as Gavi (a global vaccine organization co-founded by Gates), the Wellcome Trust (a British research foundation that collaborated with the Gates Foundation) and the Coalition for Epidemic Preparedness Innovations (an international vaccine research and development group co-created by Gates and Wellcome in 2017), have also opposed the idea.

The apparent contradiction in showing off ostensibly altruistic positions supporting global health while adopting actions that show a total lack of empathy toward the very same people supposed to be helped is difficult to make sense of. Yet, it can be better understood by delving into the realm of philanthropy and the motivations behind some actions of extremely wealthy companies and individuals. An important term often used to describe private organizations in the global health sector is "philanthrocapitalism."[83] Coined in an article in *The Economist* in 2006 and further explored in the book by Matthew Bishop and Michael Green *Philanthrocapitalism: How the Rich Can Save the World and Why We Should Let Them*, the term broadly refers to "the growing role for private sector actors in addressing the major social and environmental challenges facing the planet."[84] Mainly, it is about very wealthy individuals, driven by a sense of responsibility for the common good, who choose to dedicate a portion of their time and wealth to humanitarian actions.

Over the decades, some philanthrocapitalist associations have gained significant power, influencing political decisions made by governments and international organizations. Their influence is rooted in economic and political transformations that have occurred over the last half-century, leading to a paradigm shift in the approach to global health.[85] This transformation involved a departure from a universal approach, as embodied in the "health for all" slogan of the Declaration of Alma Ata in 1978, toward an operational model where market forces play an increasingly significant role. This shift emphasizes individual responsibility for health over a public, collective, social approach and a move from a "horizontal" approach to health interventions, which considers the complexity of health determinants beyond the biomedical model, to "vertical" programs, focusing on specific diseases or single health risk factors, often at the individual level. These programs, however, rather than supporting and integrating national health systems, often align with the interests of donor nations and pose sustainability issues due to their time-limited and externally managed nature. In addition to wielding influence over political decisions that ideally should emerge from democratic consensus and debate, private actors engage in political lobbying against laws advocating for universal healthcare coverage and regulations aimed at reducing carbon emissions.[86] As observed in an article published in Global Public Health by Katerini Storeng, a professor of global health politics at the University of Oslo, Bill Gates declared himself to be "vehemently against health systems." As he once declared "I wouldn't see a dollar or a cent of my money go to strengthening health systems."[87] In their quest to contribute to the world's pandemic strategy, the leaders of the four most influential global health philanthropic organizations have had unprecedented access to the highest levels of governments, spending at least 8.3 million dollars to lobby lawmakers and officials in the United States and Europe. As Lawrence Gostin, a professor of global health at Georgetown University, explains, "Putting it very crudely, money buys influence. And this is the worst kind of influence. Not only because it's money … but also because it's preferential access, behind closed doors." According to an investigation by Politico, Bill Gates and his partners used their power to control the global response to COVID-19, interfering with key policy decisions that were beyond their purview.[88] For example, philanthropic organizations appear to have played a central role in shaping the global COVAX response, particularly in discrediting alternative approaches to vaccine distribution. The COVAX strategy was ostensibly designed to combat COVID-19 without jeopardizing corporate and financial wealth accumulation. In fact, it actually reinforced existing mechanisms for profit making among pharmaceutical companies (failing to challenge the global trade architecture that supports them) while simultaneously opening up new opportunities (in the form of vaccine bonds) for profit.

The involvement of private actors in shaping global health policies raises critical questions about transparency, accountability and the impact of money on decision-making processes that should ideally prioritize the public good. Philanthrocapitalism does not seem to be just a benevolent gesture by ultra-rich individuals, but an avenue for the growing influence of business and private finance in global health.[89] This encroachment is a consequence of opportunism and financialization in international development, both within and beyond the realm of global health. Philanthropy, in this context, serves the crucial function of "de-risking," or, as explained by Jessica Sklair and Paul Gilbert in an article on the subject, "providing guarantees for interventions that might otherwise put private capital at risk."[90] "Philanthropic" causes must also be scrutinized in the context of the tax benefits they provide to their contributors. The tax breaks accompanying philanthropy often promote charity while downplaying the importance of economic justice policies. It's noteworthy that philanthropy is frequently accompanied by tax avoidance by large companies, impacting public money that could otherwise fund robust health systems and a more equitable global response to the pandemic. A report from the Fair Tax Foundation sheds light on the tax practices of the "Silicon Six" (Facebook, Apple, Amazon, Netflix, Google and Microsoft), revealing that from 2011 to 2020 they paid $149.4 billion less than their tax rate.[91] For instance, Microsoft Global Finance invested over $100 billion in total and paid no taxes in 2020. These figures may dispel the illusions of those who believe in the charity and generosity of philanthropists and ultra-wealthy individuals engaged in charitable activities. A closer look reveals unedifying aspects and underscores the realization that the super-rich will not save the world precisely because they cannot become a solution to the problems that they themselves have helped to create.

References

1. Chimera M. Brusegana, barista muore suicida: aveva perso il lavoro a causa del Coronavirus. Dissapore. Published online Dec 16, 2020. https://www.dissapore.com/notizie/brusegana-barista-muore-suicida-aveva-perso-il-lavoro-a-causa-del-coronavirus/ (accessed Jan 23, 2024).
2. Napoli Fanpage, Imprenditore si suicida nella sua fabbrica nel Casertano: l'azienda in crisi per il Covid. Napoli Fanpage. Published online Dec 30, 2020. https://www.fanpage.it/napoli/imprenditore-si-suicida-nella-sua-fabbrica-nel-casertano-lazienda-in-crisi-per-il-covid/ (accessed Jan 23, 2024).
3. Ricci R. 'Aveva paura di non farcela a pagare le tasse' Noto imprenditore si uccide. ContoCorrenteOnline. Published online Dec 15, 2020. https://www.contocorrenteonline.it/2020/12/15/paolo-piccardo-morto-suicida-imprenditore/ (accessed Jan 23, 2024).
4. World Bank, Global economic prospects. World Bank, Jan 2023 Washington, DC: World Bank. https://www.worldbank.org/en/publication/global-economic-prospects (accessed Jan 23, 2024).
5. International Labour Office (ILO), COVID-19 and the worlds of work. 7th edition. ILO Monitor. Published online Jan 25, 2021. http://www.ilo.org/global/topics/coronavirus/impacts-and-responses/WCMS_767028/lang–en/index.htm (accessed Jan 23, 2024).
6. PIL Italia, nel 2020 calo dell'8,8% (leggermente meglio delle stime). Redazione Economia Corriere della Sera. Economia. Published online Feb 2, 2021. https://www.corriere.it/economia/finanza/21_febbraio_02/pil-italia-2020-calo-dell-88percento-leggermente-meglio-stime-b3254410-6535-11eb-a6ae-1ce6c0f0a691.shtml (accessed Jan 23, 2024).
7. Istat, perso un milione di posti di lavoro nell'anno della pandemia. L'emorragia si stabilizza a febbraio. *la Repubblica*. Published online Apr 6, 2021. https://www.repubblica.it/economia/2021/04/06/news/istat_disoccupazione_febbraio-295230230/ (accessed Jan 23, 2024).
8. Covid Italia, Confcommercio: nel 2020 chiuse 390mila imprese. Ecco i settori più colpiti. *Il Messaggero*. Published online Dec 28, 2020. https://www.ilmessaggero.it/economia/news/confcommercio_negozi_covid_crisi_quante_imprese_chiuse_2020_dati_settori_ultime_notizie-5668998.html (accessed Jan 23, 2024).
9. Pelzer B, Schaffrath S, Vernaleken I. Coping with unemployment: the impact of unemployment on mental health, personality, and social interaction skills. *Work* 2014; **48**: 289–95.
10. De Vogli R, De Falco R, Mattei G. Excess suicides due to the global economic crisis in Italy: an update. *Epidemiologia e prevenzione* 2019; **43**: 111.
11. Tucker, J. A. Lockdown Suicide Data Reveal Predictable Tragedy. American Institute for Economic Research (AIER). Published online on May 22, 2020 (accessed on June 30, 2024) https://www.aier.org/article/lockdown-suicide-data-reveal-predictable-tragedy/
12. Pirkis J, John A, Shin S, *et al*. Suicide trends in the early months of the COVID-19 pandemic: an interrupted time-series analysis of preliminary data from 21 countries. *Lancet Psychiatry* 2021; **8**: 579–88.

13. Woolf SH, Chapman DA, Lee JH. COVID-19 as the leading cause of death in the United States. *JAMA* 2021; **325**: 123–4.
14. Fletcher R. Many assumed suicides would spike in 2020. So far, the data tells a different story. CBC News. Published online Feb 8, 2021. https://www.cbc.ca/news/canada/calgary/suicides-alberta-bc-saskatchewan-canada-2020-no-increase-1.5902908 (accessed Jan 23, 2024).
15. Rück C, Mataix-Cols D, Malki K, *et al*. Will the COVID-19 pandemic lead to a tsunami of suicides? A Swedish nationwide analysis of historical and 2020 data. MedRxiv. 2020; https://doi.org/10.1101/2020.12.10.20244699.
16. Calderon-Anyosa RJC, Kaufman JS. Impact of COVID-19 lockdown policy on homicide, suicide, and motor vehicle deaths in Peru. *Preventive Medicine* 2021; **143**: 106331.
17. Appleby L. What has been the effect of Covid-19 on suicide rates? *BMJ* 2021; **372**: n834.
18. Leske S, Kõlves K, Crompton D, Arensman E, de Leo D. Real-time suicide mortality data from police reports in Queensland, Australia, during the COVID-19 pandemic: an interrupted time-series analysis. *Lancet Psychiatry* 2021; **8**: 58–63.
19. Knudsen AKS, Stene-Larsen K, Gustavson K, *et al*. Prevalence of mental disorders, suicidal ideation and suicides in the general population before and during the COVID-19 pandemic in Norway: a population-based repeated cross-sectional analysis. *The Lancet Regional Health. Europe* 2021; **4**: 100071.
20. Berger Z, Altiery DE Jesus V, Assoumou SA, Greenhalgh T. Long COVID and health inequities: the role of primary care. *Milbank Q* 2021; **99**: 519–41. https://pubmed.ncbi.nlm.nih.gov/33783907/.
21. Istat: "Nella prima ondata Covid seconda causa di morte dopo i tumori". Aogoi. Published online Apr 21, 2021. https://www.aogoi.it/notiziario/archivio-news/covid-causa-morte/ (accessed Jan 23, 2024).
22. Pathirathna ML, Nandasena HMRKG, Atapattu AMMP, Weerasekara I. Impact of the COVID-19 pandemic on suicidal attempts and death rates: a systematic review. *BMC Psychiatry* 2022; **22**: 1–15.
23. Pirkis J, Gunnell D, Shin S, *et al*. Suicide numbers during the first 9–15 months of the COVID-19 pandemic compared with pre-existing trends: an interrupted time series analysis in 33 countries. *eClinicalMedicine* 2022; **51**. https://doi.org/10.1016/j.eclinm.2022.101573.
24. Hill RM, Rufino K, Kurian S, Saxena J, Saxena K, Williams L. Suicide ideation and attempts in a pediatric emergency department before and during COVID-19. *Pediatrics* 2021; **147**: e2020029280.
25. Wingfield-Hayes R. Covid and suicide: Japan's rise a warning to the world? BBC News. Published online Feb 18, 2021. https://www.bbc.com/news/world-asia-55837160 (accessed Jan 23, 2024).
26. Tanaka T, Okamoto S. Increase in suicide following an initial decline during the COVID-19 pandemic in Japan. *Nature Human Behaviour* 2021; **5**: 229–38.
27. Germain S, Yong A. COVID-19 highlighting inequalities in access to healthcare in England: a case study of ethnic minority and migrant women. *Feminist Legal Studies* 2020; **28**: 301–10.
28. Michela B, Emanuele K, Paola B, *et al*. Suicide spectrum among young people during the COVID-19 pandemic: a systematic review and meta-analysis. *eClinicalMedicine* 2022; **54**: 101705.
29. Yan Y, Hou J, Li Q, Yu NX. Suicide before and during the COVID-19 pandemic: a systematic review with meta-analysis. *International Journal of Environmental Research and Public Health* 2023; **20**: 3346.
30. Psychologist says 'come together effect' may have helped reduce suicides in Sask. in 2020 I CBC News. Published online Jan 8, 2021. https://www.cbc.ca/news/canada/saskatoon/suicide-come-together-effect-mccormick-saskatchewan-1.5866598 (accessed Jan 23, 2024).

31. Zeng G, Wang L, Zhang Z. Prejudice and xenophobia in COVID-19 research manuscripts. *Nature Human Behaviour* 2020; **4**: 879.

32. Chu DK, Akl EA, Duda S, *et al*. Physical distancing, face masks, and eye protection to prevent person-to-person transmission of SARS-CoV-2 and COVID-19: a systematic review and meta-analysis. *The Lancet* 2020; **395**: 1973–87.

33. COVID-19: from a PHEIC to a public mental health crisis? *The Lancet Public Health* 2020; **5**: e414.

34. Pierce M, McManus S, Jessop C, *et al*. Says who? The significance of sampling in mental health surveys during COVID-19. *The Lancet Psychiatry* 2020; **7**: 567.

35. Daly M, Sutin AR, Robinson E. Longitudinal changes in mental health and the COVID-19 pandemic: evidence from the UK Household Longitudinal Study. *Psychological medicine* 2022; **52**: 2549–58.

36. Pierce M, Hope H, Ford T, *et al*. Mental health before and during the COVID-19 pandemic: a longitudinal probability sample survey of the UK population. *Lancet Psychiatry* 2020; **7**: 883–92.

37. Ettman CK, Abdalla SM, Cohen GH, Sampson L, Vivier PM, Galea S. Prevalence of depression symptoms in US adults before and during the COVID-19 pandemic. *JAMA Network Open* 2020; **3**: e2019686.

38. Schuppe J., 'I gave this to my dad': COVID-19 survivors grapple with guilt of infecting family. NBC News. Published online May 16, 2020. https://www.nbcnews.com/news/us-news/i-gave-my-dad-covid-19-survivors-grapple-guilt-infecting-n1207921 (accessed Jan 23, 2024).

39. OECD. Health at a glance 2021: OECD indicators. Paris: Organisation for Economic Co-operation and Development, 2021. https://www.oecd-ilibrary.org/social-issues-migration-health/health-at-a-glance-2021_ae3016b9-en (accessed Jan 23, 2024).

40. van der Velden PG, Contino C, Das M, van Loon P, Bosmans MWG. Anxiety and depression symptoms, and lack of emotional support among the general population before and during the COVID-19 pandemic. a prospective national study on prevalence and risk factors. *Journal of Affective Disorders* 2020; **277**: 540–8.

41. Andersen LH, Fallesen P, Bruckner TA. Risk of stress/depression and functional impairment in Denmark immediately following a COVID-19 shutdown. *BMC Public Health* 2021; **21**: 984.

42. Taquet M, Dercon Q, Luciano S, *et al*. Incidence, co-occurrence, and evolution of long-COVID features: a 6-month retrospective cohort study of 273,618 survivors of COVID-19. *PLoS Med* 2021; **18**: e1003773.

43. Kim Y, Bae S, Chang H-H, Kim S-W. Long COVID prevalence and impact on quality of life 2 years after acute COVID-19. *Scientific Reports* 2023; **13**: 11207.

44. Unwin HJT, Hillis S, Cluver L, *et al*. Global, regional, and national minimum estimates of children affected by COVID-19-associated orphanhood and caregiver death, by age and family circumstance up to Oct 31, 2021: an updated modelling study. *The Lancet Child & Adolescent Health* 2022; **6**: 249–59.

45. Hillis SD, Blenkinsop A, Villaveces A, *et al*. COVID-19–associated orphanhood and caregiver death in the United States. *Pediatrics* 2021; **148**: e2021053760.

46. Hodgson S, Watts I, Fraser S, Roderick P, Dambha-Miller H. Loneliness, social isolation, cardiovascular disease and mortality: a synthesis of the literature and conceptual framework. *Journal of the Royal Society of Medicine* 2020; **113**: 185–92.

47. Brooks SK, Webster RK, Smith LE, *et al*. The psychological impact of quarantine and how to reduce it: rapid review of the evidence. *The Lancet* 2020; **395**: 912–20.

48. Anderson G, Frank JW, Naylor CD, Wodchis W, Feng P. Using socioeconomics to counter health disparities arising from the Covid-19 pandemic. *BMJ* 2020; **369**: m2149.
49. Long E, Patterson S, Maxwell K, *et al.* COVID-19 pandemic and its impact on social relationships and health. *Journal of Epidemiology and Community Health* 2022; **76**: 128–32.
50. Usher K, Bhullar N, Durkin J, Gyamfi N, Jackson D. Family violence and COVID-19: increased vulnerability and reduced options for support. *International Journal of Mental Health Nursing* 2020; **29**: 549–52.
51. Wang F, Gao Y, Han Z, *et al.* A systematic review and meta-analysis of 90 cohort studies of social isolation, loneliness and mortality. *Nature Human Behaviour* 2023; **7**: 1307–19.
52. Chulov M, correspondent MCME. Iran's deputy health minister: I have coronavirus. *The Guardian*. Published online Feb 25, 2020. https://www.theguardian.com/world/2020/feb/25/irans-deputy-health-minister-i-have-coronavirus (accessed Jan 23, 2024).
53. Whitcomb CG. Review of Slavoj Žižek (2020). Pandemic!: COVID-19 shakes the world. *Postdigital Science and Education* 2020; **2**: 1020–4.
54. Bentley GR. Don't blame the BAME: ethnic and structural inequalities in susceptibilities to COVID-19. *American Journal of Human Biology* 2020; **32**: e23478.
55. Hatef E, Chang H-Y, Kitchen C, Weiner J, Kharrazi H. Assessing the impact of neighborhood socioeconomic characteristics on COVID-19 prevalence across seven states in the United States. *Frontiers in Public Health* 2020; **8**. https://doi.org/10.3389/fpubh.2020.571808.
56. Bach-Mortensen AM, Degli Esposti M. Is area deprivation associated with greater impacts of COVID-19 in care homes across England? A preliminary analysis of COVID-19 outbreaks and deaths. *Journal of Epidemiology and Community Health* 2021; **75**: 624–7.
57. Mackey K, Ayers CK, Kondo KK, *et al.* Racial and ethnic disparities in COVID-19-related infections, hospitalizations, and deaths: a systematic review. *Annals of Internal Medicine* 2021; **174**: 362–73.
58. Woolf SH, Masters RK, Aron LY. Effect of the Covid-19 pandemic in 2020 on life expectancy across populations in the USA and other high income countries: simulations of provisional mortality data. *BMJ* 2021; **373**: n1343.
59. Gessa GD, Maddock J, Green MJ, *et al.* Pre-pandemic mental health and disruptions to healthcare, economic and housing outcomes during the COVID-19 pandemic: evidence from 12 UK longitudinal studies. *The British Journal of Psychiatry: The Journal of Mental Science* 2022; **220**: 21–30.
60. Rosengren A, Smyth A, Rangarajan S, *et al.* Socioeconomic status and risk of cardiovascular disease in 20 low-income, middle-income, and high-income countries: the Prospective Urban Rural Epidemiologic (PURE) study. *The Lancet. Global Health* 2019; **7**: e748–60.
61. Naylor-Wardle J, Rowland B, Kunadian V. Socioeconomic status and cardiovascular health in the COVID-19 pandemic. *Heart* 2021; **107**: 358–65.
62. Stringhini S, Carmeli C, Jokela M, *et al.* Socioeconomic status and the 25 × 25 risk factors as determinants of premature mortality: a multicohort study and meta-analysis of 1·7 million men and women. *Lancet* 2017; **389**: 1229–37.
63. Topriceanu C-C, Wong A, Moon JC, *et al.* Evaluating access to health and care services during lockdown by the COVID-19 survey in five UK national longitudinal studies. *BMJ Open* 2021; **11**: e045813.
64. Burr JA, Mutchler JE, Gerst K. Patterns of residential crowding among Hispanics in later life: immigration, assimilation, and housing market factors. *The Journals*

of Gerontology. Series B, Psychological Sciences and Social Sciences 2010; **65B**: 772–82.

65. Bettoni S. Moratti: 'Ripartire vaccini anche per Pil delle Regioni'. Speranza: 'La salute non è un privilegio'. *Corriere della Sera.* Published online Jan 18, 2021. https://milano.corriere.it/notizie/cronaca/21_gennaio_18/vaccini-anti-covid-moratti-ripartizione-anche-base-pil-regioni-7f6e1a40-59b2-11eb-89c7-29891efac2a7.shtml (accessed Jan 23, 2024).

66. Phillips N. The coronavirus is here to stay — here's what that means. *Nature* 2021; **590**: 382–4.

67. Duke Global Health Innovation Center. Africa: New study shows rich country shopping spree for Covid-19 vaccines could mean fewer vaccinations for billions in low-income countries. Published online Nov 2, 2020. https://allafrica.com/stories/202011020103.html (accessed Jan 23, 2024).

68. Costello A. The richest countries are vaccine hoarders. Try them in international court. *The Guardian.* Published online Dec 14, 2021. https://www.theguardian.com/commentisfree/2021/dec/14/richest-countries-vaccine-hoarders-international-court-millions-have-died (accessed Jan 23, 2024).

69. Ding D, Zhang R. China's COVID-19 control strategy and its impact on the global pandemic. *Front Public Health* 2022; **10**: 857003.

70. Ledford H. COVID vaccine hoarding might have cost more than a million lives. *Nature* 2022. https://doi.org/10.1038/d41586-022-03529-3.

71. Tan SY, Ponstein N. Jonas Salk (1914–1995): a vaccine against polio. *Singapore Med J* 2019; **60**: 9–10.

72. A patent waiver on COVID vaccines is right and fair. *Nature* 2021; **593**: 478–478.

73. Gerald R. Ford School of Public Policy. Policy memo: Parthasarathy on 'ensuring global access to COVID-19 vaccines.' Published online on Jan 21, 2021. https://fordschool.umich.edu/news/2021/policy-memo-parthasarathy-ensuring-global-access-covid-19-vaccines (accessed Jan 23, 2024).

74. The Independent Panelon Pandemic Preparedness and Response. COVID-19: make it the last pandemic. Published online May 2, 2021. https://recommendations.theindependentpanel.org/main-report/main-report/ (accessed Jan 23, 2024).

75. Amnesty International. A double dose of inequality: pharma companies and the Covid-19 vaccines crisis. Published online on Sep 22, 2021. https://www.amnesty.org/en/documents/pol40/4621/2021/en/ (accessed Jan 24, 2024).

76. Davies M. Covid-19: WHO efforts to bring vaccine manufacturing to Africa are undermined by the drug industry, documents show. *BMJ* 2022; **376**: o304. https://www.bmj.com/content/376/bmj.o304.

77. Gold ER. What the COVID-19 pandemic revealed about intellectual property. *Nat Biotechnol* 2022; **40**: 1428–30.

78. Covid vaccines: will drug companies make bumper profits? BBC News. Published online Dec 13, 2020. https://www.bbc.com/news/business-55170756 (accessed Jan 24, 2024).

79. Mazzucato M. State of innovation: busting the private-sector myth. *NewScientist.* Published online Aug 21, 2013. https://www.newscientist.com/article/mg21929310-200-state-of-innovation-busting-the-private-sector-myth/ (accessed Jan 24, 2024)

80. Galkina Cleary E, Beierlein JM, Khanuja NS, *et al.* Contribution of NIH funding to new drug approvals 2010–2016. *Proceedings of the National Academy of Sciences of the United States of America* 2018; **115**: 2329–34. https://doi.org/10.1073/pnas.1715368115.

81. Bill Gates: too late to vaccinate 70% of the world's population. YouTube. CNBC International. Published online Feb 18, 2022. https://www.youtube.com/watch?v=ugCrTuGXJP0 (accessed Jan 24, 2024).
82. Watson OJ, Barnsley G, Toor J, Hogan AB, Winskill P, Ghani AC. Global impact of the first year of COVID-19 vaccination: a mathematical modelling study. *The Lancet Infectious Diseases* 2022; **22**: 1293–302.
83. Haydon S, Jung T, Russell S. 'You've been framed': a critical review of academic discourse on philanthrocapitalism. *International Journal of Management Reviews* 2021; **23**: 353–75.
84. Bishop M, Green MF. Philanthrocapitalism: how the rich can save the world and why we should let them. London: A & C Black, 2008.
85. Wilson J. Philanthrocapitalism and global health. In: Benatar, S and Brock, G, (eds.) Global Health Ethical Challenges (pp. 416–28). Cambridge, UK: Cambridge University Press, 2021.
86. Butler CD. Philanthrocapitalism: promoting global health but failing planetary health. *Challenges* 2019; **10**: 24.
87. Storeng KT. The GAVI alliance and the 'Gates approach' to health system strengthening. *Global Public Health* 2014; **9**: 865–79.
88. How Bill Gates and his partners took over the global Covid pandemic response. *Politico*, Banco E, Furlong A & Lennart P. Published online Sep 14, 2022. https://www.politico.com/news/2022/09/14/global-covid-pandemic-response-bill-gates-partners-00053969 (accessed Jan 24, 2024).
89. Soskis B. Impact investing and critiques of philanthrocapitalism. Urban Institute. Published online June 30, 2021. https://www.urban.org/research/publication/impact-investing-and-critiques-philanthrocapitalism (accessed Jan 24, 2024).
90. Sklair J, Gilbert P. Giving as "de-risking": philanthropy, impact investment and the pandemic response. *Public Anthropologist* 2022; **4**: 51–77.
91. Microsoft – gaming global taxes, winning government contracts. Public Services International. Published online Oct 13, 2022. https://publicservices.international/resources/publications/microsoft—gaming-global-taxes-winning-government-contracts?id=13396&lang=en (accessed Jan 24, 2024).

PART II

Vital actions

6

PREVENTION

"In the last few days, I have witnessed people being escorted into the corridors to literally die because we are crammed everywhere. There is no space to be able to guarantee them a dignified death." This eyewitness account, shared in December 2020, echoed the sentiments of numerous healthcare workers in Veneto, as hospitals grappled with an overwhelming surge in COVID-19 cases.[1] During those weeks, desperate pleas for assistance echoed through various medical facilities, some struggling to find space for the growing number of patients.[2] Ivano Dal Dosso, the Secretary of the Association of Medical Directors in Verona, succinctly captured the dire situation, questioning the sustainability of their efforts: "we are in a situation on the verge of breaking … how long can we continue to hold on?"[3] In those dramatic days, the shock was palpable. Yet, the overwhelming situation stood in stark contrast to Veneto's earlier reputation as a model for effective pandemic management during the initial phases of the crisis. Despite being the unfortunate site of Italy's first COVID-19 fatality, during the first wave of the crisis the region had earned praise for its success in containing infections. The second wave, however, overwhelmed Veneto with the most rapid increase of COVID-19 deaths in Italy. What happened between the commendable early efforts and the overwhelming challenges faced by Veneto in December 2020? What went wrong in the intervening months, leading to a situation where hospitals were stretched to their limits and healthcare professionals were grappling with the seemingly insurmountable task of providing dignified care amid chaos?

DOI: 10.4324/9781003511977-9

Veneto: they called it "Northeast Korea"

Zero infections: the enviable achievement by Veneto's health policies on May 21, 2020, set the region apart from others in Italy.[4] It was an extraordinary result. Governor of Veneto Luca Zaia attributed this success to "my invention", an advanced regional health plan and the foresight of his health managers.[5,6] But was this really the case? Veneto, like other Italian regions, lacked a specific COVID-19 pandemic plan, relying instead on a dated influenza strategy from 2007.[7,8] What really made the difference in the first wave, however, was the adoption of local prevention strategies based on the use of swabs at the population level and prompt case isolation. During the early phase of the pandemic, Veneto's containment interventions were guided by the advice of Andrea Crisanti, at the time a professor at the University of Padova. As the expert put it, "if you want to eliminate a cluster you have to lock down the village [or neighborhood], test everybody, and isolate the positives." Crisanti's foresight was evident in January 2020 when, ahead of the curve, he secured enough reagents, funded by Imperial College London (his previous institution), to produce half a million swabs. This proactive approach gave Veneto a surplus of testing materials, allowing prompt testing across the region. As Crisanti himself underlined, without the reagents from Imperial College London, it would have taken a month and a half to develop the swabs. Crisanti received the Lion of Veneto award for his service to the region, as well as the seal of the city of Padova, and was celebrated by a special concert in Vo' Euganeo, the site where he conducted the first successful prevention activities.[9]

While the "Veneto model" in the first wave was unique in Italy, it wasn't entirely innovative. Instead, it mirrored successful approaches employed by countries such as South Korea, Vietnam and Taiwan. Yet, the success of the Veneto model was short-lived. At the end of the first wave, the "honeymoon" between Crisanti and the governor ended abruptly, and the expert was stripped of his leadership in managing the pandemic. Worse, he was denounced by the Veneto region lawyers for the "crime" of having criticized some decisions of the regional strategy. The legal case, however, turned out to be an embarrassing flop, as well as a useless expense borne by the citizens.[10] Like a boomerang, it "transformed" itself into legal proceedings against some officials of the Veneto region for "fraud and misdirection."[11]

Crisanti's departure and the sudden change of strategy were behind the debacle experienced in Veneto during the second wave. The region was totally overwhelmed by infections and thousands of excess deaths. In those dramatic weeks, Veneto, with the worst indicators of the pandemic in Italy, was transformed from a model to emulate to a disaster to avoid. Many have wondered how all this could have happened. Some have hypothesized that the crisis was caused by changes in the behavior of Veneto citizens, who, in general, adopt healthier lifestyles than the national average.[12,13] The hypothesis, however, is not very credible. During the first wave, Governor Zaia thanked the inhabitants of his region for their "extraordinary" civic responsibility,[14] but there is no evidence that the propensity of Veneto citizens to protect their own health worsened drastically during the second. Something else had gone wrong.

In November, the Ministry of Health in Italy introduced a classification system utilizing 21 indicators to determine the regional risk level for COVID-19. Each region was assigned a color – yellow, orange or red – indicating the severity of the situation. The regions designated as red zones, considered most vulnerable to overwhelming hospitalizations, faced stringent closures. A pivotal factor in determining the color designation was the probability of intensive care beds reaching critical occupancy thresholds. The number of intensive care beds, however, does not necessarily relate to success in reducing COVID-19 mortality, which is largely preventable by community health interventions. Veneto, with a substantial number of beds, managed to evade the red zone classification for weeks, despite a rapid surge in infections and hospitalizations. This traffic light system inadvertently fostered a false sense of security and created an unintended incentive to abstain from adopting more stringent prevention measures to curb contagion. The reliance on indicators that did not accurately reflect the imminent threats to public health resulted in a delayed and inadequate response to the escalating crisis.

The second major reason for Veneto's fiasco in the second wave concerns the misuse of rapid swab tests. An effective virus management strategy requires two types of tests: (a) molecular swabs to make accurate diagnoses in vulnerable populations at high risk (e.g., long-term residents in nursing homes) and (b) rapid antigenic swabs for case identification activities in the general population with low risk. These rapid tests are indeed effective tools, particularly when repeated to identify cases in the general population.[15,16] However, during the second wave in Veneto, a region that conducted a high volume of swabs, these tests were employed for both accurate diagnoses in high-risk groups and general case identification.[17] The departure of Crisanti marked a shift in approach. The new coordinators of the COVID-19 prevention strategy viewed rapid tests as being on par with molecular swabs in terms of reliability,[18] despite scientific evidence suggesting otherwise.[19] Healthcare personnel in the Veneto region, medical associations and sector experts raised concerns about their poor reliability.[20,21] Their inappropriate use had the potential to compromise prevention efforts, as individuals receiving false-negative results might mistakenly believe they were not infected, inadvertently contributing to the spread of the virus. According to Crisanti, rapid tests as they were used in Veneto during the second wave, rather than acting as a barrier to the virus, created a "Gruyere effect."[22] As an old saying explains, "if you leave a gun in the hands of someone who doesn't know how to use it, they will probably shoot themselves in the foot."

Test, trace and isolate on time: how to save lives at scale

If the inappropriate use of swabs was an obstacle to an effective prevention strategy against the virus in Veneto, ignoring their importance was even worse. Analysis on the propensity for the strategic and timely use of swabs shows that this indicator is inversely correlated with COVID-19 mortality and infections.[23,24] Countries that adopted the most effective strategies for managing the pandemic embraced a robust public health policy, encapsulated in the so-called test, trace and isolate (TTI) approach, which derives from the "test, trace and treat (3T) model" coined by the WHO for managing various infectious diseases, including malaria.[25]

Testing, tracing and isolating are closely interconnected activities, and to confront COVID-19 without these prevention tools is akin to fighting an invisible enemy. The identification and management of outbreaks hinge on the deployment of swabs to confirm potential infections, analyze outbreaks and facilitate prompt intervention. Simultaneously, a robust contact tracing system becomes imperative to work in pair with testing.[26] It is essential to identify and manage contacts of confirmed cases in order to quickly isolate any infections or test them, so as to interrupt the chain of transmission. In practice, this involves casting a wide net around each case in order to capture second-order contacts, called "contacts of contacts," to be in turn traced and subjected to isolation or quarantine if infected. As already explained, the effectiveness of preventive activities strongly depends on their timely adoption.[27] More recently, surveillance systems began to benefit from increasingly sophisticated information derived from temporal analyses of wastewaters. These tools offer valuable data on the incidence and prevalence of the virus, and they proved to be instrumental in monitoring pandemic trends and evaluating the effectiveness of interventions, providing an additional weapon in the fight against SARS-CoV-2.[28]

Some of the countries that have adopted prevention interventions based on testing, tracing and isolating in a timely manner have been called "zero-COVID nations," and they include China, Vietnam, South Korea, Taiwan, Singapore and New Zealand. These nations initially aimed to control the transmission of the COVID-19 infection to a minimal level, ideally reducing it to a few cases or even eliminating it entirely.[29-31] The overarching goal of these strategies, encapsulated in the slogan "every infection is one infection too many,"[32] reflected a very ambitious goal featured in a *Lancet* article, where an international group of scientists, comprising epidemiologists, virologists, political scientists and economists, advocated for the adoption of the zero-COVID strategy in the Eurozone too. Their big idea was to transform

Europe into a virus-free territory, establishing green zones where the virus could be kept under control.[33] The propitious moment for such a strategy was identified as the summer of 2020 when many European nations had significantly reduced infections through rigorous and prolonged lockdowns. On top of testing, tracing and isolation of infected individuals, the zero-COVID model advocated for financial and practical support for those in isolation or quarantine and preventive interventions to secure schools, workplaces and public spaces. In the United Kingdom, the Independent SAGE supported a similar approach known as the Maximum Sustainable Suppression Strategy. This approach involved testing, tracing and isolating infected individuals, providing support for those in isolation, implementing preventive measures such as ventilation in various settings and imposing strict control measures on international travel.[34]

Despite repeated calls to act vigorously against the virus, in the European Union, the United Kingdom and the United States there was limited interest and response. An analysis published in the journal *Science* highlighted that, with a few exceptions, most Western countries overlooked prevention and failed to capitalize on the window of opportunity presented during the summer of 2020.[35] The goal of completely eliminating the virus, proposed by some scientists, has sparked considerable debate, with critics presenting plausible arguments against the feasibility of such an ambitious objective. Indeed, a strategy aimed at eliminating of the virus posed significant challenges, requiring extraordinary efforts on the political, organizational, logistical and epidemiological fronts. It necessitated a focus on public health, coupled with a broad popular consensus, trust and active public participation. Acknowledging these challenges, it became evident that the goal of achieving complete virus elimination was indeed prohibitive. However, the experiences of countries that endeavored to eliminate the virus before the emergence of the Omicron variants reveal that while complete elimination might not have been achieved, the approach proved notably successful in limiting mortality, mitigating health inequalities, supporting mass vaccination strategies and diminishing the risk of new and potentially dangerous variants of concern.[36]

Lessons from the East

Taiwan

Taiwan, despite its close proximity to China and the initial risk of being overwhelmed by the virus, stands out as one of the world's most successful nations in pandemic control. The island had a valuable advantage – the experience gained from previous pandemics, including SARS and MERS. Additionally, similar to New Zealand and Australia, Taiwan has the geographical characteristic of not having highly porous land borders, which facilitated the implementation of travel restrictions and robust border control measures. However, the success of Taiwan's response goes well beyond these factors. An article that delved into Taiwan's COVID-19 experience emphasized several key elements that contributed to its effective management. The Asian country's approach involved vigorous prevention interventions, characterized by the rapid deployment of swabs and early tracing of infected individuals and the utilization of advanced digital technologies for infection identification.[37] Crucially, Taiwan also implemented effective methods of isolation and quarantine, bolstered by a robust border control system. The country demonstrated agility in responding to emerging threats through rapid and targeted lockdowns, and the widespread adoption of masks further played a role in fortifying the nation's defenses against the virus.[38,39]

The effectiveness of Taiwan's response can be attributed to a well-coordinated and multifaceted approach, driven by key public health organizational and technological assets. The direction and coordination of screening measures and epidemiological surveillance at the borders, coupled with proactive prevention programs utilizing early swab testing and robust methods of isolation and quarantine, have been pivotal. Taiwan's epidemiological intelligence benefited from collaborative relationships with internationally renowned institutions, such as the Johns Hopkins University School of Public Health. A key aspect of the strategy was the extraordinary timeliness. Thanks to efficient epidemiological information systems capable of guaranteeing the monitoring of outbreaks in real time, the coordination between actions relating to swabs, tracing and analysis of epidemiological data was fundamental in allowing officials not only to understand the phenomenon but also to make predictions on the progress of the pandemic. A national alert system was also used, capable of identifying and visualizing infections through sentinel surveillance, as well as immediate screening of the health of air passengers and digital technologies for contact tracing and monitoring of cases of both isolation and quarantine. Existing legislation in the form of the Taiwanese Infectious Disease Control Act 2007 gave officials access to data and information that facilitated pandemic control operations. This legal framework allowed people's travel history to be linked to their national health insurance card to identify potential cases in real time.[37] The national contact tracing platform, named TRACE, and the integration of data from multiple sources have enabled healthcare facilities to access patients' databases for testing and monitoring purposes.[40] In late January 2020, these types of screenings involved all passengers entering Taiwan from high-risk countries; these measures were extended in early February 2020 to all passengers regardless of their location of origin. Finally, in mid-March 2020, non-Taiwanese citizens or people with non-resident status were banned from entering.

The Taiwan Social Distancing App played a key role in the government's proactive measures, employing a digital notification system to anonymously record nearby phones and triangulate the geographic locations of potential cases.[41] Stringent quarantine measures were implemented for travelers from high-risk countries and close contacts of confirmed cases, ensuring a two-week isolation period. Throughout this duration, individuals in quarantine were closely monitored through telephone messages inquiring about health and occasional in-person checks. The effectiveness of electronic monitoring during home quarantine was enhanced by geolocation systems, enabling the identification of possible violations and imposition of fines.[42] As the Omicron variants posed new challenges, Taiwan faced a resurgence of cases, prompting the adjustment of prevention measures, especially in areas like Taipei. Despite the late start of the vaccination campaign and a relatively low emphasis on vaccines, Taiwan's public health-centric approach, based on early testing, tracing and isolation, allowed it to maintain its status as one of the nations with the lowest COVID-19 mortality rates globally.[43] Taiwan will also go down in history as the nation that temporarily achieved zero COVID-19 cases without a lockdown.[44]

South Korea

Much like Taiwan, South Korea has implemented a robust strategy centered around testing, tracing and isolation, leveraging geolocation data from smartphones, credit cards and closed-circuit television (CCTV). The effective coordination and management of data have been integral to the adoption of digital technologies, seamlessly integrating them into COVID-19 containment and mitigation activities. These activities include epidemiological surveillance, mass swab testing, contact tracing and quarantine, with centralized guidance from the government.[45] South Korea shares another key aspect of its strategy with Taiwan – early restrictions on international travel, defying initial WHO advice and implementing stringent measures even in the very first weeks of the crisis. Rigorous screening, including possible quarantine for passengers arriving from Wuhan, showcased the government's proactive stance. Timeliness was a hallmark of South Korea's response, marked by the early adoption of massive swab campaigns to anticipate and address the formation of the first infection clusters. The country also established an extensive network of contact tracers, granting them access to diverse data sources beyond direct interviews with individuals. Innovative testing strategies further characterized South Korea's approach. The deployment of mobile drive-through stations allowed for convenient and contact-free swab testing, conducted directly in the tested subjects' cars. Walk-through stations provided the means for testing in public spaces, minimizing direct contact between operators and potentially infected individuals.[46,47] Moreover, to prevent the spread of the virus within healthcare settings, COVID-19 screening clinics were strategically placed outside hospital entrances.[48]

Similar to Taiwan, South Korea's approach to combating the pandemic was characterized by a high-tech strategy involving the collection and management of data on digital platforms. This technological emphasis played a crucial role in efficient tracing, testing and information dissemination and the swift delivery of test results to individuals. South Korea's technological prowess is underscored by having the fastest internet in the world, boasting a bandwidth speed four times greater than that of the United States. A key legislative measure, enacted in response to the MERS outbreak in 2015, empowered authorities to utilize data from credit cards, cell phones and closed-circuit television to track individuals' movements and identify potential exposures to the virus. The country's commitment to expanding epidemiological intelligence further fortified the response. Rapid training initiatives in numerous public health centers around the nation, recruitment of hundreds of epidemiologists and collaboration with non-governmental organizations to train additional personnel contributed to an efficient and well-prepared workforce. This approach facilitated early diagnoses of cases, maintained a low rate of new infections and prevented both hospital overcrowding and infections among high-risk populations.

The South Korean app, Corona100m, played a crucial role in swiftly collecting relevant data for identifying outbreaks, informing citizens about areas with a high number of infections and providing support to those forced into isolation. This digital tool became an essential component of the country's strategy for managing the pandemic, contributing to the prompt dissemination of information and aiding in containment efforts. However, as the Omicron variants spread, the effectiveness of South Korea's initial strategy began to wane. With the relaxation of measures, the government shifted its focus and resources toward protecting the most vulnerable populations only. While this change created dissatisfaction among some citizens accustomed to rigid measures, the country's adoption of a robust mass vaccination campaign proved instrumental in preventing the healthcare system from being overwhelmed. Despite the challenges posed by the rapid waves of Omicron variants, South Korea, with one of the highest population densities globally, stands among nations with a low rate of COVID-19 deaths per million inhabitants.[49]

Vietnam

Among the most virtuous countries in managing the COVID-19 pandemic, there is also Vietnam, a lower-middle-income country with a dense population of 95.5 million in a limited territory. Praised by experts and international organizations like the IMF, Vietnam's success has been acknowledged as a roadmap not only for developing countries but also for wealthier and technologically advanced nations.[6, 50] Key elements contributing to Vietnam's success include rapid and decisive action in identifying infections through public health strategies, with an effective use of swabs and contact tracing.[50,51] As highlighted in the journal *Nature*, the country's success in managing the virus can be attributed to early preparation, contact tracing, isolation, testing, timely border closures, physical distancing and a commitment to community health adherence.[52] An article in the *American Journal of Public Health* also underscored Vietnam's success factors, emphasizing the importance of testing, tracing, isolating and a public health-oriented healthcare system equipped with emergency operations centers and territorial surveillance systems.[51]

Vietnam's proactive approach included conducting mass swab testing and extensive contact tracing. This strategy was supported by the dedication of "boots on the ground," such as contact tracing teams who contacted secondary contacts. Unlike countries where contact tracing has never managed to cover a large percentage of the population, Vietnam, in the early stages of the pandemic, had a very low percentage of infections from unknown sources. Contact tracing teams interviewed people face-to-face, using additional surveillance data to obtain more information, including movement and location details from smartphones. The timely search for every positive case and all of that person's possible contacts, an activity overlooked in Western countries, makes Vietnam one of the nations that have best withstood the blows inflicted by the pandemic. Of course, the challenge created by the Omicron variants created numerous obstacles to the Vietnamese strategy: the shift from a zero-COVID approach to a "new normal" was insidious and cost human lives. Nevertheless, public health scientists recognize the importance of Vietnam's approach, widely appreciated for its rigor and consistency.[53] Undoubtedly, the country had an advantage: it had learned important lessons from the past SARS and avian flu experiences. These pandemics had shaped the health system in terms of its ability to face new crises, but the Vietnamese government and its people managed to learn lessons from these events. As Ho Chi Minh, national hero and father of the Vietnamese nation, said, "the storm is a good opportunity for the pine and cypress to show their strength and stability."[54]

New Zealand

"Zero COVID has cost New Zealand dearly," argued a professor of medicine from Stanford University, a supporter of the mass infection/herd immunity strategy and first signer of the Great Barrington Declaration. Epidemiology, a subject that made him famous, proved him utterly wrong: when COVID deaths per million people are looked at, New Zealand stands out as another exemplary country in managing the COVID-19 pandemic.[55] Guess what? The elements contributing to its success align precisely with those observed in Taiwan, South Korea and Vietnam. The key to New Zealand's strategy lies in prompt and decisive government action, in stark contrast to the initial denialism of the danger of the virus observed in some European Union, UK, and US responses. Learning from the experiences of other nations, particularly witnessing the severity of the pandemic in Europe, provided valuable insights for New Zealand's pandemic managers. Despite not having faced deadly pandemics like SARS and MERS in the past, New Zealand acted swiftly and efficiently, demonstrating a proactive approach. The government's rapid response was instrumental in curbing the spread of the virus within its borders. New Zealand, much like Taiwan and South Korea, took a bold stance on border control, diverging even from WHO advice. The country implemented restrictive policies on international travel, temporarily closing its borders and mandating a two-week self-isolation period for travelers arriving from other countries. For citizens and residents repatriating who couldn't safely isolate themselves, New Zealand established special quarantine facilities that ensured rigorous testing, check-ups and health monitoring to safeguard public health.

Michael Baker, government advisor and professor of public health at the University of Otago, emphasized a pandemic management strategy that rejected the idea of coexistence with the virus and opted for its elimination, aiming to reduce infections to zero through targeted interventions that quickly interrupted the chain of contagion.[56] The country's commitment to timely interventions, stringent border control measures and isolation and quarantine protocols has positioned it as a global example of effective pandemic management, showcasing the significance of proactive and science-driven policies.[57,58] Former Prime Minister Jacinda Ardern's decisive governance and reliance on expert advisors in public health and epidemiology, such as Director of Health Ashley Bloomfield, have played a pivotal role in New Zealand's successful pandemic response. Ardern's leadership was particularly effective when she made the strategic decision to "go hard and go early" in the face of her country's unpreparedness.[31, 59]

Clear communication through a decisive information campaign was another key aspect of New Zealand's success not only to inform the population but also to foster collective participation in national strategies against a "common enemy" – the virus. Ardern's administration garnered high credit and trust from citizens, though discontent with health policies grew after the arrival of the virtually unstoppable Omicron variants. This may have led to her resignation in January 2023. However, New Zealand relaxed preventive measures only after a successful vaccination campaign.[60] Though criticized in the West, New Zealand's approach avoided a worse health scenario and a high number of COVID-19 deaths. Of course, the goal of the elimination strategy has never been reached. Yet, as Ardern noted, "even if prevention will never achieve zero infections, a virus elimination approach will save lives."[61] Evidence proved her right.

Singapore

Singapore, with the highest population density among nations with at least 1 million inhabitants, stands out as another exemplary case of a virtuous country in managing the COVID-19 pandemic. Following in the footsteps of Taiwan and South Korea, Singapore swiftly imposed restrictions on air travel from China in the early stages of the pandemic and implemented an effective program encompassing testing, contact tracing and quarantine surveillance.[62] The emphasis on public health, the significance of community medicine and the deployment of thousands of community workers played a pivotal role in Singapore's effective response against SARS-CoV-2.[63] The country's strategy was strengthened by communication grounded in scientific evidence and systematic countering of COVID-19 misinformation.[62]

At the core of these successful strategies in Singapore, however, there was a profound sense of civic responsibility, fostering a high level of collaboration between citizens, who prioritized the common good over personal interest. Although Singapore's high social cohesion played a crucial role in its success, it was the effect of systematic, swift and well-planned prevention interventions such as mass swabs and contact tracing that strongly limited infections and deaths.[64] The success of the TraceTogether app, downloaded by about four out of five citizens, might not have lived up to the claim of being "the most effective contact tracing program in the world," as stated by Foreign Minister Vivian Balakrishnan.[65] Yet, the app likely contributed to identifying a substantial number of infections, encouraging preventive behaviors and containing mortality. Singapore also demonstrated a high level of commitment to adopting timely prevention strategies against SARS-CoV-2, including targeted and short lockdowns after a few infections. Despite facing very difficult challenges against Omicron, Singapore can brag about having one of the lowest COVID-19 mortality rates per capita globally.

Japan

Japan too, despite having one of the world's oldest populations and a very high population density, has successfully avoided being overwhelmed by COVID-19. Several factors contributed to Japan's resilience, including a high proportion of healthy individuals compared to other high-income nations. For example, the prevalence of obesity, a significant risk factor for severe SARS-CoV-2 effects, is around 6% in Japan, contrasting with over 36% in the United States. In addition to pre-existing health factors, the contribution of an effective community health system (based on over 8,000 public health nurses in 400 public health centers) played a crucial role in conducting contact tracing activities and identifying transmission clusters early on. Japan also serves as an example of a virtuous country waging a successful vaccination campaign that covered a large proportion of its population.

Yet, Japan's approach to prevention, which has been very effective in avoiding excessive mortality and public discontent, was not rigid and never included the option of a national lockdown. It has largely been informed by an awareness that SARS-CoV-2 is primarily airborne. The government's strategy, as highlighted in *Nature*, emphasized the "3Cs" (sanmitsu) to avoid: closed environments, crowded conditions and close contacts. While other countries prioritized disinfection and hand hygiene, Japan's emphasis on preventing airborne transmission proved to be very effective.[66] The government has also emphasized common risk factors associated with super-spreader events, delivering messages and precautions to the public based on this awareness and made significant efforts to improve ventilation in buildings.[67,68] Furthermore, Japan focused on creating a barrier against airborne virus transmission through the widespread use of masks.

Despite the challenges posed by the Omicron variants and their rapid transmission, Japan's proactive prevention strategies, implemented before widespread vaccine distribution, have been successful in preventing millions of deaths, aligning with the experiences of other virtuous nations (Figure 6.1).

Failures of the West: app flops

The vital role of contact tracing in preventing infections and deaths cannot be underestimated, as underscored by the experiences of nations that widely adopted this intervention.[69,70] While contact tracing is not a panacea, it has proven especially useful at the onset of the pandemic, when vaccines were unavailable. Tracing apps serve to notify contacts almost instantly and aid in outbreak containment by tracing contacts up to 15 days before infection. This strategy known as "backward tracing" requires meticulous monitoring of people's movements, gatherings and flows. To implement this strategy optimally, the development of surveillance systems for identifying outbreaks and electronic monitoring of at-risk individuals, utilizing technologies like smartphone apps, is essential.[71] Early in the pandemic, experts suggested that more than 60% of the population needed to use a contact tracing app to effectively contain the virus.[72] Unfortunately, only a few countries were able to achieve this goal. In the West, the strategy failed completely. Experts attribute the main causes of these app flops to concerns over privacy violations. However, investigations into the issue reveal that the primary determinant of low app usage was governments' inability to establish working alliances with citizens through open and collaborative communication. The United States, for instance, did not have a nationwide app for tracking infections, and most Western countries saw low citizen participation rates, making the

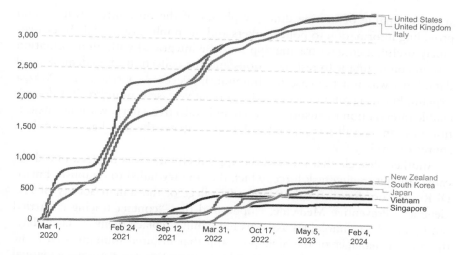

FIGURE 6.1 Lessons from the East, failures of the West: cumulative confirmed COVID-19 deaths per million people in the United States, United Kingdom, Italy, New Zealand, South Korea, Japan, Vietnam and Singapore (March 1, 2020 – February 4, 2024)

Sources: WHO COVID-19 Dashboard – processed by Our World in Data. "Total deaths (per 1M)" [dataset]. WHO COVID-19 Dashboard [original data].

Retrieved Feb 14, 2024 from https://ourworldindata.org/explorers/coronavirus-data-explorer? zoomToSelection=true&time=2020-03-01.latest&facet=none&country=USA~GBR~ITA~ VNM~SGP~JPN~KOR~NZL&pickerSort=asc&pickerMetric=location&hideControls= false&Metric=Confirmed+deaths&Interval=Cumulative&Relative+to+Population=true& Color+by+test+positivity=false

use of contact tracing apps practically ineffective. In Italy, the current Prime Minister, Giorgia Meloni, and the Governor of Veneto, Luca Zaia, openly encouraged citizens to boycott contact tracing activities that were implemented by the previous administration.[73]

In some instances, such as in the United Kingdom, instead of encouraging citizen participation to strengthen contact tracing capacity, the government's scientific advisors even suggested halting the practice of contact tracing when cases surged – a recommendation that left epidemiologists in the dark about new infection details.[74]

An emblematic failure in adopting a contact tracing strategy regards the Italian software Immuni, which was downloaded by less than one in five Italians.[75] The disorganization of the national awareness campaign on the use of this tool, coupled with citizens' distrust of government institutions, proved fatal to its adoption.[76] According to Andrea Crisanti and Michele Mazza in their book *Alla Caccia del Virus*, the Immuni app represents the epitome of improvisation and amateurism in managing the pandemic. Health information systems capable of uniting different phases of the preventive strategy and providing information to policymakers and the public are crucial. To be genuinely useful, a contact tracing app must be integrated with an information system connecting it to testing actions and the collection of epidemiological data. This was not the case for Immuni, however. As Crisanti and Mazza explain, knowing about encountering a positive case is pointless if it doesn't enable intervention to ensure personal and collective safety; without integration into an overall testing and isolation strategy, the app becomes only a source of anxiety for users.[77]

Another obstacle that reduced the app's usefulness was the lack of a dedicated contact tracing task force, which the country failed to establish. Enrico Di Rosa, Coordinator of the National College of the Italian Society of Hygiene and Preventive Medicine, emphasized that "contact tracing is carried out by people; technologies assist us but cannot replace them."[78] Jason Bay, the project manager of the Singapore app that inspired Immuni, shares the same opinion, observing that no digital tracing system can replace the manual one and countries effectively adopting contact tracing are usually "equipped" with thousands of tracers.[79] Based on the recommendations of the European Center for Disease Prevention and Control (ECDC), ensuring effective tracing requires at least one contact tracer per 10,000 inhabitants. The Center for Health Security at Johns Hopkins University estimated that during the peaks of contagion, at least three times more contact tracers were needed.[80] In Italy, instead of hiring new employees for contact tracing, the task was assigned to healthcare workers, who were already overwhelmed with job duties due to the pandemic. Moreover, no or insufficient training was provided. According to one of the developers of the Immuni app, this was a huge mistake and significantly contributed to the ineffectiveness of the entire strategy.[79, 81]

Strengthening epidemiological surveillance technologies is key. As the Italian Association of Epidemiology (AIE) explains, standardized national information systems are needed to collect and share data on deaths, hospitalizations and emergency room records. They are also essential to generate ad hoc surveys to analyze the contexts of infections (school, family, work, transport) and consolidate the data into a governance system to support health policies.[81, 82] Epidemiological data management systems could greatly benefit from the information regularly collected by private multinational companies such as Google, Apple, Facebook, Instagram and WhatsApp.[83] However, even in the face of millions of deaths, these companies and governments of the world's richest countries have not considered making these data available to enhance epidemiological surveillance systems.

The primary concerns about privacy and the possibility that these data could "fall into the wrong hands" were serious. The ethical dilemma was the balance between individual freedoms and the collective responsibility to prevent the deaths of millions of people. Yet, possible strategies were in place to appropriately anonymize information during the monitoring and containment phases of outbreaks without compromising privacy rights. An OECD report titled "Testing for Covid-19: A Way to Lift Confinement Restrictions" highlighted the pan-European privacy-preserving proximity tracing initiative (PEPP-PT), which mandated the encryption of data on contact tracing. This system would have ensured that neither the infected person nor the exposed individuals could be identified.[84] Data from epidemiological surveillance systems, obtained through GPS and Bluetooth technologies, could also undergo similar processes to remove personally identifiable information, incorporating protection mechanisms with anonymized data. Additionally, the use of data could be temporally limited, and measures could be implemented to erase any digital information once the monitoring phase of the pandemic was concluded.[45]

Perhaps the most paradoxical aspect of this debate is the decision to forgo adopting life-saving contact tracing activities due to privacy concerns in a society where most citizens have long since given up their privacy. Citizens of the most technologically and economically advanced countries provide enormous amounts of sensitive information in real-time to private companies or the so-called web giants. Apps and smartphones are used for daily activities, such as purchasing consumer goods, watching movies, reading newspapers, or immersing in video games. The main private actors in global technology geo-reference our movements every day, bypassing laws and government regulations to collect large amounts of data from our cell phones. If the most digitized and surveilled civilization ever, with the most violated personal information of all time, revolted against using an app that would have saved millions of lives for privacy reasons, it remains to be understood why it is not protesting against the indiscriminate use of its sensitive information by private powers without any democratic control.

"Schools are safe, hands off the kids!"

"Death is a difficult event to contemplate, and when a flower, a vital and sweet young lady, passes away, the mind becomes cloudy, and sorrow takes over." These are the words of the mayor of Polignano a Mare, a beautiful town in the province of Bari in southern Italy. They are referring to Giustina, a 39-year-old teacher who died after contracting the virus at the kindergarten where she worked. Once she was hospitalized, her condition worsened, and she never left the ICU until her death. She left behind a child, her husband and all those who loved her. The death of teachers like Giustina, who were infected while carrying out their school duties, reflects the profound pain caused by the pandemic, which has affected all aspects of society including schools. While individual stories are poignant, investigating the role played by schools in the spread of COVID-19 requires a scientific examination.[85] Were schools really safe?

Many were absolutely certain.

"You are ill-thinking!!" the Italian Education Minister Lucia Azzolina exclaimed, smiling, while she was personally testing what in her opinion could become an insurmountable bulwark against COVID-19 infections in schools: a desk with wheels.[86] Her government had just decided to invest more than 100 million euros in this prevention measure.[87] According to her view, the decision had made use of the position of authoritative voices in the field of public health, such as that of a member of the Italian CTS, who assured everyone that schools are "not a place of risk."[88] Another well-known figure on the same committee, as well as the president of the Superior Council of Health, reiterated the same idea: "The school is safe. No more lies."[89] An immunologist from the University of Padova joined the chorus and guaranteed that the school "is not a source of infections."[90] Even the president of the Italian Society of Pediatrics agreed: "School is the safest place because there are precise rules and there are those who enforce them."[91]

We do not have precise estimates about fatalities among schoolchildren in Italy, but as already noted, COVID-19 was a leading cause of death among children in the United States[51] and UNICEF estimated a total number of 17, 491 children's fatalities due to COVID-19 in a sample of 95 countries.[52] How about their teachers? Reports of school staff dying from COVID are scarce. A Norwegian study found that teachers weren't at increased risk compared to the general population in the first wave. A study from Wales, however, showed exactly the opposite, indicating an elevated risk of COVID-19 amongst younger teaching staff in primary schools.[92] Research from the United States showed that, at the end of December 2023, 1,308 active and retired educators had succumbed to the virus.[93]

These deaths and countless studies in the literature indicate that schools were not necessarily safe. Moreover, evidence shows that teenagers and children, though less susceptible to severe cases of COVID-19, have contributed to the transmission of the virus.[94] A systematic review revealed that school outbreaks primarily occurred in secondary schools. The population most exposed to infections from children and adolescents, as confirmed by earlier studies, is the family where they reside.[95,96] Within the home, adolescents were identified as more likely to spread the virus than adults and younger children.[97] An English study highlighted that schools, along with nursing homes, were the most high-risk environments for new acute respiratory diseases.[98] An ecological longitudinal study across 37 OECD countries demonstrated that the early implementation of school closures significantly reduced COVID-19 mortality during the initial wave of the pandemic, indicating a clear role for schools in the contagion.[99]

In effect, expecting schools and students not to contribute to the infection was unrealistic. Scientific evidence published in journals such as *Science*, *Nature*, and *The Lancet* has highlighted their potential danger.[100–103] Despite emotional responses fueled by slogans such as "hands off the kids," as observed by a report of the European Center for Disease Control (ECDC), the prevalence of COVID-19 within schools is inevitably influenced, by the prevalence in the community. In other words, in situations with high community transmission, schools contribute to contagion.[104] Of course, avoiding school closures must be a priority to avoid negative effects on the psychological well-being, socialization and health-related behaviors of children, especially those living in disadvantaged socioeconomic conditions.[105] Some argue with some merit that closing schools was ethically and socially indefensible, emphasizing the need to protect the right to education "at all costs." However, this assertion raises another question: what is really meant by "all cost"? According to an Italian professor who teaches at a US university, it was acceptable to endure some deaths to prevent the damage caused to students by school closures.[106] Yet, this perspective prompts reflection on the families of school staff who lost their lives due to infections within school premises. What would they say to the idea that the lives of their loved ones had to be sacrificed uphold the right to education?

Was there a viable way to prevent these deaths while simultaneously ensuring students' right to study? We do not know. What we do know, however, is that in regions where community-based containment strategies significantly reduced transmission, schools remained relatively safe. A South Korean study observed no sudden surge in pediatric cases after schools were reopened between April and June 2020, employing a phased reopening approach alongside a robust national infection containment strategy.[107] Similarly, a Finnish study reported no increase in pediatric hospital visits following the reopening of nurseries, reflecting the country's effective pandemic management compared to that of other European nations.[108] Another research project from North Carolina also demonstrated that schools could reopen without triggering excessive transmission of infections when the reopening was complemented by appropriate prevention interventions.[109] Contrary to slogans such as "schools are safe," international scientific literature emphasized specific conditions and interventions essential for ensuring genuine safety in schools.[110,111] According to a *Lancet* contribution, the key to reopening schools safely lies not in mere assurances but in emphasizing preventive interventions.[112] Multiple analyses in the literature echoed similar conclusions.[113,114] As highlighted by a study from New Jersey, to make schools safe, multiple strategies were needed which included rapid swabs, contact tracing, isolation and mandatory screening for all positive cases before arriving at school, as well as behavioral agreements with students.[115] Emphasizing a data-driven approach, Independent SAGE stressed that the reopening of schools must be guided by rigorous monitoring of infections using epidemiological surveillance technologies.[116] Action was also needed to improve the safety of public transport used by students.

In addition to these preventive measures, a crucial aspect that deserved significant investment and action was the ventilation of school classrooms.[117]

Mounting scientific evidence has unequivocally demonstrated that SARS-CoV-2 is an airborne pathogen, requiring targeted measures such as indoor ventilation and air filtration. Despite clear evidence that the majority of infections occur indoors, most resources have been allocated to outdoor activities. During the first wave in Italy, there was a misguided tendency to search for scapegoats. First, runners and joggers were blamed as "plague spreaders," diverting attention from critical indoor measures. Then, the blame was directed at random citizens who were outdoors alone. The height of absurdity was probably reached when an Italian citizen sunbathing alone on the beach was confronted by the police with a helicopter. While even some Italian epidemiologists expressed doubts about the suitability of ventilation and CO_2 detectors in school settings,[118] scientific evidence has clearly demonstrated their significant potential to reduce infection risks in classrooms.[119] A systematic review of 32 studies indicated that increasing the ventilation rate was significantly associated with a reduction in infections.[120] Simple measures such as adopting air exchange methods proved to be relevant. Experts also highlighted that alterations in the internal configuration of spaces, including the size and number of windows, their location and the position of extraction and supply air vents, could impact contagion.

A group of Italian teachers, activists and experts advocated for the mandatory provision of carbon monoxide detectors in Italian classrooms, a measure already implemented in countries like Belgium and France.[121] The importance of ventilation goes beyond schools. It is also key to improving air quality in workplaces, hospitals, nursing homes and other indoor environments. Ventilation can mitigate not only SARS-CoV-2 infections but also other respiratory diseases and toxic effects from volatile organic compounds.[122] In addition to the immediate health benefits, alterations in building design, including changes to ventilation and air filtration systems, can also contribute to reducing CO_2 emissions.

The former Italian Minister of Education was right when she pointed out that school students should not be "the ones to pay the highest price for this emergency."[123] Public health sciences have shown that there are interventions that can be used to safeguard students' right to in-person learning without jeopardizing the lives of school workers, but none of them require the use of a desk with wheels. Moreover, if schools were truly safe, why invest more than 100 million euros in this useless tool?

References

1. Verona. 'In ospedale è il caos. Morti anche in corridoio'. Denuncia shock. Rainews. Published online on Dec 14, 2020. https://www.rainews.it/tgr/veneto/video/2020/12/ven-Ospedale-Verona-Borgo-Trento-Morti-Malati-Coronavirus-Allarme-f95a31fa-a612-422e-9fb5-fdab69469aa7.html (accessed Jan 24, 2024).

2. Oggi Treviso. Covid: l'ospedale di Montebelluna è al collasso non si sa più dove mettere i malati. Published online on December 17, 2020. https://www.oggitreviso.it/node/243660 (accessed Jan 24, 2024).

3. Bonifacio S, Rotta A, Dal Dosso I. 'Ospedali al collasso, cosa succede in Veneto?'. La rabbia dei medici. L'Arena. Published online Dec 13, 2020. https://www.larena.it/news/veneto/posti-finiti-paziente-covid-mandato-da-san-bonifacio-a-belluno-cosa-succede-in-veneto-la-rabbia-dei-medici-1.8385881 (accessed Jan 24, 2024).

4. Sarsini D. Zero contagi in Veneto. 'Il modello funziona'; AGI. Published online Jan 24, 2024. https://www.agi.it/cronaca/news/2020-05-21/zero-contagi-in-veneto-coronavirus-8689495/ (accessed Jan 24, 2024).

5. Libero Quotidiano. Francesca Russo, la dottoressa siciliana che ha salvato il Veneto: coronavirus, piano pronto già il 31 gennaio. Published online on May 18, 2020. https://www.liberoquotidiano.it/news/scienze-tech/22680318/francesca_russo_dottoressa_siciliana_salvato_veneto_coronavirus_luca_zaia.html (accessed Jan 24, 2024).

6. Zaia: 'I tamponi a tutti, una mia invenzione. Io premier? Ma no, vengo dalla campagna'. *la Repubblica*. Published online May 15, 2020. https://www.repubblica.it/politica/2020/05/15/news/zaia_i_tamponi_a_tutti_una_mia_invenzione_io_premier_ma_no_vengono_dalla_campagna_-301030860/ (accessed Jan 24, 2024).

7. La confessione: 'Il piano anti Covid è del 2006'. Ora rischiano il posto i ricercatori Veneti. Corriere del Veneto. Published online Dec 2, 2020. https://corrieredelveneto.corriere.it/veneto/politica/20_dicembre_02/confessione-il-piano-anti-covid-2006-ora-rischiano-posto-ricercatori-veneti-73a3fbfe-3481-11eb-ab4d-d12e341be9b9.shtml (accessed Jan 24, 2024).

8. Il Mattino. Crisanti contro la collega Russo: 'Il piano tamponi una bagginata'. La replica: 'Lui voleva farli solo ai cinesi'. Published online May 23, 2020. https://www.ilmattino.it/primopiano/cronaca/coronavirus_piano_tamponi_veneto_crisanti_polemica_russo_zaia-5245572.html (accessed Jan 24, 2024).

9. Starr D. How Italy's 'father of the swabs' fought the coronavirus. Science. https://www.science.org/content/article/how-italy-s-father-swabs-fought-coronavirus?fbclid=IwAR3hPPzDTzvvsRTT49ZpSnxcSh8ldg-vuB-YR032eZUZqMAGhtAmXDwymhME (accessed Jan 24, 2024).

10. L'Espresso. L'autogol della Regione Veneto: paga 27mila euro per fare causa a Crisanti ma la Procura chiede l'archiviazione e vuole valutare le spese. Published online May 2, 2022. https://lespresso.it/c/attualita/2022/5/2/lautogol-della-regione-veneto-paga-27mila-euro-per-fare-causa-a-crisanti-ma-la-procura-chiede-larchiviazione-e-vuole-valutare-le-spese/12628 (accessed Jan 24, 2024).

11. L'Espresso. Vi ricordate i tamponi rapidi del Veneto? Il super esperto è a giudizio per false attestazioni sui test. Published online July 21, 2022. https://lespresso.it/c/attualita/2022/7/21/vi-ricordate-i-tamponi-rapidi-del-veneto-il-super-esperto-e-a-giudizio-per-false-attestazioni-sui-test/12763 (accessed Jan 24, 2024).

12. EpiCentro. Attività fisica – Sorveglianza Passi. Istituto Superiore di Sanità. https://www.epicentro.iss.it/passi/dati/attivita-oms (accessed Jan 24, 2024).

13. EpiCentro. Abitudine al fumo dati sorveglianza Passi. Istituto Superiore di Sanità. https://www.epicentro.iss.it/passi/dati/fumo (accessed Jan 24, 2024).

14. Giorgi A. Zaia e il modello Veneto: 'Così siamo riusciti a contenere il coronavirus'. Il Giornale. Published online Apr 6, 2020. https://www.ilgiornale.it/news/politica/zaia-e-modello-veneto-cos-siamo-riusciti-contenere-1850760.html?fbclid=IwAR25_6RNAmL-ZJUMcQixAXFbEu9ydDvhKEF6qVwgHmGrcL2fQ8SLqr4GBRM (accessed Jan 24, 2024).

15. Guglielmi G. Rapid coronavirus tests: a guide for the perplexed. *Nature* 2021; 590: 202–5.

16. Ramdas K, Darzi A, Jain S. 'Test, re-test, re-test': using inaccurate tests to greatly increase the accuracy of COVID-19 testing. *Nature Medicine* 2020; **26**: 810–1.

17. Parlaveneto. Test rapidi Covid, Veneto che Vogliamo: "Zaia ha sbagliato tutto, circolare ministero ci boccia". Vipiù. Published online Jan 11, 2021. https://www.vipiu.it/leggi/test-rapidi-covid-veneto-che-vogliamo-zaia-ha-sbagliato-tutto-circolare-ministero-ci-boccia/ (accessed Jan 24, 2024).

18. Covid Veneto, inchiesta test rapidi: Rigoli e Simionato rinviati a giudizio. Udienza nel 2024. Il Resto del Carlino. Published online Feb 10, 2023. https://www.ilrestodelcarlino.it/veneto/cronaca/covid-test-rapidi-rigoli-simionato-tmnvbsq7 (accessed Jan 24, 2024).

19. Drain PK, Ampajwala M, Chappel C, *et al.* A rapid, high-sensitivity SARS-CoV-2 nucleocapsid immunoassay to aid diagnosis of acute COVID-19 at the point of care: a clinical performance study. *Infectious Diseases and Therapy* 2021; **10**: 753–61.

20. Rainews. Il test rapido non individua la positività: i familiari si contagiano. Published online Dec 10, 2020. https://www.rainews.it/tgr/veneto/video/2020/12/ven-Covid19-Coronavirus-Padova-il-test-rapido-non-individua-la-positivita-i-familiari-si-contagiano-e56e15ac-e954-474f-9281-bdb6cb3b26df.html (accessed Jan 24, 2024).

21. Covid. No ai test rapidi per la biosorveglianza del personale sanitario, Anaao Veneto diffida i vertici delle Aulss. Quotidiano Sanità. https://www.quotidianosanita.it/veneto/articolo.php?articolo_id=91460 (accessed Jan 24, 2024).

22. Ruccia G., Crisanti: 'In Veneto uso inappropriato dei test rapidi, non da barriera ma da gruviera. Natale? Sì a zona rossa in tutta Italia ma con negozi aperti'. *Il Fatto Quotidiano.* Published online Dec 17, 2020. https://www.ilfattoquotidiano.it/2020/12/17/crisanti-in-veneto-uso-inappropriato-dei-test-rapidi-non-da-barriera-ma-da-gruviera-natale-si-a-zona-rossa-in-tutta-italia-ma-con-negozi-aperti/6040232/ (accessed Jan 24, 2024).

23. De Vogli R, Buio MD, De Falco R. [Effects of the COVID-19 pandemic on health inequalities and mental health: effective public policies]. *Epidemiologia e prevenzione* 2021; **45**: 588–97.

24. Liang L-L, Tseng C-H, Ho HJ, Wu C-Y. Covid-19 mortality is negatively associated with test number and government effectiveness. *Scientific Reports* 2020; **10**: 12567.

25. Contreras S, Dehning J, Loidolt M, *et al.* The challenges of containing SARS-CoV-2 via test-trace-and-isolate. *Nature Communications* 2021; **12**: 378. https://doi.org/10.1038/s41467-020-20699-8.

26. ECDC. Contact tracing in the European Union: public health management of persons, including healthcare workers, who have had contact with COVID-19 cases – fourth update. Published online Oct 28, 2021. https://www.ecdc.europa.eu/en/covid-19-contact-tracing-public-health-management (accessed Jan 24, 2024).

27. Kretzschmar ME, Rozhnova G, Bootsma MCJ, van Boven M, van de Wijgert JHHM, Bonten MJM. Impact of delays on effectiveness of contact tracing strategies for COVID-19: a modelling study. *Lancet Public Health* 2020; **5**: e452–9.

28. Varkila MRJ, Montez-Rath ME, Salomon JA, *et al.* Use of wastewater metrics to track COVID-19 in the US. *JAMA Network Open* 2023; **6**: e2325591.

29. Hassan I, Mukaigawara M, King L, *et al.* Hindsight is 2020? Lessons in global health governance one year into the pandemic. *Nature Medicine* 2021; **27**: 396–400. https://doi.org/10.1038/s41591-021-01272-2.

30. Dickens BL, Koo JR, Lim JT, *et al.* Modelling lockdown and exit strategies for COVID-19 in Singapore. *The Lancet Regional Health – Western Pacific* 2020; **1**: 100004. https://doi.org/10.1016/j.lanwpc.2020.100004.

31. Jefferies S, French N, Gilkison C, *et al.* COVID-19 in New Zealand and the impact of the national response: A descriptive epidemiological study. *The Lancet Public Health* 2020; 5: e612–23.
32. Horton R. Offline: the case for No-COVID. *The Lancet* 2021; **397**: 359.
33. Priesemann V, Brinkmann MM, Ciesek S, *et al.* Calling for pan-European commitment for rapid and sustained reduction in SARS-CoV-2 infections. *The Lancet* 2021; **397**: 92–3.
34. A 'sustainable suppression' strategy for keeping society open. Lockdowns, mitigation measures, COVID-19 strategy. Independent SAGE. Published online Feb 19, 2021. https://www.independentsage.org/a-sustainable-suppression-strategy-for-keeping-society-open/ (accessed Jan 24, 2024).
35. Blasimme A, Vayena E. What's next for COVID-19 apps? Governance and oversight. *Science* 2020; **370**: 760–2.
36. Baker M. & McKee M. All countries should pursue a Covid-19 elimination strategy: here are 16 reasons why. *The Guardian.* Published online Jan 28, 2021. https://www.theguardian.com/world/commentisfree/2021/jan/28/all-countries-should-pursue-a-covid-19-elimination-strategy-here-are-16-reasons-why (accessed Jan 24, 2024).
37. Summers J, Cheng H-Y, Lin H-H, *et al.* Potential lessons from the Taiwan and New Zealand health responses to the COVID-19 pandemic. *The Lancet Regional Health – Western Pacific* 2020; **4**: 100044.
38. Wang CJ, Ng CY, Brook RH. Response to COVID-19 in Taiwan: big data analytics, new technology, and proactive testing. *JAMA* 2020; **323**: 1341–2.
39. Lai C-C, Lee P-I, Hsueh P-R. How Taiwan has responded to COVID-19 and how COVID-19 has affected Taiwan, 2020–2022. *Journal of Microbiology, Immunology, and Infection* 2023; **56**: 433.
40. Jian S-W, Cheng H-Y, Huang X-T, Liu D-P. Contact tracing with digital assistance in Taiwan's COVID-19 outbreak response. *International Journal of Infectious Diseases* 2020; **101**: 348–52.
41. Garrett PM, Wang Y-W, White JP, Kashima Y, Dennis S, Yang C-T. High acceptance of COVID-19 tracing technologies in Taiwan: a nationally representative survey analysis. *International Journal of Environmental Research and Public Health* 2022; **19**: 3323.
42. Coronavirus: under surveillance and confined at home in Taiwan. BBC News. Published online Mar 24, 2020. https://www.bbc.com/news/technology-52017993 (accessed Jan 24, 2024).
43. Fitzpatrick P. How Taiwan beat COVID-19 – new study reveals clues to its success. *The Conversation.* Published online Apr 15, 2021. http://theconversation.com/how-taiwan-beat-covid-19-new-study-reveals-clues-to-its-success-158900 (accessed Jan 24, 2024).
44. Chen Y-H, Fang C-T. Achieving COVID-19 zero without lockdown, January 2020 to March 2022: the Taiwan model explained. *Journal of the Formosan Medical Association* 2024; **123**: S8–16.
45. Whitelaw S, Mamas MA, Topol E, Spall HGCV. Applications of digital technology in COVID-19 pandemic planning and response. *The Lancet Digital Health* 2020; **2**: e435–40.
46. Palaniappan A, Dave U, Gosine B. Comparing South Korea and Italy's healthcare systems and initiatives to combat COVID-19. *Revista Panamericana de Salud Pública* 2020; **44**: e53.
47. Kang S-J, Kim S, Park K-H, *et al.* Successful control of COVID-19 outbreak through tracing, testing, and isolation: lessons learned from the outbreak control efforts made in a metropolitan city of South Korea. *Journal of Infection and Public Health* 2021; **14**: 1151–4.

48. Terhune T, Levine D, Hyunjoo J, Lee JL. Special report: how Korea trounced U.S. in race to test people for coronavirus. *Reuters*. Published online March 18, 2020. https://www.reuters.com/article/idUSKBN2153CF/ (accessed Jan 24, 2024).

49. Lim S, Sohn M. How to cope with emerging viral diseases: lessons from South Korea's strategy for COVID-19, and collateral damage to cardiometabolic health. *The Lancet Regional Health - Western Pacific* 2023; 30: 100581.

50. Tran TPT, Le TH, Nguyen TNP, Hoang VM. Rapid response to the COVID-19 pandemic: Vietnam government's experience and preliminary success. *Journal of Global Health* 2020; 10: 020502. https://doi.org/10.7189/jogh.10.020502.

51. Trevisan M, Le LC, Le AV. The COVID-19 pandemic: a view from Vietnam. *American Journal of Public Health* 2020; 110: 1152–3.

52. Van Tan L. COVID-19 control in Vietnam. *Nature Immunology* 2021; 22: 261.

53. Toan DTT, Pham TH, Nguyen KC, *et al*. Shift from a Zero-COVID strategy to a new-normal strategy for controlling SARS-COV-2 infections in Vietnam. *Epidemiology and Infection* 2023; 151: e117.

54. Dabla-Norris E, Gulde-Wolf A-M, Painchaud F, IMF Asia and Pacific Department. Vietnam's success in containing COVID-19 offers roadmap for other developing ountries. IMF News. https://www.imf.org/en/News/Articles/2020/06/29/na062920-vietnams-success-in-containing-covid19-offers-roadmap-for-other-developing-countries (accessed Jan 24, 2024).

55. Battacharya J., Zero Covid has cost New Zealand dearly. Spiked. Published online Aug 7, 2022. https://www.spiked-online.com/2022/08/07/zero-covid-has-cost-new-zealand-dearly/ (accessed Jan 29, 2024).

56. Baker MG, Wilson N, Blakely T. Elimination could be the optimal response strategy for Covid-19 and other emerging pandemic diseases. *BMJ* 2020; 371: m4907.

57. COVID-19 Government Response Tracker. University of Oxford. Published online March 18, 2020. https://www.bsg.ox.ac.uk/research/covid-19-government-response-tracker (accessed Jan 24, 2024).

58. Robert A. Lessons from New Zealand's COVID-19 outbreak response. *Lancet Public Health* 2020; 5: e569–70.

59. Stockman J. How New Zealand eliminated COVID-19. LSE COVID-19. LSE Blogs. Published online Jan 4, 2021. https://blogs.lse.ac.uk/covid19/2021/01/04/how-new-zealand-eliminated-covid-19/ (accessed Jan 24, 2024).

60. Geoghegan JL, Moreland NJ, Le Gros G, Ussher JE. New Zealand's science-led response to the SARS-CoV-2 pandemic. *Nature Immunology* 2021; 22: 262–3.

61. Devi Shridar. Preventable: How a Pandemic Changed the World & How to Stop the Next One. Viking, New York 2023.

62. Yip W, Ge L, Ho AHY, Heng BH, Tan WS. Building community resilience beyond COVID-19: the Singapore way. *The Lancet Regional Health – Western Pacific* 2021; 7. https://doi.org/10.1016/j.lanwpc.2020.100091.

63. Venkatachalam I, Conceicao EP, Aung MK, *et al*. Healthcare workers as a sentinel surveillance population in the early phase of the COVID-19 pandemic. *Singapore Medical Journal* 2022; 63: 577.

64. Singapore's Covid success isn't easily replicated. Bloomberg. Published online Jan 3, 2021. https://www.bloomberg.com/view/articles/2021-01-03/singapore-s-covid-success-isn-t-easily-replicated (accessed Jan 24, 2024).

65. Wamsley L. Singapore says COVID-19 contact-tracing data can be requested by police. NPR. Published online Jan 5, 2021. https://www.npr.org/sections/coronavirus-live-updates/2021/01/05/953604553/singapore-says-covid-19-contact-tracing-data-can-be-requested-by-police (accessed Jan 24, 2024).

66. Oshitani H. COVID lessons from Japan: the right messaging empowers citizens. *Nature* 2022; **605**: 589.
67. Matsuyama K, Mayger J. How Japan achieved one of the world's lowest COVID-19 death rates. *The Japan Times*. Published online June 18, 2022. https://www.japantimes.co.jp/news/2022/06/18/national/science-health/japan-coronavirus-deaths-low/ (accessed Jan 24, 2024).
68. A breath of fresh air for public health messaging. Nature 2023. https://www.nature.com/articles/d42473-023-00186-6 (accessed Jan 24, 2024).
69. Keeling MJ, Hollingsworth TD, Read JM. Efficacy of contact tracing for the containment of the 2019 novel coronavirus (COVID-19). *Journal of Epidemiology and Community Health* 2020; **74**: 861–6.
70. Lewis D. Why many countries failed at COVID contact-tracing — but some got it right. *Nature* 2020; **588**: 384–7.
71. Mbunge E, Akinnuwesi B, Fashoto SG, Metfula AS, Mashwama P. A critical review of emerging technologies for tackling COVID-19 pandemic. *Human Behavior and Emerging Technologies* 2021; **3**: 25–39.
72. Fraser C. Digital contact tracing can slow or even stop coronavirus transmission and ease us out of lockdown. University of Oxford. Published online Apr 16, 2020. https://www.research.ox.ac.uk/article/2020-04-16-digital-contact-tracing-can-slow-or-even-stop-coronavirus-transmission-and-ease-us-out-of-lockdown (accessed Jan 24, 2024).
73. Ròciola A. La parabola di Immuni. Storia dell'app di contact tracing, dall'inizio. AGI. Published online Jan 24, 2024. https://www.agi.it/economia/news/2020-11-01/immuni-app-contact-tracing-storia-10138862/ (accessed Jan 24, 2024).
74. Scala A. The mathematics of multiple lockdowns. *Scientific Reports*. 2021; **11**: 8078. https://doi.org/10.1038/s41598-021-87556-6
75. Zoppi B. Immuni: come funziona e si scarica l'app coronavirus per Android e iPhone. Agenda Digitale. Published online Apr 9, 2021. https://www.agenda-digitale.eu/cultura-digitale/immuni-come-funziona-lapp-italiana-contro-il-coronavirus/ (accessed Jan 24, 2024).
76. Luna R. Lo spettacolare fallimento delle app contro il coronavirus. la Repubblica. Published online July 8, 2020. https://www.repubblica.it/dossier/stazione-futuro-riccardo-luna/2020/07/09/news/lo_spettacolare_fallimento_delle_app_contro_il_coronavirus-261374292/ (accessed Jan 24, 2024).
77. Crisanti A, Mazza M. Caccia al virus. Rosso e Nero, 2021.
78. Baratta L. Il fallimento delle tre T | Il governo si accorge solo ora che le Regioni non si sono attrezzate a dovere per il tracciamento dei contagi. Linkiesta. Published online Oct 28, 2020. https://www.linkiesta.it/2020/10/tracciamento-contatti-dati-regioni-governo/ (accessed Jan 24, 2024).
79. Baratta L. Misteri della fase due | Non è scomparsa solo Immuni, mancano anche seimila tracciatori di contatti. Linkiesta. Published online May 23, 2020. https://www.linkiesta.it/2020/05/immuni-tracciatori-di-contatti-contact-tracing/ (accessed Jan 24, 2024).
80. Watson C & Mullen L. Center for Health Security/NPR state survey. Johns Hopkins Coronavirus Resource Center. Published online March 2021. https://coronavirus.jhu.edu/contact-tracing/state-survey-march-2021 (accessed Jan 24, 2024).
81. Epidemiologia. E' urgente un Piano per una strategia nazionale dei test COVID-19. Associazione Italiana di Epidemiologia. www.epidemiologia.it. Published online Oct 10, 2020. https://www.epidemiologia.it/6565 (accessed Jan 24, 2024).
82. Epidemiologia. A cosa serve un piano pandemico? Associazione Italiana di Epidemiologia. Published online Jan 16, 2021. https://www.epidemiologia.it/6576 (accessed Jan 24, 2024).

83. Pasqualetto A. Crisanti: 'I tracciatori adesso sono inutili. Serve la banca dati di Google'. Corriere della Sera. Published online Nov 10, 2020. https://www.corriere.it/cronache/20_novembre_10/crisanti-ora-tracciatori-non-servono-piu-sfruttiamo-banca-dati-google-17709ff6-22a0-11eb-bd01-ee72f0d01280.shtml (accessed Jan 24, 2024).

84. Testing for COVID-19: A way to lift confinement restrictions. OECD. Published May 4, 2020. https://www.oecd.org/coronavirus/policy-responses/testing-for-covid-19-a-way-to-lift-confinement-restrictions-89756248/ (accessed Jan 23, 2024).

85. Di Zanni C. Coronavirus, Giustina si era contagiata all'asilo: la collaboratrice scolastica di Polignano è morta a 39 anni. *la Repubblica*. Published online Dec 7, 2020. https://bari.repubblica.it/cronaca/2020/12/07/news/coronavirus_brigida_si_era_contagiata_a_scuola_la_collaboratrice_scolastica_di_polignano_e_morta_a_39_anni-277380258/ (accessed Jan 24, 2024).

86. Lucia Azzolina, test in diretta tv del banco con le rotelle: 'Voi siete malpensanti'. Il video della prova. Informazione – Notizie a Confronto. Published online July 24, 2020. https://www.informazione.it/a/A047120E-98FD-4F07-955D-8160F460A2E0/Lucia-Azzolina-test-in-diretta-tv-del-banco-con-le-rotelle-Voi-siete-malpensanti-Il-video-della-prova (accessed Jan 24, 2024).

87. Di redazione. Forza Italia: 2,4 milioni di banchi e gli studenti a casa. Non era forse meglio investire i 500mln per i trasporti? Orizzonte Scuola Notizie. Published online Dec 6, 2020. https://www.orizzontescuola.it/forza-italia-24-milioni-di-banchi-e-gli-studenti-a-casa-non-era-forse-meglio-investire-i-500mln-per-i-trasporti/ (accessed Jan 24, 2024).

88. Di redazione. Miozzo (Cts): la scuola non è luogo di rischio con le dovute precauzioni, priorità riaprire. Orizzonte Scuola Notizie. Published online Nov 22, 2020. https://www.orizzontescuola.it/miozzo-cts-la-scuola-non-e-luogo-di-rischio-con-le-dovute-precauzioni-priorita-riaprire/ (accessed Jan 24, 2024).

89. Di redazione. Coronavirus, Locatelli: 'La scuola è sicura. Basta bugie. Chiudere significa condannare i ragazzi alla deprivazione culturale e affettiva'. Orizzonte Scuola Notizie. Published online Nov 17, 2020. https://www.orizzontescuola.it/coronavirus-locatelli-la-scuola-e-sicura-basta-bugie-chiudere-significa-condannare-i-ragazzi-alla-deprivazione-culturale-e-affettiva/ (accessed Jan 24, 2024).

90. De Angelis F. La scuola è sicura, non si chiude. L'immunologa Viola: 'Non è fonte di contagi'. Tecnica della Scuola. Published online Oct 21, 2020. https://www.tecnicadellascuola.it/la-scuola-e-sicura-non-si-chiude-limmunologa-viola-non-e-fonte-di-contagi (accessed Jan 24, 2024).

91. Di redazione. Il pediatra Villani: 'La scuola è il posto più sicuro perché ci sono regole precise e c'è chi le fa rispettare'. Orizzonte Scuola Notizie. Published online Oct 16, 2020. https://www.orizzontescuola.it/il-pediatra-villani-la-scuola-e-il-posto-piu-sicuro-perche-ci-sono-regole-precise-e-ce-chi-le-fa-rispettare/ (accessed Jan 24, 2024).

92. Thomas F, Fedeli A, Steggall E, *et al*. SARS-CoV-2 incidence among teaching staff in primary and secondary schools – Wales, 2020–2021. *BMC Public Health* 2023; **23**: 922.

93. Maxwell LA. Over 1,000 educators died from COVID. Here's the story of one. *Education Week*. Published online Dec 19, 2022. https://www.edweek.org/teaching-learning/over-1-000-educators-died-from-covid-heres-the-story-of-one/2022/12 (accessed Jan 29, 2024).

94. Li F, Li Y-Y, Liu M-J, *et al*. Household transmission of SARS-CoV-2 and risk factors for susceptibility and infectivity in Wuhan: a retrospective observational study. *The Lancet Infectious Diseases* 2021; **21**: 617–28.

95. Lessler J, Grabowski MK, Grantz KH, *et al.* Household COVID-19 risk and in-person schooling. *Science* 2021; 372: 1092–7.
96. Silverberg SL, Zhang BY, Li SNJ, *et al.* Child transmission of SARS-CoV-2: a systematic review and meta-analysis. *BMC Pediatrics* 2022; 22: 172.
97. Park YJ, Choe YJ, Park O, *et al.* Contact tracing during coronavirus disease outbreak, South Korea, 2020. *Emerging Infectious Diseases* 2020; 26: 2465–8. https://doi.org/10.3201/eid2610.201315.
98. ECDC. Weekly surveillance report on COVID-19. Published online May 15, 2020. https://www.ecdc.europa.eu/en/covid-19/surveillance/weekly-surveillance-report (accessed Jan 24, 2024).
99. Piovani D, Christodoulou MN, Hadjidemetriou A, *et al.* Effect of early application of social distancing interventions on COVID-19 mortality over the first pandemic wave: an analysis of longitudinal data from 37 countries. *Journal of Infectious Diseases* 2021; 82: 133–42.
100. Brauner JM, Mindermann S, Sharma M, *et al.* Inferring the effectiveness of government interventions against COVID-19. *Science* 2021; 371: eabd9338.
101. Haug N, Geyrhofer L, Londei A, *et al.* Ranking the effectiveness of worldwide COVID-19 government interventions. *Nature Human Behaviour* 2020; 4: 1303–12.
102. Li Y, Campbell H, Kulkarni D, *et al.* The temporal association of introducing and lifting non-pharmaceutical interventions with the time-varying reproduction number (R) of SARS-CoV-2: a modelling study across 131 countries. *The Lancet Infectious Diseases* 2021; 21: 193–202.
103. Auger KA, Shah SS, Richardson T, *et al.* Association between statewide school closure and COVID-19 incidence and mortality in the US. *JAMA* 2020; 324: 859–70.
104. COVID-19 in children and the role of school settings in transmission – second update. ECDC. Published online July 8, 2021. https://www.ecdc.europa.eu/en/publications-data/children-and-school-settings-covid-19-transmission (accessed Jan 24, 2024).
105. Sheen A, Ro G, Holani K, Santos ACZPD, Kagadkar F, Zeshan M. 51.7 impact of Covid-19–related school closures on children and adolescents worldwide: a literature review. *Journal of the American Academy of Child & Adolescent Psychiatry* 2020; 59: S253.
106. Nepi M., Scuole, Silvestri: "Tornare in presenza, anche con il rischio di qualche morto in più". TPI. Published online Jan 10, 2022. https://www.tpi.it/cronaca/scuole-silvestri-tornare-in-presenza-anche-con-il-rischio-di-qualche-morto-in-piu-20220110857411/ (accessed Jan 24, 2024).
107. Yoon Y, Kim KR, Park H, Kim S, Kim YJ. Stepwise school opening and an impact on the epidemiology of COVID-19 in the children. *Journal of Korean Medical Science* 2020; 35: e414. https://doi.org/10.3346/jkms.2020.35.e414.
108. Kuitunen I, Haapanen M, Artama M, Renko M. Closing Finnish schools and day care centres had a greater impact on primary care than secondary care emergency department visits. *Acta Paediatrica* 2021; 110: 937–8.
109. Zimmerman KO, Akinboyo IC, Brookhart MA, *et al.* Incidence and secondary transmission of SARS-CoV-2 infections in schools. *Pediatrics* 2021; 147: e2020048090. https://doi.org/10.1542/peds.2020-048090.
110. Vogel G. School risk calculations scrambled by fast-spreading virus strains. Science. Published online Jan 19, 2021. https://www.science.org/content/article/new-coronavirus-variant-scrambles-school-risk-calculations (accessed Jan 24, 2024).
111. Torjesen I. What do we know about lateral flow tests and mass testing in schools? *BMJ* 2021; 372: n706.

112. Panovska-Griffiths J, Kerr CC, Stuart RM, *et al*. Determining the optimal strategy for reopening schools, the impact of test and trace interventions, and the risk of occurrence of a second COVID-19 epidemic wave in the UK: a modelling study. *The Lancet Child & Adolescent Health* 2020; **4**: 817–27.

113. Ziauddeen N, Woods-Townsend K, Saxena S, Gilbert R, Alwan NA. Schools and COVID-19: reopening Pandora's box? *Public Health in Practice (Oxford)* 2020; **1**: 100039.

114. Larosa E, Djuric O, Cassinadri M, *et al*. Secondary transmission of COVID-19 in preschool and school settings in northern Italy after their reopening in September 2020: a population-based study. *Eurosurveillance* 2020; **25**: 2001911.

115. Volpp KG. Minimal SARS-CoV-2 transmission after implementation of a comprehensive mitigation strategy at a school — New Jersey, August 20–November 27, 2020. *Morbidity and Mortality Weekly Report* 2021; **70**. https://doi.org/10.15585/mmwr.mm7011a2.

116. The return to school: a consultation document. Independent SAGE. Published online Feb 5, 2021. https://www.independentsage.org/the-return-to-school-a-consultation-document/ (accessed Jan 24, 2024).

117. [Withdrawn] Actions for schools during the coronavirus outbreak. UK Government Department of Education. Published online April 1, 2022. https://www.gov.uk/government/publications/actions-for-schools-during-the-coronavirus-outbreak (accessed Jan 24, 2024).

118. De Angelis D. Rientro in classe, l'AIE: 'Le misure funzionano, non serve la chiusura scuole. L'apertura delle finestre in aula è più efficace dei sistemi meccanici' [INTERVISTA]. Orizzonte Scuola Notizie. Published online Dec 29, 2021. https://www.orizzontescuola.it/rientro-in-classe-laie-le-misure-funzionano-non-serve-la-chiusura-scuola-lapertura-delle-finestre-in-aula-e-piu-efficace-dei-sistemi-meccanici-intervista/ (accessed Jan 24, 2024).

119. McLeod RS, Hopfe CJ, Bodenschatz E, *et al*. A multi-layered strategy for COVID-19 infection prophylaxis in schools: a review of the evidence for masks, distancing, and ventilation. *Indoor Air* 2022; **32**: e13142.

120. Thornton GM, Fleck BA, Kroeker E, *et al*. The impact of heating, ventilation, and air conditioning design features on the transmission of viruses, including the 2019 novel coronavirus: a systematic review of ventilation and coronavirus. *PloS Global Public Health* 2022; **2**: e0000552.

121. I lettori ci scrivono. IdeaScuola: firmate per richiedere i rilevatori di CO2 nelle aule scolastiche. Tecnica della Scuola. Published online Jan 13, 2023. https://www.tecnicadellascuola.it/ideascuola-firmate-per-richiedere-i-rilevatori-di-co2-nelle-aule-scolastiche (accessed Jan 24, 2024).

122. Dowell D, Lindsley WG, Brooks JT. Reducing SARS-CoV-2 in shared indoor air. *JAMA* 2022; **328**: 141–2.

123. Da Azzolina a Locatelli, il fronte della scuola aperta: 'È sicura'. HuffPost Italia. Published online Nov 17, 2020. https://www.huffingtonpost.it/politica/2020/11/17/news/da_azzolina_a_locatelli_il_fronte_della_scuola_aperta_e_sicura_-5352817/ (accessed Jan 24, 2024).

7

IMMUNIZATION

9 November 2020. The companies Pfizer and BioNTech announced the results of the phase 3 study of the BNT162b2 mRNA vaccine. The results were extraordinary, and the vaccine showed very high efficacy, especially in avoiding serious illnesses and death in those who have been infected. Subsequent studies unveiled additional effective vaccines, sparking a ray of hope in the battle against the virus. Despite the spread of new variants capable of drastically reducing the ability to contain infections, these breakthroughs have completely transformed the evolution of the pandemic. Yet, in numerous mass media and social media outlets, misinformation on the topic became unstoppable. On July 9, 2022, a well-known Italian newspaper headlined its front page article "Vaccinated people die, not anti-vaxxers."[1] This sensational claim added fuel to the growing litany of fake news circulating in the public domain. Amidst all these false statements, the Italian Undersecretary for Health Marcello Gemmato cast doubt on the effectiveness of the vaccination campaign directed by his very own government, saying, "there is no proof that without vaccines we would have been worse off."[2]

SARS-CoV-2 vaccines: killers or saviors?

A few days after Gemmato's statements, the Istituto Superiore di Sanità published a report evaluating the impact of the Italian vaccination campaign: the mortality rate for unvaccinated Italians was almost 3 to 9.5 times higher than that of vaccinated individuals.[3] This comes as no surprise. Previous analyses had already underscored the significant disparities in hospitalization rates between vaccinated and unvaccinated individuals. In May–June 2022, the standardized hospitalization rate for those aged over 12 years was more than

DOI: 10.4324/9781003511977-10

3.5 times higher for the unvaccinated than for those with full vaccination and a booster dose. Additionally, in April–May 2022, the standardized mortality rate for the unvaccinated was roughly 6.5 times higher than for those with a complete cycle of vaccination and additional/booster dose.[3]

Similar robust evidence emerged from other countries. According to the CDC in the United States, unvaccinated citizens faced a mortality rate 6 times higher than those who received at least the first vaccine dose, with individuals aged 50 or over being 12 times more likely to die if unvaccinated than their peers with one or more boosters.[4] A 2022 study from the United Kingdom indicated that two-dose vaccination reduced the likelihood of death by 93%.[5] A systematic literature search involving over 50 studies highlighted a strong inverse relationship between vaccination and mortality in various contexts, emphasizing a "dose-response" pattern wherein mortality rates were lower for those with two doses than for those with only one.[6] Systematic reviews, meta-analyses, and studies conducted by the Imperial College London, the Institute for Health Metrics and Evaluation and other institutions consistently demonstrated the high effectiveness of vaccines in preventing hospitalizations and deaths.[7-9] Imperial College London's analysis showed that vaccines provided by the global COVAX initiative had prevented 2.7 million deaths in 92 low-income countries.[10] A study based on mathematical modeling for 185 countries estimated that globally COVID-19 vaccination has substantially altered the pandemic's trajectory, saving an estimated 14.4 million lives.[11]

Despite the wealth of scientific evidence supporting the lifesaving effectiveness of vaccines, the widespread support for these health technologies continued to face obstacles in mass media and social media. In an interview with Radio Radio TV, which garnered over 80,000 views on YouTube alone, an *endocrinologist* analyzed a single study on excess mortality in Germany suggesting that the results demonstrated a peak in deaths in 2022, implying a connection to the introduction of mass vaccination. During the same interview, a well-known psychiatrist implied the prospect of terrifying mortality increases among vaccinated people, stating that the same study's results would have been even more poignant with the release of 2023 data. He did not even realize that such data were already available,[12] and they showed, in fact, exactly the opposite.[13,14]

Regrettably, in the confusion created by misinformation spread by loud and captivating voices, solid knowledge derived from meticulous scientific research is often overlooked or dismissed. The stark consequences of falling victim to false news about vaccine effectiveness have been most strikingly evident in the United States leading to significant disparities in mortality rates between unvaccinated and vaccinated cohorts (Figure 7.1). Varying levels of vaccine hesitancy among American states inadvertently served as the empirical basis for natural experiments, shedding light on the lethal impact

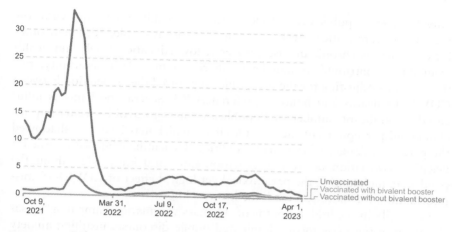

FIGURE 7.1   Lifesaving vaccination in the United States: COVID-19 weekly death rate by vaccination status (October 9, 2021 – April 1, 2023)

Note: Death rates are calculated as the number of deaths in each group divided by the total number of people in this group. Numbers given are per 100,000 people. The mortality rate for the "All ages" group is age-standardized to account for the different vaccination rates of older and younger people.

Source: Centers for Disease Control and Prevention, Vaccine Breakthrough/Surveillance and Analytics Team – processed by Our World in Data. "Unvaccinated" [dataset]. Centers for Disease Control and Prevention, Vaccine Breakthrough/Surveillance and Analytics Team [original data]. Retrieved Feb 14, 2024 from https://ourworldindata.org/grapher/united-states-rates-of-covid-19-deaths-by-vaccination-status

of misinformation.[15,16] Even in the early stages of the American vaccination campaign, solid evidence emerged about vaccines' effectiveness in preventing death and hospitalization.[17] However, vaccine misinformation led a significant portion of citizens to make self-harming decisions. A glaring example is Texas, where nearly half of COVID-19 deaths recorded through August 24, 2022, occurred after May 1, 2021, when vaccines were already available. The study showed that 85% of COVID-19 deaths in 2021 happened among the unvaccinated, and during the Omicron wave in the first three months of 2022 death rates were 20 times higher among the unvaccinated than among those with booster shots.[18]

The "Texas tragedy" is just the tip of the iceberg. Various other studies have pointed out disparities in COVID-19 mortality rates and different prevalences of vaccination across American states. Those with political preferences favoring Republican candidates were particularly affected.[19] Notably, supporters of the Republican Party, influenced by figures like Donald Trump, who is known for spreading pandemic-related hoaxes, exhibited a greater propensity to spread and believe fake news about COVID-19 vaccines.[20,21] An empirical study highlighted a gap in COVID-19 excess death rates between Republicans and Democrats, especially in counties with low vaccination rates, after vaccines became widely available. Although other factors, such as chronic diseases, poverty, low education levels and health inequalities contribute to state-level differences in COVID mortality, further analyses adjusting for these variables supported the association between COVID-19 deaths and political preferences.[22-26] Several mechanisms influenced a significant number of Republican voters to avoid vaccination, including misperceptions of vaccine side effects which may have overshadowed the perceived danger of the virus. Additional scientific evidence revealed a negative association between vaccination rates and knowledge about the pandemic, highlighting the paradoxical yet logical effect of COVID-19 misinformation: the more you read, the less you know.[15, 27]

Especially in the initial months of the mass vaccination campaign, sensationalism in the mass media dominated public discourse, instilling anxiety and concern regarding vaccine administration. Some newspapers even dedicated front-page coverage to discussing the perceived serious adverse effects of vaccines, often relying on anecdotes or incomplete data.[28] The most commonly reported systemic adverse events after SARS-CoV-2 vaccine administration are fever, fatigue, headache and swelling or redness at the injection site. However, a few tragic cases did occur and nothing can ease the pain of losing a loved one. Scientists consistently maintain a unanimous stance, however: collectively the benefits of vaccination far outweigh the risks. A study published in *Nature* examined the effects of COVID-19 vaccines on adverse events such as myocarditis and pericarditis. Results highlighted that the risks of these events were lower among vaccinated individuals than among those who had tested positive for SARS-CoV-2.[29] Another study in *JAMA* found that full vaccination against COVID-19 was associated with a reduced risk of myocardial infarction and ischemic stroke after contracting COVID-19.[30] In late December 2022, the Cochrane Library published an extensive literature review on the effectiveness and safety of COVID-19 vaccines before the emergence of the Omicron variants. Analyzing data from 41 randomized controlled trials of 12 different COVID-19 vaccines involving nearly half a million people worldwide, the report concluded that, compared to a placebo, most vaccines reduced the most severe effects of COVID-19. Regarding serious adverse effects, no significant differences were found between most vaccines and the placebo effect, although findings could not be generalized to pregnant women or immunocompromised individuals.[31]

To reduce avoidable mortality due to vaccine hesitancy, it became imperative for government agencies and policymakers to address misinformation about the vaccine's potential adverse effects. Several issues contributed to the reluctance of many undecided individuals to get vaccinated. First, the swift development of vaccines raised concerns that the validation of scientific evidence had been rushed. However, a substantial body of highly credible scientific evidence has been meticulously produced in support of the safety and effectiveness of vaccines. Second, the novelty of mRNA vaccine technology, with no previously approved vaccines of this kind, led to uncertainty and doubt. Nevertheless, scientific analyses have provided ample assurances regarding the safety and effectiveness of this approach too. Third, vaccine hesitancy is the outcome of the relentless dissemination of fake news and conspiracy theories about vaccines, propagated by highly organized anti-vaccination movements. They produced tragic consequences. Dr. Brytney Cobia, a physician from Alabama, described several instances of young patients in critical conditions who, "before being intubated," pleaded to receive the vaccine when it was already "too late."[32]

Many scientists and public health experts acknowledge the need for more initiatives to increase public knowledge and awareness of these crucial preventive measures. Communication strategies could be enhanced by leveraging community commitment through the involvement of influential leaders and addressing the population's concerns. Research underscores the importance of public trust in both COVID-19 vaccines and those administering them. Policymakers, in their efforts to enhance trust and combat misinformation, must also address the needs of the most disadvantaged social groups. These groups often report lower levels of trust in the medical community and institutions, stemming from experiences of neglect and discrimination.[33] The literature stresses the crucial importance of communication strategies that avoid criminalizing those who refuse the vaccine. To effectively reduce vaccine hesitancy, research suggests that top-down approaches give way to programs involving local populations and communities in the decision to get vaccinated.[34,35] A dynamic and ongoing dialogue about vaccines is essential, particularly given the changing nature of vaccine hesitancy in the context of the pandemic. Expert analyses on the topic emphasize the fluidity of people's opinions, reject rigid categorizations and stress the persuasive power of communication based on scientific evidence.[36]

Frequently, those advocating for the effectiveness of COVID-19 vaccines have found themselves accused of unquestioningly "believing" in science, as if adhering to it were akin to religious conviction. In more extreme cases, individuals have been unfairly labeled as part of a power structure defending the interests of "Big Pharma." In my case, I have never received a penny from Big Pharma. On the contrary, my written contributions have often challenged policies that prioritize the profit of large pharmaceutical companies and harm public health. I have often critiqued intellectual property laws when they limit access to lifesaving tools such as vaccines, especially in economically disadvantaged countries.[37] Furthermore, my critical analyses have extended to free trade agreements like the TTIP (Transatlantic Trade and Investment Partnership USA-EU) and the legal clauses (notably the ISDS) frequently used by pharmaceutical multinationals to sue governments when regulations safeguarding public health indirectly affect their profits.[38]

"Natural" immunity?

One of the most important pieces of resistance embraced by anti-vaxxers is the argument of "natural" immunity. Here again, it is crucial to dispel myths and misconceptions surrounding the topic, acknowledging that, currently, there are no miracle solutions for fortifying the immune system. Many self-proclaimed naturalists and influencers have misinformed the public, offering a myriad of products and advice, from brewed coffee to protein powder and mystical roots from the Amazon rainforest to vitamin pills, all claimed to confer superhero-like immunity. Yet, scientific understanding of the immune system's optimal functioning is still very limited. Key questions, such as the types of cells required, their necessary activity levels and the precise quantity needed for optimal immune function, remain unanswered. Anyone asserting definitive knowledge on these aspects could be either misinformed or attempting to sell and promote unrealistic products or cures. It's crucial to approach claims of "immune system enhancement" with a high degree of skepticism and rely only on solid evidence-based knowledge. As of now, there are no magic pills that can enhance the immune system's resilience against viruses.[39]

Nevertheless, public health science must strive to comprehend why, given similar age, prior illnesses and viral load, some individuals succumbed to SARS-CoV-2 while others remained totally unaffected and even asymptomatic. Scientists aim to discern why certain individuals, in a metaphorical sense, "behave like bats," acting as exceptional viral reservoirs without suffering severe health consequences. In effect, bats exhibit unique immune responses, maintaining effective defenses without succumbing to excessive or self-destructive immune reactions, common in severe COVID-19 cases in humans. Bats showcase a "peaceful coexistence" with viruses, seemingly impervious to the harmful responses, like uncontrolled inflammation, rapid viral replication or organ damage, seen in severe human COVID-19 cases. Most research on "natural" immunity has primarily investigated the protection resulting from prior COVID-19 infections. Yet, what does science reveal about the natural immunity of individuals who, despite being infected and perhaps harboring a high viral load, not only avoid the severe effects of SARS-CoV-2 but also remain unaware of their infection?

Individual responses to infections are poorly understood and yet influenced by a myriad of factors, including genetic predispositions that can modulate the immune response to viruses. Each person's immune system varies, with some individuals being more adept at fighting viruses while others excel against bacteria. Understanding the specific biological mechanisms behind systemic inflammation associated with severe SARS-CoV-2 effects is crucial. Numerous studies have explored elements capable of improving the immune system. An article in the journal *Nature Immunology*, for instance, investigated the role of T lymphocytes in vaccine response.[40] Scientific evidence indicates that the response of T lymphocytes, often referred to as "killer cells" targeting viruses, is a critical component of immune protection against the SARS-CoV-2 virus. SARS-CoV-2-specific T cell responses are deemed essential for robust memory and for recognizing viral variants, and T lymphocytes, activated after vaccination, play a pivotal role in providing exceptional protection against hospitalization and death. Moreover, they feature prominently in the interplay between lifestyles and vaccination, influencing the biological response to the virus.

Scientific research has also investigated the role of risk or protective factors that predispose people to be more or less vulnerable to the manifestations of severe disease and post-acute sequelae of SARS-CoV-2.[41] Age, chronic diseases and pre-existing risk factors such as hypertension and obesity are established contributors to worse COVID-19 outcomes, although the precise mechanisms leading to severe outcomes are not entirely clear. According to a very large and detailed review of the scientific literature published in the *American Journal of Lifestyle Medicine*, there are three major biological mechanisms in the manifestations of severe disease and post-acute sequelae of SARS-CoV-2: (a) chronic non-resolvable inflammation, (b) alterations of the intestinal microbiome (dysbiosis and loss of beneficial microorganisms) and (c) compromised viral defenses. Aging, chronic diseases and pre-existing risk factors are all linked to a progressively less resolvable state of chronic inflammation. These conditions also seem to foster a dysbiotic gut microbiome, involving the loss of beneficial microorganisms crucial for maintaining intestinal barrier integrity and preventing unresolvable inflammation. In cases of severe COVID-19 outcomes, pre-existing conditions of inflammation and dysbiosis may be exacerbated by SARS-CoV-2, leading to systemic and uncontrolled inflammation, compromised immune defenses and a weakened viral control system unable to contain virus replication.

Despite the importance of genetic factors, age, previous diseases and other pre-existing risk factors in generating severe SARS-CoV-2 outcomes, an important part of this variability in response to the virus is linked to lifestyles and behaviors such as an unbalanced diet, physical inactivity, chronic psychological stress and exposure to environmental pollutants.[42] These factors act in synergy with each other and SARS-CoV-2 and seem to contribute to non-resolvable inflammation mechanisms with consequent compromise of immunity against pathogens. A prospective cohort study involving 1,981 women who tested positive for SARS-CoV-2 from April 2020 to November 2021 revealed that maintaining a healthy lifestyle, characterized by a normal body mass index, not smoking, a high-quality diet, moderate alcohol intake, regular exercise and consistent sleep patterns before SARS-CoV-2 infection offered protection against the long-term effects of COVID-19 disease.[43]

An adequate diet is necessary for the cells of the immune system to respond effectively to infections and phenomena such as chronic non-resolvable inflammation and dysbiosis. Some micronutrients, for example, appear to play a fundamental role in adaptive immune responses to viral infections, in particular in the regulation of pro- and anti-inflammatory responses. On the contrary, an unhealthy and unbalanced diet weakens adaptive immune responses through various mechanisms. While regular consumption of ultra-processed, excessively energy-dense, micronutrient-deficient foods promotes unresolvable inflammation, a diet low in fruits, vegetables, seeds and whole grains does not provide sufficient anti-inflammatory micronutrients. Furthermore, a diet predominantly based on ultra-processed foods is deficient in prebiotic dietary components, which are necessary to maintain the integrity of the intestinal barrier, to counteract unresolved inflammation and to support other vital functions. Finally, the accumulation of excess fat in a deep layer around the waist (visceral fat) is associated with dysfunctional immune defences against viruses such as SARS-CoV-2, as well as uncontrolled systemic inflammation.

Just like a healthy diet, regular exercise can be a critical factor in an individual's ability to reduce inflammatory markers and improve the efficiency of the immune system against the severe effects of COVID-19 disease.[44] Physical inactivity has been linked to dysbiosis of the gut microbiome, compromised integrity of the intestinal barrier and non-resolvable inflammation. A cohort study of 387,109 adults in the UK showed that physical inactivity increased the risk of hospitalization for COVID-19 by 32%. Another population-based study of 48,440 individuals in the United States showed that participants who were consistently inactive had a higher risk of hospitalization, intensive care unit admission and death than those who exercised regularly. A retrospective study of 552 patients hospitalized with COVID-19 in Spain estimated that a sedentary lifestyle was associated with an approximately 6-fold increase in mortality risk. Similar results were obtained from a nationwide cohort study of 12,768 adults in South Korea.[45] A case-control study of 196,444 participants also showed that regular physical activity was associated with improved vaccine efficacy against COVID-19 hospitalization, with higher levels of physical activity associated with greater vaccine efficacy.[46]

In addition to health-related behavioral factors such as diet and exercise, epidemiological research has also highlighted plausible links between chronic stress and the biological response to the virus. Stress responses seem to be implicated in the biological alterations that predispose to serious outcomes of the COVID-19 disease. Although there are no randomized experimental studies on behavioral and psychosocial factors related to the immune response to the COVID-19 virus, there is significant scientific evidence suggesting a possible link between these risk factors and COVID-19 outcomes. Using a national sample of US older adults, a study published in *PNAS* showed that exposure to social stress was associated with the distribution of T cells indicative of accelerated immune aging.[47] Stress can worsen immune defenses and induce the release of hormones such as cortisol and adrenaline, which are associated with insufficient immune regulation and contribute to the non-resolution of inflammation and alterations of the microbiome. Stressful living conditions interact with environmental factors such as urban air pollution to trigger inflammatory and oxidative stress pathways that increase the risk of severe COVID-19.[48] Chronic stress is also associated with a worsening of lifestyle and unhealthy behaviors such as an unbalanced diet, alcohol use and tobacco smoking, which can be conceptualized as self-medication or maladaptive coping strategies.

We already know our immune system's defenses can be influenced by vaccinations and previous infections. However, can it also be strengthened by interventions that modify our diet, exercise, chronic stress and living conditions in our everyday lives? Can interventions improving our lifestyles be complementary to virus containment and vaccination? Although the practice of strengthening the immune system does not automatically guarantee protection against the more serious effects caused by viruses such as SARS-CoV-2, evidence seems to suggest that the likelihood and severity of many viral infections can be significantly reduced if appropriate measures are taken to improve the effectiveness of the immune response to invading organisms.[42] Anti-inflammatory diets, rich in fiber, legumes, fruits and vegetables, seem to support the lung and intestinal microbiome and improve defenses against viral diseases. A diet rich in fiber and fruits and vegetables and high levels of omega-3 fatty acids can improve symptoms in individuals with severe effects of COVID-19 disease and reduce inflammation. It still seems unclear whether dietary supplements can help people maintain a healthier immune system. Available data, however, seem to suggest that the association of the unpredictable presence of new viral pathogens with a micronutrient deficiency represents a dual threat to health.[49]

The scientific evidence supporting the hypothesis that regular physical activity reduces the likelihood of non-resolving inflammation and promotes a healthy gut microbiome composition while reducing the severity of COVID-19 is equally promising. It is perhaps no coincidence that most athletes presented had a very low likelihood of experiencing severe SARS-CoV-2 health outcomes. While disinformation on the topic must still be fought, there is increasing scientific interest in systemic interventions against infectious diseases that consider "pre-existing health behaviors," including nutrition, physical exercise and the reduction of chronic stress, as complementary actions to the prevention and vaccination phases. Systematic reviews and meta-analyses of available studies also indicate that stress-reduction interventions such as cognitive-behavioral therapy, or stress reduction may help reduce non-resolving inflammation, a key predisposing factor for the sequelae of serious COVID-19 effects.[50–53]

While intervening in areas of diet, physical activity and stress may contribute to the prevalence of chronic conditions that significantly affect COVID-19 outcomes,[54] it's essential to recognize that these behavioral and psychosocial factors are influenced by the social, economic and environmental conditions in which individuals are born, live and work.[55–57] As concluded in a meta-analysis based on 43 studies, socioeconomic conditions are strong predictors of inflammatory markers such as CRP and IL-6. The study also showed that proinflammatory pathways are important mechanisms for understanding how socioeconomic inequalities translate into health inequalities.[58] Even contextual factors such as social cohesion and economic inequality seem to be involved in the association between individual-level socioeconomic position and inflammation.[59] Public policies affecting income, employment, housing, exposure to environmental agents can play a crucial role in shaping people's lifestyles and stress levels. Lifestyle and stress are not only resulting from individual choices but are substantially influenced by broader social and societal factors.[60] The disease burden of COVID-19 for example, has been shown to be more prevalent in countries with a higher level of economic inequalities.[61,62] These inequities can act as "causes of the causes" explaining why disenfranchised communities may be more susceptible to non-resolvable inflammation, microbiome dysbiosis and a higher risk of severe COVID-19, which, in turn, increases their risk of severe SARS-CoV-2 outcomes.

Effectively tackling a pandemic necessitates addressing these inequalities in lifestyle, stress and environmental exposure. Structural changes are vital to facilitate healthy lifestyles and reduce chronic stress for all members of society. This, for example, includes initiatives to lower the cost and increase access to health-promoting foods like fruits and vegetables.[63] Creating more green spaces, along with accessible walking and bicycle paths, can encourage physical activity. Policies that reduce stress, poverty and inequalities in health can also offer lasting benefits in improving mental and physical health.[64,65] Examples of structural interventions include social protection policies, guaranteed minimum income, unemployment benefits and regulations against environmental pollution.[66]

Endemic but still lethal

If some of the key shortcomings in pandemic management were inadequate prevention and vaccination and a lack of interventions to address social inequalities in health and health behaviors, another was the misconception of vaccines as magic bullets. Alongside suboptimal responses such as allowing the virus to spread ("laissez-faire the virus" strategy) or underestimating the importance of vaccines ("prevention only" strategy), the exclusive reliance on vaccination ("only vax" strategy") reduced the potential to save lives. While some countries adopted non-pharmaceutical interventions to curtail cases, hospitalizations and deaths, others opted to rely primarily on vaccines.[67] As emphasized repeatedly, vaccination undeniably stood as one of the crucial elements in COVID-19 containment measures. Yet, this strategy needed to be preceded and supported by infection control interventions and efforts to address social inequalities and access to vaccines.[68] In essence, prevention interventions and vaccination demanded equal attention in mitigating COVID-19 mortality as complementary strategies: while vaccination played a pivotal role in the latter stages of pandemic management, prevention emerged as the primary weapon to contain the impact of the virus, especially during the initial phases.[69]

Absolute faith in the capacity of vaccines to single-handedly solve the pandemic has led to false promises and illusions about their efficacy. During the early stages of the vaccination campaign, CDC Director Rochelle Walensky asserted that "the data suggest that ... vaccinated people do not transmit the virus."[70] This was an unrealistic expectation. Experts also spoke of vaccines as capable of "eliminating the correlation between infections and hospitalizations." However, evidence indicated that vaccines could only weaken, not eliminate, this association.[71] With the emergence of Omicron variants, vaccines, though effective in reducing mortality and hospitalization, proved largely ineffective in reducing infections. In some instances, they even fostered a false sense of security among vaccinated individuals, who could both contract and transmit the virus. As Professor Chris Goodnow from the Garvan Institute of Medical Research in Sydney emphasized, the belief that "variant-specific vaccines were the answer" to defeating the virus corresponded to an ambitious, yet quite unrealistic expectation.[72]

In January 2021, a survey published in *Nature* asked more than 100 immunologists, infectious disease researchers and virologists whether the coronavirus could be eradicated. Almost 90% of them responded that it would become endemic, circulating globally for years. Epidemiologist Michael Osterholm stated that eradicating the virus from the world was like "trying to plan to build a steppingstone path to the Moon. It's not realistic."[73]

Despite the awareness of not having been able to eliminate SARS-CoV-2, the optimistic perspective that the virus would become less lethal through a combination of vaccination and acquired immunity, however, proved to be correct. In September 2022, with SARS-CoV-2 still claiming approximately 500 lives per day in the United States, President Joe Biden "declared the pandemic over." Christian Drosten, head of virology at the Charité University Hospital in Berlin, shared a similar view,[74] and the same sentiment was expressed in Italy by the president of the Italian Medicines Association (AIFA).[75] As underlined in an editorial in the *New York Times* entitled "A Positive Covid Milestone,"[76] the decision to declare the "end of the pandemic" could be perhaps justified for at least two reasons: (a) observed decreasing trends in SARS-CoV-2 mortality, which in the first half of 2023 showed a clear reduction at a global level, and (b) historical series on excess mortality, which had returned to "quasi-normal" values compared to the number of deaths observed in the five-year period (2015–2019) preceding the pandemic.

Rather than declaring the end of the pandemic, cautious commentators emphasized the transition from "pandemic" to "endemic." The WHO defines pandemics, epidemics and endemic diseases based on the rate at which they spread. While an epidemic is characterized by an unexpected increase in the number of disease cases in a specific geographic area, a pandemic crosses international borders. This vast geographic reach is what causes pandemics to produce large-scale social upheaval, economic losses and general hardship. A virus is declared a pandemic when it produces large-scale social upheaval, economic losses and general hardship and covers a large area, affecting several countries and populations; a disease outbreak is endemic when it is constantly present but limited to a particular region, with predictable rates of disease spread.[77]

Although mortality data for SARS-CoV-2 in the first half of 2023 indicated a notable global reduction, as highlighted in the title of an editorial in *Nature*, "endemic doesn't mean harmless."[78] In September 2022, at the time the virus was declared "over," it continued to claim a significant number of lives in most of the world's regions. In the same year, despite the availability of vaccines highly effective in preventing COVID-19 deaths, official statistics reported nearly 1.2 million deaths. This made the pathogen milder but still more lethal than the regular flu, which, according to the Global Pandemic Mortality Project II, causes between 294,000 and 518,000 deaths globally each year.[79] Clinical epidemiologist Deepti Gurdasani from Queen Mary University of London aptly explained, "I think endemicity is one of the least understood and most misused terms by many scientists who have suggested that endemicity is somehow a good thing. Endemicity is essentially what we see for many diseases now, including malaria. And malaria kills millions of people."[80]

Undoubtedly, the effects of mass vaccination and immunity acquired through previous infections changed the face of the pandemic and significantly reduced the mortality burden of COVID-19. However, the enthusiasm for these achievements was tempered by at least three types of arguments. First, in the early months of 2023, many countries stopped counting or changed the way they recorded COVID-19 deaths, making it much more difficult to discern the true impact of the pandemic. Second, although the 2023 excess mortality in countries such as the United States aligns with that of the previous five years, it's important to note that these preceding years include the worst mortality crisis since the Second World War. Globally, when considering the five-year period from 2015 to 2019, data from 2023 indicated a 5% increase in excess mortality compared to the pre-pandemic period, resulting in 3 million excess deaths.[81] Third, the choice to declare "the end of the pandemic" and let the virus spread globally led to an explosion of infections and cases of long COVID. As estimated in an article published in *Nature*, approximately one in five people infected with the virus developed long COVID, and globally, as of January 2023, at least 65 million people suffered from this debilitating condition.[82] While the desire to "go back to normal" was understandable, the reality was that even if the virus was declared over, it didn't know it. As argued by WHO officials, there are many Omicron subvariants circulating around the world, but "the virus is not gone. It is changing. It is still killing."[83] Rather than learning "to live with the virus," it would be more appropriate to say that we have simply surrendered to it.

Variants of concern and nation "super spreaders"

A common piece of misinformation circulating among anti-vaxxers is the attribution of the spread of new variants to vaccines. While Omicron variants reduced the effectiveness of vaccines in slowing infections,[84] the assertion that vaccines are the major causes of new variants lacks any support in scientific literature. Quite the contrary, evidence shows that vaccines, by preventing transmission, have helped to reduce, not increase, the risk of new mutations.[85] Yet, an important question remains: where did all these new variants come from? Evolutionary biologists and infectious disease epidemiologists at the University of Pittsburgh have studied this phenomenon by tracing the evolution of pathogens like the coronavirus. Their analyses concluded that the emergence of new contagious variants has been mainly driven by uncontrolled transmission of infections. Such conclusions align with findings that appeared in another article in the New England Journal of Medicine (NEJM), emphasizing the link between high transmission and the increased likelihood of mutations. It is like playing Russian roulette with the virus. Allowing it to spread without making any attempt at prevention creates new opportunities for mutations. Although the latest pandemic waves have indeed become milder in line with more optimistic predictions, it has been a dangerous gamble to assume that viruses necessarily evolve toward less lethality.

If the rapid spread of the virus is the key driver of new variants, the most important way to limit their development is to reduce the number of cases through non-pharmacological interventions.[86] Prevention actions not only reduce infections but also contribute to the effectiveness of mass vaccination campaigns. An article published in *Cell* supports this hypothesis, emphasizing that to prevent the rapid spread of potentially more transmissible SARS-CoV-2 variants key interventions include the use of masks, reduction of social contacts, effective testing and tracing, outbreak identification and control, support for isolation and quarantine and vaccination.[87] Vaccination, however, had to be supported by global solidarity and a cosmopolitan effort aimed at reaching populations with greater socioeconomic difficulties, especially in developing countries.[88,89] Unfortunately, as already stated, rather than investing in prevention and global aid to ensure greater vaccination coverage in poor nations, high-income countries pursued policies protecting their national interests and the profit motives of "Big Pharma." Determining whether, for example, the first Omicron variant that originated in Botswana and South Africa has been facilitated by these nations' poor vaccination coverage is difficult.[90] In March 2021, Oxfam International reported the results of a survey of global epidemiology experts, with the vast majority acknowledging that persistent low vaccination coverage in many countries increased the likelihood of vaccine-resistant mutations.

Understanding whether global inequalities in access to vaccines, on top of having allowed the virus to spread, contributed to the proliferation of new variants, is a challenging task.[33] Yet, it is even more difficult to examine how this "vaccine apartheid" interacted with the "laissez-faire approach to the virus" in producing these outcomes. Devi Sridhar, Professor of Global Public Health at the University of Edinburgh, emphasized, "The more the virus circulates, the more likely it is that mutations and variants will emerge, which could render our current vaccines ineffective. At the same time, poor countries have been left behind without vaccines ..."[91] A paper published in *Nature*, echoed the same idea arguing that countries that have opted to "live with the virus" and abandoned prevention measures seem to have significantly contributed to the proliferation of new variants.[92] The topic has also been addressed in an editorial by Ngaire Woods and Anna Petherick, both at the Blavatnik School of Government, University of Oxford. According to the two academics, many G20 countries acted as "COVID-19 super spreaders" in the initial phases of the pandemic when, by failing to contain the virus through effective policies, they contributed to its worldwide spread. "Had they acted sooner," the authors added, "they could have at least slowed its transmission to poorer countries. Worse still, their failure to commit to vaccinating the whole world as quickly as possible has created a self-defeating cycle where more transmissible and harmful variants of the virus are likely to be unleashed."[93]

Indeed, the Western world's collective reluctance to cooperate in the global fight against the virus has been remarkable. While the zero-COVID strategy helped to avert the emergence of new variants of concern, it proved unsustainable without international solidarity, particularly from the world's wealthiest and most influential nations. Rather than joining forces to safeguard global health, some nations acted as inadvertent "super spreaders," a term typically reserved for individuals who disproportionately contribute to infecting large populations and accelerate the pace and severity of an outbreak. Examining the origins of major variants provides some intriguing insights: the Alpha variant originated in the UK, Beta in South Africa, Gamma in Brazil, Delta in India, Omicron in South Africa and the XBB.1.5 variant in the United States. Is it mere coincidence that these mutations emerged from highly populated countries with significant COVID-19 infections and outbreaks? Maybe. Furthermore, it is noteworthy that countries that prioritized stringent measures to contain the virus, such as Singapore, Vietnam, Japan, New Zealand, Australia, and South Korea, have not been sources of major variants of concern. Another coincidence?

"Catapulting infections"

After the declaration of "the end of the pandemic" or the "surrender to the virus," the "laissez-faire the virus" approach went global. The advocates of the herd immunity mirage declared victory. For them, preventive measures were useless. In their opinion, the significant number of deaths caused by Omicron variants in the very same "healthy nations" that adopted effective prevention policies in the early phases of the pandemic proved the futility of their approach.

A notable case of a virtuous nation struggling with the overwhelming impact of Omicron variants has been Hong Kong. Hong Kong, a special administrative region of China, is an interesting case because in the early phases of the pandemic it adopted a zero-COVID policy, resulting in one of the world's lowest COVID-19 mortality indicators. With the emergence of the Omicron variants, however, death rates increased rapidly, making Hong Kong one of the most afflicted countries by COVID-19 mortality rates in East Asia. Critics of the zero-COVID strategy maintain that early testing, tracing and isolation activities adopted in Hong Kong have only postponed the inevitable impact of the virus. However, this argument lacks epidemiological support. Despite the Omicron waves, "virtuous states" that adopted these activities continued to exhibit significantly lower COVID-19 deaths per million population than nations that neglected prevention interventions.

To understand what happened in Hong Kong, it is crucial to analyze the management of the COVID-19 pandemic in two distinct phases: the (pre-vaccine) prevention phase and the vaccination phase. In the initial stages of the pandemic, preventive strategies such as testing, tracing and isolation, along with strict border controls, were key to controlling the virus. These interventions were successfully employed in various countries, including Hong Kong, and there is substantial evidence supporting their effectiveness. However, the landscape changed with the emergence of new variants with highly transmissible characteristics, particularly Omicron. Fortunately, these variants turned out to be less deadly and became dominant at a time when vaccinations were widely available. Yet, while some countries effectively managed both phases of the pandemic (prevention in the early phase and vaccination later), countries such as Hong Kong faced challenges in transitioning between the two. Despite successful management in the prevention phase, the nation struggled to capitalize on its earlier successes.[94] When the Omicron variants became dominant, over half of Hong Kong's elderly population had not completed the full vaccination course, including booster doses. Moreover, the vaccines administered in Hong Kong, primarily produced in China, demonstrated lower efficacy than those distributed in Europe and the United States. As emphasized in an article published in *Emerging Microbes & Infections*, the exceptionally high mortality rate during the fifth wave of COVID-19 in Hong Kong can be attributed to the tragic loss of elderly individuals (many in nursing homes) who were either unvaccinated or not fully or effectively vaccinated.[95] The case of Hong Kong not only stressed the importance of combining prevention and vaccination efforts in a complementary way but also dispelled the misconception of comparing Omicron to a common cold. As highlighted by Martin Hibberd, a professor of emerging infectious diseases, Omicron can be mild for those who are vaccinated, but deadly for those who are not.[96]

The Hong Kong case also underscores the importance of a coordinated international response, emphasizing cooperation, solidarity and collective responsibility for public health among nations. The excellent management of the pandemic by some virtuous nations in the early phases of the pandemic did not guarantee protection from the virus later on because of the high transmissibility of the new variants. While Hong Kong did its best to reduce the chance of mutations by adopting rigorous prevention interventions, its efforts could not do much against Omicron. The nation paid dearly for the ineptitude of those nations that allowed the virus to mutate rapidly. It is a typical example of the "tragedy of the commons," a situation where individuals use a common good for their own interests and end up harming the larger community they belong to. As noted by Rob Wallace during a webinar organized in my global health course at the University of Padova, by providing greater opportunities for the virus to replicate and create mutations, "super-spreader countries" have metaphorically "catapulted their dead bodies into the fortresses of virtuous countries," making preventive actions ineffective in containing new infections. The metaphor refers to a historical episode of bacteriological warfare during the siege of Caffa, a prosperous Genoese colony on the route to the East, by the Tatar and Mongol tribes. Leading the nomadic armies was Ganī Bek, a descendant of Genghis Khan. The soldiers of the Golden Horde were already infected with a deadly virus. Aware that time was running out to win the war, the khan made a cruel, lethal, and ingenious decision: he ordered his men's infected corpses to be tied to catapults and launched into the fortress of Caffa, thereby spreading the deadly virus within the enemy city. This event marked the onset of the Black Death in the year 1346.

References

1. De Vogli R. Covid, tra le prove sull'efficacia dei vaccini e le opinioni di alcuni c'è un mare di disinformazione. Il Fatto Quotidiano. Published online Dec 9, 2022. https://www.ilfattoquotidiano.it/2022/12/09/covid-tra-le-prove-sullefficacia-dei-vaccini-e-le-opinioni-di-alcuni-ce-un-mare-di-disinformazione/6897597/ (accessed Jan 24, 2024).
2. Redazione. Bufera sul sottosegretario alla Salute Gemmato: 'Non c'è la prova che senza vaccini saremmo stati peggio'. Letta (Pd): 'Ora si dimetta'. E lui fa retromarcia. Open. Published online Nov 15, 2022. https://www.open.online/2022/11/15/governo-meloni-marcello-gemmato-vaccini/ (accessed Jan 24, 2024).
3. EpiCentro. Sorveglianza integrata COVID-19: i principali dati nazionali. Istituto Superiore di Sanità. https://www.epicentro.iss.it/coronavirus/sars-cov-2-sorveglianza-dati (accessed Jan 24, 2024).
4. Mathieu E, Roser M. How do death rates from COVID-19 differ between people who are vaccinated and those who are not? *Our World in Data*. Published online Dec 28, 2023. https://ourworldindata.org/covid-deaths-by-vaccination (accessed Jan 24, 2024).
5. Schreiber M. Who is dying from COVID now and why. Scientific American. https://www.scientificamerican.com/article/who-is-dying-from-covid-now-and-why/ (accessed Jan 24, 2024).
6. Rahmani K, Shavaleh R, Forouhi M, *et al.* The effectiveness of COVID-19 vaccines in reducing the incidence, hospitalization, and mortality from COVID-19: a systematic review and meta-analysis. *Frontiers in Public Health* 2022; **10**. https://doi.org/10.3389/fpubh.2022.873596.
7. Ssentongo P, Ssentongo AE, Voleti N, *et al.* SARS-CoV-2 vaccine effectiveness against infection, symptomatic and severe COVID-19: a systematic review and meta-analysis. *BMC Infectious Diseases* 2022; **22**: 439.
8. Korang SK, Rohden E von, Veroniki AA, *et al.* Vaccines to prevent COVID-19: a living systematic review with trial sequential analysis and network meta-analysis of randomized clinical trials. *PLoS One* 2022; **17**: e0260733.
9. COVID-19 vaccine efficacy summary. Institute for Health Metrics and Evaluation. Published online Nov 18, 2022. https://www.healthdata.org/research-analysis/diseases-injuries/covid/covid-19-vaccine-efficacy-summary (accessed Jan 24, 2024).

10. Watson OJ, Barnsley G, Toor J, Hogan AB, Winskill P, Ghani AC. A preliminary assessment of COVAX's impact in lower-income countries. May, 2023. https://www.gavi.org/news-resources/knowledge-products/preliminary-assessment-covaxs-impact-lower-income-countries (accessed Jan 24, 2024).
11. Watson OJ, Barnsley G, Toor J, Hogan AB, Winskill P, Ghani AC. Global impact of the first year of COVID-19 vaccination: a mathematical modelling study. *The Lancet Infectious Diseases* 2022; **22**: 1293–302.
12. Radio Radio. Frajese presenta lo studio Cureus che fa luce sui morti in eccesso. Guardate i dati manipolati. Published online on Aug 6, 2023. https://www.radio-radio.it/2023/08/frajese-studio-cureus-nature-morti-germania/
13. EU excess mortality above the baseline in May 2023. Products Eurostat News. Published online July 14, 2023. https://ec.europa.eu/eurostat/web/products-euro-stat-news/w/ddn-20230714-2 (accessed Jan 24, 2024).
14. Excess deaths associated with COVID-19. Centers for Disease Control (CDC). Published online Sept 28, 2023. https://www.cdc.gov/nchs/nvss/vsrr/covid19/ex-cess_deaths.htm (accessed Jan 24, 2024).
15. Pierri F, Perry BL, DeVerna MR, *et al.* Online misinformation is linked to early COVID-19 vaccination hesitancy and refusal. *Scientific Reports* 2022; **12**: 5966.
16. de Albuquerque Veloso Machado M, Roberts B, Wong BLH, van Kessel R, Mossialos E. The relationship between the COVID-19 pandemic and vaccine hesitancy: a scoping review of literature until August 2021. *Frontiers in Public Health* 2021; **9**. https://doi.org/10.3389/fpubh.2021.747787.
17. Chen X, Huang H, Ju J, Sun R, Zhang J. Impact of vaccination on the COVID-19 pandemic in U.S. states. *Scientific Reports* 2022; **12**: 1554.
18. Hotez PJ. The great Texas COVID tragedy. *PLOS Global Public Health* 2022; **2**: e0001173.
19. Wallace J, Goldsmith-Pinkham P, Schwartz JL. Excess death rates for Republican and Democratic registered voters in Florida and Ohio during the COVID-19 pandemic. *JAMA Internal Medicine* 2023; **183**: 916–23.
20. Guess A, Nagler J, Tucker J. Less than you think: prevalence and predictors of fake news dissemination on Facebook. *Science Advances* 2019; **5**: eaau4586.
21. Calvillo DP, Ross BJ, Garcia RJB, Smelter TJ, Rutchick AM. Political ideology predicts perceptions of the threat of COVID-19 (and susceptibility to fake news about it). *Social Psychological and Personality Science* 2020; **11**: 1119–28. https://doi.org/10.1177/1948550620940539.
22. Parzuchowski AS, Peters AT, Johnson-Sasso CP, Rydland KJ, Feinglass JM. County-level association of COVID-19 mortality with 2020 United States presidential voting. *Public Health* 2021; **198**: 114–7.
23. Gao J, Radford BJ. Death by political party: The relationship between COVID-19 deaths and political party affiliation in the United States. *World Medical & Health Policy* 2021; **13**: 224–49.
24. Liebl D, Schüwer U. Pro-Trump partisanship and COVID-19 mortality: a model-based counterfactual analysis. Published online Oct 26, 2021. https://doi.org/10.2139/ssrn.3924620.
25. Cegan JC, Trump BD, Cibulsky SM, *et al.* Can comorbidity data explain cross-state and cross-national difference in COVID-19 death rates? *Risk Management and Healthcare Policy* 2021; **14**: 2877–85.
26. Morris DS. Polarization, partisanship, and pandemic: the relationship between county-level support for Donald Trump and the spread of Covid-19 during the spring and summer of 2020. *Social Science Quarterly* 2021; **102**: 2412–31.
27. Hoffman YSG, Levin Y, Palgi Y, Goodwin R, Ben-Ezra M, Greenblatt-Kimron L. Vaccine hesitancy prospectively predicts nocebo side-effects following COVID-19 vaccination. *Scientific Reports* 2022; **12**: 20018.

28. Davies C. Harm to AstraZeneca jab's reputation 'probably killed thousands'. The Guardian. Published online Feb 7, 2022. https://www.theguardian.com/society/2022/feb/07/doubts-cast-over-astrazeneca-jab-probably-killed-thousands-covid-vaccine (accessed Jan 24, 2024).

29. Patone M, Mei XW, Handunnetthi L, et al. Risks of myocarditis, pericarditis, and cardiac arrhythmias associated with COVID-19 vaccination or SARS-CoV-2 infection. *Nature Medicine* 2022; **28**: 410–22.

30. Kim Y-E, Huh K, Park Y-J, Peck KR, Jung J. Association between vaccination and acute myocardial infarction and ischemic stroke after COVID-19 infection. *JAMA* 2022; **328**: 887–9.

31. Efficacy and safety of COVID-19 vaccines. Cochrane. Dec 7, 2022. https://www.cochrane.org/news/cochrane-review-covid-19-vaccines-shows-they-are-effective (accessed Jan 24, 2024).

32. Diaz N. "Younger, sicker, quicker": Doctors plead for vaccinations as US hospitals fill with young patients. World Socialist Web Site. Published online Aug 9, 2021. https://www.wsws.org/en/articles/2021/08/09/yout-a09.html (accessed Jan 24, 2024).

33. Wouters OJ, Shadlen KC, Salcher-Konrad M, et al. Challenges in ensuring global access to COVID-19 vaccines: production, affordability, allocation, and deployment. *The Lancet* 2021; **397**: 1023–34.

34. Wells K, Moore KL, Bednarczyk R. Supporting immunization programs to address COVID-19 vaccine hesitancy: recommendations for national and community-based stakeholders. *Vaccine* 2022; **40**: 2819–22.

35. Berdzuli N, Datta SS. How to tackle inequitable access, vaccine hesitancy, and other barriers to achieve high vaccine uptake. *BMJ* 2022; **377**: o1094.

36. Larson HJ, Gakidou E, Murray CJL. The vaccine-hesitant moment. *New England Journal of Medicine* 2022; **387**: 58–65.

37. Roberto De Vogli Blog | Vaccino Covid, sui brevetti vince il diritto al profitto di pochi. Il Fatto Quotidiano. Published online June 24, 2021. https://www.ilfattoquotidiano.it/2021/06/24/vaccino-covid-sui-brevetti-vince-il-diritto-al-profitto-di-pochi/6239703/ (accessed Jan 24, 2024).

38. De Vogli R, Renzetti N. The potential impact of the Transatlantic Trade and Investment Partnership (TTIP) on public health. *Epidemiologia e Prevenzione* 2016; **40**: 95–102.

39. The myth of a 'super-charged' immune system. BBC News. Published online Feb 1, 2022. https://www.bbc.com/news/health-60171592 (accessed Jan 24, 2024).

40. Moss P. The T cell immune response against SARS-CoV-2. *Nature Immunology* 2022; **23**: 186–93.

41. Enichen E, Harvey C, Demmig-Adams B. COVID-19 spotlights connections between disease and multiple lifestyle factors. *American Journal of Lifestyle Medicine* 2022; **17**: 231–57.

42. Monye I, Adelowo AB. Strengthening immunity through healthy lifestyle practices: recommendations for lifestyle interventions in the management of COVID-19. *Lifestyle Medicine* 2020; **1**: e7.

43. Wang S, Li Y, Yue Y, et al. Adherence to healthy lifestyle prior to infection and risk of post–COVID-19 condition. *JAMA Internal Medicine* 2023; **183**: 232–41.

44. Thirupathi A, Wang M, Lin JK, et al. Effect of different exercise modalities on oxidative stress: a systematic review. *BioMed Research International* 2021; **2021**: 1947928.

45. Gualano B. Evidence-based physical activity for COVID-19: what do we know and what do we need to know? *British Journal of Sports Medicine* 2022; **56**: 653–4. https://bjsm.bmj.com/content/56/12/653.

46. Collie S, Saggers RT, Bandini R, *et al.* Association between regular physical activity and the protective effect of vaccination against SARS-CoV-2 in a South African case-control study. *British Journal of Sports Medicine* 2023; 57: 205–11.
47. Klopack ET, Crimmins EM, Cole SW, Seeman TE, Carroll JE. Social stressors associated with age-related T lymphocyte percentages in older US adults: evidence from the US Health and Retirement Study. *Proceedings of the National Academy of Sciences* 2022; **119**: e2202780119.
48. Vogel CFA, Van Winkle LS, Esser C, Haarmann-Stemmann T. The aryl hydrocarbon receptor as a target of environmental stressors - Implications for pollution mediated stress and inflammatory responses. *Redox Biology* 2020; **34**: 101530.
49. Gorji A, Khaleghi Ghadiri M. Potential roles of micronutrient deficiency and immune system dysfunction in the coronavirus disease 2019 (COVID-19) pandemic. *Nutrition* 2021; **82**: 111047. https://doi.org/10.1016/j.nut.2020.111047.
50. Djalilova DM, Schulz PS, Berger AM, Case AJ, Kupzyk KA, Ross AC. Impact of yoga on inflammatory biomarkers: a systematic review. *Biological Research for Nursing* 2019; **21**: 198–209.
51. Moreira FP, Cardoso T de A, Mondin TC, *et al.* The effect of proinflammatory cytokines in cognitive behavioral therapy. *Journal of Neuroimmunology* 2015; **285**: 143–6.
52. Pascoe MC, Thompson DR, Jenkins ZM, Ski CF. Mindfulness mediates the physiological markers of stress: systematic review and meta-analysis. *Journal of Psychiatric Research* 2017; **95**: 156–78.
53. Sanada K, Montero-Marin J, Barceló-Soler A, *et al.* Effects of mindfulness-based interventions on biomarkers and low-grade inflammation in patients with psychiatric disorders: a meta-analytic review. *International Journal of Molecular Sciences* 2020; **21**: 2484.
54. LeWine H. How to boost your immune system. Harvard Health. Published online, March 28, 2024. https://www.health.harvard.edu/staying-healthy/how-to-boost-your-immune-system (accessed July 1, 2024).
55. De Vogli R, Brunner E, Marmot MG. Unfairness and the social gradient of metabolic syndrome in the Whitehall II Study. *Journal of Psychosomatic Research* 2007; **63**: 413–9.
56. Gimeno D, Delclos GL, Ferrie JE, *et al.* Association of CRP and IL-6 with lung function in a middle-aged population initially free from self-reported respiratory problems: the Whitehall II Study. *European Journal of Epidemiology* 2011; **26**: 135–44.
57. De Vogli R, Ferrie JE, Chandola T, Kivimäki M, Marmot MG. Unfairness and health: evidence from the Whitehall II Study. *Journal of Epidemiology and Community Health* 2007; **61**: 513–8.
58. Muscatell KA, Brosso SN, Humphreys KL. Socioeconomic status and inflammation: a meta-analysis. *Molecular Psychiatry* 2020; **25**: 2189–99.
59. Oberndorfer M, Leyland AH, Pearce J, Grabovac I, Hannah MK, Dorner TE. Unequally unequal? Contextual-level status inequality and social cohesion moderating the association between individual-level socioeconomic position and systemic chronic inflammation. *Social Science & Medicine* 2023; **333**: 116185.
60. Institute of Medicine (US) Committee on Capitalizing on Social Science and Behavioral Research to Improve the Public's Health; Smedley BD, Syme SL. Legal and public policy interventions to advance the population's health. In: *Promoting Health: Intervention Strategies from Social and Behavioral Research*. National Academies Press (US), 2000. https://www.ncbi.nlm.nih.gov/books/NBK222835/ (accessed Jan 24, 2024).
61. Su D, Alshehri K, Pagán J. Income inequality and the disease burden of COVID-19: survival analysis of data from 74 countries. *Preventive Medicine Reports* 2022; **27**: 101828.

62. Ataguba JE-O, Birungi C, Cunial S, Kavanagh M. Income inequality and pandemics: insights from HIV/AIDS and COVID-19 – a multicountry observational study. *BMJ Glob Health* 2023; **8**: e013703.
63. Siddiqui F, Salam RA, Lassi ZS, Das JK. The intertwined relationship between malnutrition and poverty. *Frontiers in Public Health* 2020; **8**: 453.
64. Sfm C, Van Cauwenberg J, Maenhout L, Cardon G, Lambert EV, Van Dyck D. Inequality in physical activity, global trends by income inequality and gender in adults. *The International Journal of Behavioral Nutrition and Physical Activity* 2020; **17**: 142.
65. Andrea SB, Messer LC, Marino M, Goodman JM, Boone-Heinonen J. The tipping point: could increasing the subminimum wage reduce poverty-related antenatal stressors in U.S. women? *Annals of Epidemiology* 2020; **45**: 47–53.e6.
66. Ferrarini T, Nelson K, Sjöberg O. Decomposing the effect of social policies on population health and inequalities: an empirical example of unemployment benefits. *Scandinavian Journal of Public Health* 2014; **42**: 635–42.
67. Diseases TLI. The COVID-19 exit strategy – why we need to aim low. *The Lancet Infectious Diseases* 2021; **21**: 297.
68. Bowie C, Friston K. A 12-month projection to September 2022 of the COVID-19 epidemic in the UK using a dynamic causal model. *Frontiers in Public Health* 2022; **10**. https://www.frontiersin.org/articles/10.3389/fpubh.2022.999210.
69. Bollyky TJ, Castro E, Aravkin AY, *et al.* Assessing COVID-19 pandemic policies and behaviours and their economic and educational trade-offs across US states from Jan 1, 2020, to July 31, 2022: an observational analysis. *The Lancet* 2023; **401**: 1341–60. https://doi.org/10.1016/S0140-6736(23)00461-0.
70. Brueck AH Hilary. CDC director says data 'suggests that vaccinated people do not carry the virus'. Business Insider. https://www.businessinsider.com/cdc-director-data-vaccinated-people-do-not-carry-covid-19-2021-3 (accessed Jan 24, 2024).
71. Indie_SAGE. YouTube. Published online Aug 13, 2021. https://www.youtube.com/watch?v=OQCwJfEh5Ds (accessed Jan 24, 2024).
72. Three myths about COVID-19 — and the biggest challenge that lies ahead. ABC News. https://www.abc.net.au/news/health/2022-07-29/covid-19-three-myths-challenge-lies-ahead/101274980 (accessed Jan 24, 2024).
73. Phillips N. The coronavirus is here to stay — here's what that means. *Nature* 2021; **590**: 382–4.
74. Deutsche Welle. Top German virologist says COVID-19 pandemic is over. DW. Published online Dec 26, 2022. https://www.dw.com/en/top-german-virologist-says-covid-19-pandemic-is-over/a-64214994 (accessed Jan 24, 2024).
75. Bucci E. Caro Palù, ma quale fine della pandemia? Un ripasso di Darwin. Il Foglio. Published online Dec 21, 2022. https://www.ilfoglio.it/scienza/2022/12/21/news/caro-palu-ma-quale-fine-della-pandemia-un-ripasso-di-darwin-4782448/ (accessed Jan 24, 2024).
76. Leonhart D. A positive Covid milestone. *The New York Times*. Published online July 17, 2023. https://www.nytimes.com/2023/07/17/briefing/covid.html (accessed Jan 24, 2024).
77. Epidemic, endemic, pandemic: what are the differences? Columbia University Mailman School of Public Health. Published online Feb 19, 2021. https://www.publichealth.columbia.edu/news/epidemic-endemic-pandemic-what-are-differences (accessed Jan 24, 2024).
78. Katzourakis A. COVID-19: endemic doesn't mean harmless. *Nature* 2022; **601**: 485–485.
79. Paget J, Spreeuwenberg P, Charu V, *et al.* Global mortality associated with seasonal influenza epidemics: new burden estimates and predictors from the GLaMOR Project. *Journal of Global Health* 2019; **9**: 020421.

80. Mateus B. "This is a virus that we need to eliminate" – Dr. Deepti Gurdasani condemns "herd immunity" policies. World Socialist Web Site. Published online Aug 2, 2021 https://www.wsws.org/en/articles/2021/08/02/gurd-a02.html

81. The Economist. Our model suggests that global deaths remain 5% above pre-Covid forecasts. Published online on May 23, 2023. https://www.economist.com/graphic-detail/2023/05/23/our-model-suggests-that-global-deaths-remain-5-above-pre-covid-forecasts#

82. Davis HE, McCorkell L, Vogel JM, Topol EJ. Long COVID: major findings, mechanisms and recommendations. *Nature Reviews Microbiology* 2023; **21**: 133–46.

83. Chadwick L. "It's not gone. It's changing. It's killing": The COVID variants the WHO is watching closely. Euro News. Published online Nov 24, 2023 https://www.euronews.com/health/2023/11/24/its-not-gone-its-changing-its-killing-the-covid-variants-who-is-watching-closely (accessed Feb 2, 2024).

84. Stokel-Walker C. What do we know about Covid vaccines and preventing transmission? *BMJ* 2022; **376**: o298.

85. Lowe D. Vaccines will not produce worse variants. Science. Published online Sep 10, 2021. https://www.science.org/content/blog-post/vaccines-will-not-produce-worse-variants (accessed Jan 24, 2024).

86. Cooper V., Harrison L. What is causing all these new coronavirus variants? Is It the COVID-19 vaccines? SciTechDaily. Published online Sept 11, 2021. https://scitechdaily.com/what-is-causing-all-these-new-coronavirus-variants-is-it-the-covid-19-vaccines/ (accessed Jan 24, 2024).

87. Grubaugh ND, Hodcroft EB, Fauver JR, Phelan AL, Cevik M. Public health actions to control new SARS-CoV-2 variants. *Cell* 2021; **184**: 1127–32.

88. Sands P, Steiner A. Safely reopening requires testing, tracing and isolation, not just vaccines. Scientific American. https://www.scientificamerican.com/article/safely-reopening-requires-testing-tracing-and-isolation-not-just-vaccines/ (accessed Jan 24, 2024).

89. Krause PR, Fleming TR, Longini IM, *et al*. SARS-CoV-2 variants and vaccines. *The New England Journal of Medicine* 2021; **385**: 179–86.

90. Callaway E. What Omicron's BA.4 and BA.5 variants mean for the pandemic. *Nature* 2022; **606**: 848–9.

91. Two-thirds of epidemiologists warn mutations could render current COVID vaccines ineffective in a year or less. Oxfam International. Published online Mar 30, 2021. https://www.oxfam.org/en/press-releases/two-thirds-epidemiologists-warn-mutations-could-render-current-covid-vaccines (accessed Jan 24, 2024).

92. Markov PV, Katzourakis A, Stilianakis NI. Antigenic evolution will lead to new SARS-CoV-2 variants with unpredictable severity. *Nature Reviews Microbiology* 2022; **20**: 251–2.

93. Woods N, Petherick A. The rich world's super-spreader shame. Project Syndicate. Published online Aug 11, 2021. https://www.project-syndicate.org/commentary/g20-countries-are-covid19-super-spreaders-by-ngaire-woods-and-anna-petherick-2021-08 (accessed Feb 2, 2024).

94. Taylor L. Covid-19: Hong Kong reports world's highest death rate as zero Covid strategy fails. *BMJ* 2022; **376**: o707.

95. Cheung P-HH, Chan C-P, Jin D-Y. Lessons learned from the fifth wave of COVID-19 in Hong Kong in early 2022. *Emerging Microbes & Infections* 2022; **11**: 1072–8.

96. Burki T. Dynamic zero COVID policy in the fight against COVID. *The Lancet Respiratory Medicine* 2022; **10**: e58–9.

8
SUPPORT

"The coronavirus pandemic is a human tragedy of potentially biblical proportions … It's the proper role of the state to deploy its balance sheet to protect citizens and the economy … The priority must not only be providing basic income … We must protect people from losing their jobs in the first place … [and] fully mobilize the entire financial system … a change in mindset is as necessary in this crisis as it would be in times of war. Loss of income is not the fault of those who suffer from it. The cost of hesitation can be irreversible."[1] These are the words of the former head of the European Central Bank, Mario Draghi, in a famous editorial that appeared in the *Financial Times* in early 2020. Months later he would become the prime minister of Italy. In the first months of his mandate, his government would receive hundreds of billions of euros from European financial institutions for the country's economic recovery. If Draghi's initial intentions made one think of an economic revolution, the reforms adopted by his government have instead brought everyone back to reality. The pandemic required vigorous interventions capable of cushioning the impact of the crisis on the lives of the people most affected, but Draghi's government's policies did not live up to the expectations raised by his speech.

The importance of socioeconomic support during the pandemic found resonance elsewhere, though. In Taiwan, for example, interventions supporting both the population and the economy have been taken more seriously. The government stressed that free access to prevention tools such as swabs and providing people with economic guarantees regarding their livelihoods during isolation and quarantine increased adherence to prevention measures and compliance with self-isolation rules. As noted by Vice President of Taiwan

DOI: 10.4324/9781003511977-11

and epidemiology expert Chien Chien-Jen, socioeconomic supports were as important as containment strategies in fighting the pandemic.[2]

To self-isolate or not to self-isolate? Inequity is the problem

In the ongoing battle against the virus, the efficacy of preventive measures has hinged on a crucial factor: the willingness of individuals to self-isolate after testing positive and notify their close contacts. Despite prevention efforts, the Achilles' heel of many national strategies lay in the suboptimal rates of self-isolation, especially evident in Europe, the United States and the United Kingdom. During the most tragic months of the pandemic, studies revealed alarmingly low adherence rates, with English research indicating self-reported compliance below 20%.[3] Understanding the dynamics of citizens' adherence to preventive measures and self-isolation is intricate, influenced by multiple factors including culture, environment, social dynamics and political conditions. Refusal of self-isolation is more likely among males, youth, parents and those employed in critical occupational sectors. However, socioeconomic conditions emerge as pivotal.[4] A cross-national study spanning China, Italy, Japan, South Korea, the United Kingdom and the United States underscored that individuals with lower socioeconomic status exhibited less willingness to comply with government-mandated preventive measures. Moreover, people living in countries characterized by high economic inequality were less likely to adhere to such measures.[5]

Neglecting socioeconomic disparities by presuming that "we are all in this together" has severely undermined the lifesaving potential of preventive measures against the virus. The key obstacle to self-isolation wasn't the lack of motivation to self-isolate but the ability to do so.[6] Adherence to isolation rules is contingent on suitable living arrangements and economic resources. In numerous countries, national pandemic management strategies have not adequately accounted for the obstacles to self-isolation, including living conditions, financial constraints and unstable economic prospects. Asking workers in occupations completely devoid of social protection or asking the homeless population to "stay at home" after contracting the virus, without providing them with feasible options to do so, was a policy destined for failure. Furthermore, temporary workers, seasonal laborers and those working in risky environments like long-term care facilities, which often endure low pay, and lack of vacation and sickness coverage, faced similar challenges.[7] Another group of workers that faced the harsh reality of having to work despite being infected, includes self-employed individuals who could not afford business closures, those in job categories that lacked paid holidays and workers who feared upsetting unsympathetic employers.[8]

Effective management of the pandemic clearly requires addressing financial barriers to self-isolation and implementing robust social protection measures to assist those in need. In addition to reducing inequalities caused by the pandemic, these measures are essential for preventing the spread of the virus among the general population.[9] As elaborated in an article published in the *BMJ*, what we truly needed were comprehensive interventions founded on the principle that "everyone matters" and can contribute to safeguarding the collective welfare. Scientific evidence has convincingly demonstrated that community infection rates decline when the economic burden of self-isolation is kept to a minimum.[6] One approach to encourage symptomatic infected individuals to self-isolate is, for instance, compensating them for staying at home, possibly through government subsidies and sick leave provisions. Research conducted in Israel highlighted that citizens' adherence to self-isolation measures during the pandemic was significantly influenced by their knowledge of whether lost wages would be reimbursed by the government. When economic support was assured, compliance with preventive measures soared from 57% to 94%.[10]

The antidote of solidarity

Adherence to public health guidelines during the pandemic could have been improved through various types of inclusive interventions, including financial assistance for self-isolation, tangible support and proactive efforts to identify and address individuals' practical needs such as access to food or assistance for elderly relatives. Additionally, there should have been informative and emotional support interventions, such as increased access to social and psychological counseling for those in need.[11] The pandemic has generated severe effects on mental health and required providing psychological support for the most affected groups during the crisis.[12] This would have helped individuals cope with the most severe of the pandemic's psychosocial effects, including anxiety, depression and loneliness.

Despite the importance of practical and psychosocial interventions to make self-isolation feasible and desirable, only a few lonely voices have forcefully called for vigorous social protection policies. Notable exceptions are the repeated appeals of the UK Independent SAGE, which considered support measures to be indispensable and complementary to prevention and vaccination.[13] Jay Patel and colleagues, as highlighted in a *BMJ* article, stressed the need for compassionate policies that acknowledge the challenges faced by the most vulnerable, rejecting exclusive reliance on punitive measures as counterproductive. The authors advocated for support policies as well as clear, easily accessible communication messages delivered in multiple languages and tailored to varying levels of health literacy.[14]

As already stated, some countries took financial support measures for people affected by the pandemic seriously, offering self-isolation payments to people who tested positive and their contacts and work-related compensation measures or forms of practical support, including home care visits or tangible aid such as free food, free medicines and free (rapid) antigen tests. In Norway and Finland, governments adopted vigorous financial support measures for those who had to self-isolate: Finland offered 100% of the income lost during self-isolation, while Norway offered 80% of salary up to £50,000.[15] Germany provided significant financial assistance to individuals and businesses facing economic problems, especially during the lockdown. Among generous schemes, the Australian government paid up to $1,200 for each citizen in isolation. Given the high risk of household transmission in large, crowded households, countries such as Denmark and Norway have provided free accommodations to anyone unable to isolate at home. In East Asia, South Korea also stood out for having supported its inhabitants with generous economic and practical support measures for individuals who needed to self-isolate: people forced into quarantine, in addition to one-off payments, received basic necessities and healthcare kits.[14] Even medium-income countries like Taiwan found the resources to provide free masks for all citizens and adopt economic support measures, for example by offering 25 pounds for each day spent in isolation to infected people and their healthcare providers. Local government centers in Taiwan also provided help in the form of transportation services, food delivery, medical care, household services and housing for homeless people.

In Europe, the United Kingdom and the United States, the lack of redistributive policies and strong social protection resulted in further increases in economic inequalities.[16] Inequality, as eloquently shown by Richard Wilkinson and Kate Pickett in *The Spirit Level*, has negative repercussions for health, quality of life and a long list of social conditions.[17] The economic gap between rich and poor was already high even before the pandemic, after almost half a century of regressive policies that benefited the very wealthy and large corporations (Figure 8.1).[18] The pandemic, however, has intensified these social dynamics. In light of these trends, there was an urgent need for vigorous political and economic strategies to mitigate the adverse social outcomes caused by these socioeconomic gaps and poverty. Essential support was required for small businesses and individuals who lost their jobs during the lockdown, including those in tourism, catering and the arts, who were left without aid. Although many governments adopted countercyclical macroeconomic policies, increasing public spending and using central banks to prevent bankruptcies and wage suspensions, these measures were insufficient.[19] For instance, Italy's Recovery Fund, aimed at revitalizing the economy and countering the pandemic's impact, fell short in addressing the growing socioeconomic disparities. In the first year of the pandemic, more

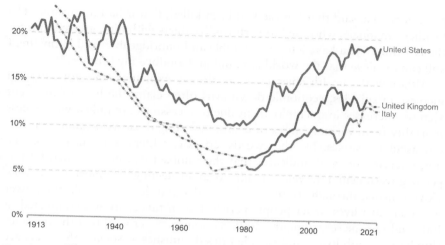

FIGURE 8.1   The revolution in reverse: income share of the richest 1% in the United States, the United Kingdom and Italy (1913–2021)

Note: In the share of income received by the richest 1% of the population, income is measured before the payment of taxes and non-pension benefits but after the payment of public and private pensions. The dotted lines represent extrapolations due to limited data availability.

Source: World Inequality Database (WID.world) (2023) – processed by Our World in Data. "Top 1% - Share (Pretax) (Estimated) – World Inequality Database – Before tax" [dataset]. World Inequality Database (WID.world), "World Inequality Database" [original data]. https://ourworldindata.org/grapher/income-share-top-1-before-tax-wid-extrapolations?time=1912.latest&country=USA~ITA~GBR

than half of the *population* experienced a significant drop in household income, while some social groups remained unaffected.[20] This situation has further strained the financial stability of the less affluent, fostering a sense of injustice among those most affected by the crisis. Such sentiments also posed serious challenges to preventive efforts, which heavily rely on social cohesion, mutual cooperation and a strong sense of public health responsibility.

The myth of scarce resources

In early 2021, a heart attack claimed the life of Adriano, a jazz pianist who had been profoundly impacted by the pandemic crisis and the subsequent Italian government's decision to ban music concerts.[21] He was forced to earn a living by working as a rider. Tragically, while on duty, pushing his broken-down car used for deliveries, Adriano suffered a heart attack and passed away at the age of 41. His sudden death was not just a personal loss but also a symbol of the struggles and sacrifices artists had to endure during these challenging times. The loss of faith in being able to work as a musician had dealt a fatal blow to his dignity, identity and talent, and he had become increasingly pessimistic. He said that "music had been killed, that it had no future." His brother Emanuele, who used to perform live duets with him, greeted him for the last time: "you have left an incredible and unbridgeable void in my life, I still can't believe that the world is so unfair. Goodbye my brother!"[22]

Although the health emergency, as already explained, did not cause an increase in suicides, economic downturns often claim the lives of innocent victims. Increases in unemployment due to recessions are linked with excess mortality from various causes of death, including those associated with cardiovascular diseases. In other words, crises can literally break our hearts. Yet, scientific research indicates that their impact can be mitigated by targeted government interventions aimed at protecting the most vulnerable. Governments, through strategic policy and social decisions, hold the power to either save lives or let people perish. For instance, studies conducted in Italy and Europe regarding the 2008 economic crisis reveal that the relationship between job losses and suicide rates diminishes as social safety nets are strengthened.[23]

There were ample policy options to respond to the socioeconomic crisis caused by COVID-19, including the development and reinforcement of guaranteed minimum income schemes. Bold, targeted social protection measures could be essential for populations and businesses hit hard by the pandemic's economic fallout. Funding for these initiatives, like supporting disadvantaged communities and establishing a COVID-19 relief fund, could be sourced from increased tax progressivity, returning to policies already adopted during the post-war period. Comprehensive global reforms to tackle inequality and prevent capital flight to tax havens could also replenish depleted government budgets for healthcare, education and social welfare. Some countries did attempt some redistributive reforms. For instance, Belgium implemented a millionaire's tax to fund public health initiatives, and Spain adopted a similar approach.[24] In Italy, a proposed solidarity contribution on incomes over 80,000 euros aimed to create a COVID-19 emergency fund to support citizens and entrepreneurs economically impacted by the pandemic. However, the proposal faced fierce opposition from the majority of both center-right and center-left political parties, which, despite their usual divisions, seemed united in their reluctance to address the problem. The Italian magazine *Il Sole 24* reported that the proposed tax mechanism would have involved a small 4–8% contribution from the five highest income brackets (ranging from 80,000 to over 1 million euros in taxable income) for 2020 and 2021. To illustrate, the 200,000 taxpayers earning above 80,000 euros per year would have had to contribute less than 10 euros per month over two years.[25] Despite the modesty of this contribution, the proposal was ultimately dismissed.

A level of resistance similar to that faced by proposals to use progressive taxation to help individuals severely affected by the pandemic has been encountered by the suggestion to have central banks distribute money directly to citizens and companies impacted by the crisis. This concept, known as "helicopter money," has faced significant opposition from the majority of conventional economists and mainstream experts. Interestingly, it has, garnered support from non-governmental organizations and appeared as a possible suggestion in an editorial in the *Financial Times*.[26] It's a paradox that in the past economists with significantly different political and economic views, like John Maynard Keynes and Milton Friedman, have expressed some interest and potential support for the idea of central banks directly issuing money to citizens.[27] Yet, regressive economic policies have prevailed.

The reluctance of governments to protect the less fortunate in society is often rationalized using two main arguments. The first is the so-called moral hazard of promoting idleness, a concern that providing public funds might encourage people to avoid work, a concept sometimes referred to as the "Malibu surfer" problem. The second argument revolves around the notion of scarce resources, suggesting that while social protection policies might be beneficial, they are unfeasible due to lack of financial support. The latter justification is particularly curious. Historical patterns reveal that when governments prioritize an issue, "scarce" resources suddenly become "abundant." For example, in the years following the 2008 crisis, governments engaged in massive quantitative easing (QE) operations, injecting over 22 trillion dollars of liquidity into the financial system. This figure is staggering, especially when compared to the global GDP in 2017, which was around 80 trillion dollars. To add injury to insult, these QE operations had a minimal impact on the "real" economy, small businesses, families and those hardest hit by the crisis. In the UK, for instance, the Bank of England's QE program of 375 billion pounds, which equates to about 6,000 pounds per person, resulted in only 8 pence of every pound created reaching the non-financial, "real" economy.[28] The argument that resources are insufficient to assist people and companies affected by the pandemic seems particularly weak when contrasted with the economic actions taken in March 2020. During this period, the central banks of the G7 countries decided to inject approximately 9 trillion dollars into their banks. This move appeared contradictory when considering the insufficient resources claimed for vaccinating poorer countries, an initiative the IMF estimated would cost around 39 billion dollars.[29] Yet, in the field of mainstream economics, ideologically driven double standards are not uncommon. Lawrence Summers, a former US Treasury Secretary and proud supporter of the deregulation policies that caused the 2008 financial collapse, critiqued the American government's proposal to distribute a $2,000 check to each citizen. He argued that such an intervention could "overheat" the economy.[30]

The pandemic offered a unique chance to reform the global economic and financial system, with a focus on measures that could address inequalities even at the global level. Among policies that have an effect on this social problem, some have proposed reforms to restrict capital flight to tax havens, where 36 trillion dollars is held.[31,32] Annually, tax havens result in a loss of 500–600 billion dollars in tax revenue for governments worldwide.[33] Taxation of large corporations and ultra-wealthy individuals in rich countries is at an all-time low since the post-war period.[34] In 2018, 60 multinational companies such as Amazon, Netflix, IBM and General Motors did not pay any taxes.[35] Tax havens, however, don't just benefit corporations; they are also used by the world's wealthiest individuals to transfer vast sums of money to low-tax jurisdictions. The non-governmental organization ProPublica published an analysis that revealed that in 2007 and 2011, Jeff Bezos, one of the richest men in the world, reportedly paid no federal income taxes. Similar instances were noted in 2018 with Elon Musk, then the second-richest person, along with other billionaires like Michael Bloomberg and George Soros, who also paid no federal income taxes for several years.[34] Another research analysis confirmed that the richest individuals in the United States paid on average less than 5% in taxes on their wealth growth.[36] In Italy, while small businesses and medium-low incomes are over-taxed, the maximum personal income tax for incomes comparable to 258 thousand euros a year and above has fallen from 72% in 1974 to 43% today.

In the years following the beginning of the pandemic, the combined wealth of the world's ten richest billionaires increased by about 500 billion dollars.[37] Tax havens contribute significantly to the increasing inequality. Estimates produced by the report "The State of Tax Justice 2020" showed that Italy lost over 12 billion dollars in revenue annually: 8.8 billion dollars from corporate tax avoidance and approximately 3.8 billion dollars from offshore tax evasion by individuals. These lost funds could have been instrumental in mitigating the impact of the health crisis on vulnerable populations and in reducing economic inequalities, which are linked to adverse social and health outcomes.[38] To put this into perspective, the revenues lost to tax havens are about 9% of Italy's annual healthcare spending and could cover the annual salaries of approximately 379,380 nurses.[39] These figures highlight a stark contrast: while the wealthy continue to accumulate vast fortunes, those hailed as "heroes" during the pandemic, including doctors, nurses, healthcare workers, supermarket staff and front office personnel who risked their lives to keep society functioning during lockdowns, have not received adequate compensation for their sacrifices.

The pandemic has not only impacted those who lost their jobs or closed their businesses but also posed a threat to social cohesion. During the pandemic, social unrest was mitigated somewhat due to reduced mobility, yet the combination of income loss, joblessness and business shutdowns created a volatile mix of social discontent. In a report titled "Vicious Circle: How Pandemics Lead to Economic Despair and Social Unrest," IMF researchers explored the connections between health crises and the role of economic inequality in fueling social anger. The study indicates that economic crises exacerbate social unrest by hampering economic growth and widening social disparities.[40]

Recently, international financial institutions have been considering progressive policies because of their pragmatic importance.

The World Bank underscored the need to mitigate the economic and health consequences of the pandemic through vigorous fiscal policies aiming at shared prosperity and poverty reduction.[41] The IMF proposed a recovery contribution imposed on high incomes or substantial assets to finance the necessary expenses and support for combating the pandemic's crisis.[42] These "solidarity calls," however, remained unfulfilled due to a lack of political will and public support. Tragicomically, it's not just the ultra-wealthy who resist economic redistribution measures but also large numbers of voters and individuals from less affluent classes who, perhaps unknowingly, act against their own interests and defend the privileges for the already privileged. This situation brings to mind the words of anti-apartheid activist Steve Biko, when he said that "the greatest weapon in the hand of the oppressor is the mind of the oppressed."[43]

United we stand, divided we fall ill

If material support from progressive economic policies could significantly contribute to cushioning the effects of the pandemic, another form of help comes from interpersonal relationships. During the health emergency, social relations were revealed to be both a challenge and a source of comfort. Psychologists often recommend surrounding ourselves with "positive" people, yet the pandemic changed almost everything, even the collective conceptualization of the term "positive." Staying away from people has turned into a life and death choice. Finnish writer Philip Teir, speaking to the French magazine *Le Monde*, attributed Finland's effective pandemic response to its cultural norm of social distancing, with less physical affection like kissing and hugging.[44] Conversely, Italy, which displays a totally different dynamic in social behaviors, seems to have paid a significant toll. For example, a notable characteristic of Italian culture is having a high proportion of adults aged 30 to 49 who live with their own parents. This may have led to more frequent and close contact among elderly Italians and their family members than in countries like Finland and Norway, creating contrasting effects: potentially increasing social support but also the risk of infection.[45] Indeed, some research during the first wave of the pandemic suggested a positive correlation between the prevalence of 30–49-year-olds living with parents and the COVID-19 fatality rate across different countries.[46]

Of interpersonal factors that contributed to improving the response of societies to SARS-CoV-2, strong civic sense and cultural collectivism played a significant role. These dimensions appear to have played a role in the success of Asian countries such as Japan (which has a higher proportion of young adults living with parents than Italy, but reported much lower COVID-19 death rates per million people) in containing the virus and fostering citizen collaboration with government efforts.[47] A study encompassing 67 nations and over 2 million respondents examined attitudes toward actions preventing COVID-19 spread, revealing significant differences between countries like the United States and Japan.[48] Results showed that, in the United States, marked by high individualism and low trust in institutions, there was less emphasis on undertaking preventive actions for personal and communal safety. Conversely, Japan, known for its social cohesion and high level of interpersonal respect, showed an opposite outcome. A key aspect of Japan's strategy, setting it apart even from other countries that managed the pandemic well, was the populace's adherence to preventive measures without even the need for stringent mandates. Japan's approach seems to have largely depended on voluntary compliance with social distancing guidelines, particularly during case surges. Despite relatively moderate government-imposed measures, the Japanese population spontaneously adhered to infection control practices, such as avoiding crowds and poorly ventilated areas. The Institute for Health Metrics and Evaluation noted that mask usage in Japan consistently remained above 90%, a level rarely achieved in other countries. Remarkably, the widespread use of masks, which was initially mandatory in Japan, continued even after the mandates were relaxed.

While Japan is often cited as an exemplary case, it alone does not provide sufficient evidence to support the significance of cultural factors in pandemic management. However, the situation in Japan is not merely a coincidence. Research has consistently shown that the cultural characteristic of collectivism is associated with better outcomes in managing pandemics. In contrast, individualism, more common in Western countries, has been associated with limited compliance with preventive measures, posing challenges to effective pandemic management.[49] Moreover, in societies with high levels of individualism, there has been frequent criticism of prevention measures and strong accusations of governments unduly restricting individual freedoms. This cultural trait promotes the tendency to view preventive behaviors as personal choices, disregarding the collective responsibility for health and hindering the efficacy of national pandemic strategies. Drawing from the lyrics of Pink Floyd's mesmerizing song, "Hey You," one can say that "united we stand, divided we fall ill."

Another key social variable that was revealed to be very important in effective pandemic management is trust. Often likened to the "glue that holds the civic fabric of society together," trust has been paramount. Two forms of trust have been particularly influential during the pandemic: trust in others and trust in institutions. These types of trust, often interlinked, are associated with higher compliance with public health mandates and recommendations set by health and government authorities.[50] A study published in *The Lancet* indicated that if all countries had the same levels of trust as Denmark, SARS-CoV-2 infection rates would have been significantly lower than what was observed.[51] Trusting others during a crisis is crucial for a united response against the virus. Trust fosters a strong sense of community and mutual aid and is closely linked to the perception of preventive measures as necessary for the common good. For instance, infected individuals are more inclined to self-isolate if they believe their actions help contain the spread and save lives, especially when they perceive others as equally committed to community health recommendations. However, citizens' levels of trust do not vary randomly. This social quality is significantly influenced by contextual social conditions, such as socioeconomic inequalities.[52]

Trust is also essential with regard to the relationships between citizens and scientific institutions. International studies have shown that people are more likely to follow prevention measures if they trust the science and the scientists who developed these guidelines.[53] Moreover, institutional trust is a predictor of compliance with quarantine and isolation rules, as well as vaccine acceptance. Although adherence to governments' public health requirements can be ensured through rules and penalties, research suggests that the best approach is not stringent laws and punitive systems. Instead, promoting a sense of collective responsibility in each citizen to combat infection is more effective. In some autocratic countries like China, strong enforcement has been used to ensure compliance with self-isolation. Yet, without the population's active cooperation, authoritarian measures can backfire, creating resentment and decreasing the public's willingness to follow health measures.

Another factor that may have influenced adherence to preventive and public health measures is social support. This refers to how much a person can rely on other people – family, friends or community members – for care or assistance both emotionally and practically.[54] Numerous studies have shown that social support is critical to a person's decision or predisposition to adhere to healthy behaviors. A survey that investigated COVID-19 preventive behaviors confirmed this link. The study showed that South Korea, a country that was relatively successful in handling the pandemic, had a higher level of perceived social support compared to Italy, which faced critical challenges in containing the virus.[55]

Lessons from the pandemic: letting the dead speak

Like all crises, the pandemic has been a learning opportunity. While the exact number of lives that could have been saved by effective prevention interventions remains unknown, it's clear that more could have been done. In September 2022, the Lancet Commission on the COVID-19 Response, comprising 28 global experts, identified major shortcomings contributing to what they defined as a "profound human tragedy" and a "multi-layered global failure."[56] These errors include the following:

1 Lack of timely notification of the onset of the COVID-19 outbreak
2 Delays in recognizing that SARS-CoV-2 spreads by aerosol and in implementing adequate public health mitigation measures nationally and internationally
3 An absence of coordination between countries to suppress viral transmission
4 The failure of governments to review the evidence and adopt best practices for controlling the pandemic and managing the economic and social fallout from other countries
5 A lack of global financing for low- and middle-income countries
6 Failure to ensure adequate supplies and equitable distribution of key resources such as protective personal equipment, diagnostic tests, drugs, medical devices and vaccines, particularly for low- and middle-income countries
7 A lack of timely, accurate and systematic data on infections, deaths, virus variants, health system responses and indirect health consequences
8 Biosafety regulations
9 A failure to combat misinformation
10 The lack of global and national safety nets to protect vulnerable populations

In late 2022, I had the opportunity to appear on the Italian TV channel Rai 3 to talk about a qualitative study published in *Nature*.[57] The study, based on a multinational Delphi consensus method, involved an extensive analysis of recommendations and suggestions for enhancing pandemic response, gathered from over 386 health professionals across 112 countries. Findings of this research effort were organized into six key domains, each representing a crucial area of improvement in pandemic management:[58]

1 Communicate effectively
2 Strengthen health systems
3 Improve vaccination
4 Promote preventive behaviors
5 Improve treatments
6 Reduce social inequalities

The first domain highlighted the importance of effective communication. The study's authors argued that public institutions needed to enhance citizen cooperation through trust- and science-based communication strategies.

Additionally, to combat the infodemic, national governments needed to actively monitor and debunk misinformation and address those responsible for its spread. The second domain focused on strengthening health systems, which are crucial for responding effectively to the COVID-19 pandemic. To alleviate hospital burdens, it is necessary to reinforce primary healthcare resources and prioritize healthcare workers' well-being. Overcoming economic barriers to accessing SARS-CoV-2 testing, personal protective equipment, treatment and care is also essential. This could be achieved by investing in health systems and establishing regional production centers for swabs, treatments and vaccines. The third domain emphasized vaccinations as a key part of prevention. The authors suggested redoubling efforts to reduce vaccine hesitancy through community leader engagement and local organizations. They also recommended enhancing the dissemination of accurate vaccine information and addressing public concerns with targeted, trust-inspiring communications. The fourth domain proposed promoting preventive behaviors. Countries were advised to adopt a holistic approach, combining COVID-19 vaccination with other prevention and treatment measures, and providing financial support for those unable to self-isolate. Governments need to incentivize structural prevention measures like improving ventilation and air filtration, especially in enclosed spaces such as workplaces, schools and shopping centers. In the fifth domain, improving treatments, the focus was on all aspects of treatment and care to cure or mitigate COVID-19's harmful effects. However, when asked about prioritizing treatment over prevention, only 7% of the surveyed professionals agreed. The sixth and final domain, decreasing inequalities, addressed the challenges posed by pre-existing social policies and social stratification. The authors called for increased efforts to make vaccines, tests and treatments more accessible to the less wealthy and to distribute vaccines for free in low- and middle-income countries.

The six domains identified in the *Nature* study resonate with themes highlighted in a previous *BMJ* editorial, where four key lessons from pandemic management were emphasized:[52]

1 The influence of trust in institutions
2 The value of commitment to reducing social inequalities
3 The necessity for clear and coherent risk communication
4 The importance of robust social protection policies

A recurring theme across these domains, echoed in various discussions about the pandemic's management, is the emphasis on health determinants beyond healthcare and the fundamental value of a preventive health approach over a purely curative one. According to the authors of the study, to effectively manage future pandemics, it is crucial to leverage community resources to reduce virus transmission and mitigate the impact of social inequalities.

Richard Horton warned, "the SAR-CoV-2 pandemic is likely neither the last nor the worst health crisis of this century." The Pandemic Preparedness and the Role of Science report suggests that to prepare for upcoming pandemics, G20 governments should enhance global epidemiological intelligence and establish a transnational surveillance network to quickly identify unusual spikes in morbidity, mortality and hospital admissions, facilitating prompt outbreak response.[59] The same topic has been reiterated in an editorial in *Nature* where the authors argued that improving warning systems for rapid government response to pandemics begins with smarter surveillance. As Jeremy Farrar, Director of the Wellcome Trust and author of *Spike: The Virus vs the People – the Inside Story*, put it, "if you don't look, you don't see. If you don't see, you will always respond too late."[60]

Proposals designed to create or strengthen national centers for epidemic prediction and global surveillance networks are commendable, but there's a need for a broader reevaluation of public health's role in the economic and political spheres. The pandemic has highlighted the shortcomings of a medicalized, specialist approach, which failed to grasp the complexity of diseases and their determinants. Western countries should critically assess not just the efficacy of their hospital-centric health systems but also the heavy reliance on pharmaceutical interventions and the pursuit of technological solutions to public health issues. Preparing for future pandemics requires shifting toward new approaches that engage with the complex interplay of social, economic, environmental and political health determinants. This necessitates embracing multidisciplinary perspectives and a systemic view of health, strengthening local medicine and reorienting health systems toward health promotion.

Throughout the pandemic, despite an estimated 27 million deaths caused by COVID-19, Western media have seen commentators who consistently downplayed or denied the seriousness of SARS-CoV-2 attempting to recast the emergency response as an overreaction. In such discussions, it would be worth considering the perspective of the pandemic's victims. Would they agree that governments' response was an overreaction to a supposedly weak virus? Certainly, the narrative of those who survived the pandemic could in fact be very different from that of those who did not. Based on the knowledge that the crisis could and should have been managed better and that our failures have cost the lives of millions of people, there is a duty toward these victims who were left not only breathless but also voiceless. The duty is to make sure their voices are heard. The absence of their opinions has created what Robert Wallace called the "fallacy of silent evidence," or the simple realization that people who have lost their lives to SARS-CoV-2 do not have a say.[61] Our analyses are therefore affected by two biases: the "survival bias," when we only pay attention to the successes and ignore the failures of an event, and the "presence bias," precisely because those who paid the highest price for these failures are no longer here.

Effectively addressing a pandemic demands not only an improved surveillance system and a new health promotion model that abandons the narrow biomedical approach to diseases but also a new way to do politics and economics, ensuring that health considerations are integral to these fields. As pharmacologist and founder and president of the prestigious Mario Negri Institute Silvio Garattini put it in the title of his recent book, *Prevention Is Revolution.*[62] In the same vein, Rudolph Virchow, one of the founders of epidemiology and public health, observed that "politics is medicine on a large scale."[63] Health decisions and economic policies can kill or save lives. It is up to us to ensure that lifesaving measures become consolidated realities. This would refute the criticism that the only thing we have learned from the pandemic is that we have learned nothing from the pandemic.

References

1. Draghi M. Draghi: we face a war against coronavirus and must mobilise accordingly. Financial Times. Published online Mar 25, 2020. https://www.ft.com/content/c6d2de3a-6ec5-11ea-89df-41bea055720b (accessed Jan 24, 2024).
2. Chen Chien-jen: Solidarity the key to Taiwan's successful pandemic fight. Politics & Society. Published online 09–04, 2020. *CommonWealth Magazine.* https://english.cw.com.tw/article/article.action?id=2794 (accessed Jan 24, 2024).
3. Smith LE, Potts HWW, Amlôt R, Fear NT, Michie S, Rubin GJ. Adherence to the test, trace, and isolate system in the UK: results from 37 nationally representative surveys. *BMJ* 2021; **372**: n608.
4. Lee GB, Jung SJ, Yiyi Y, Yang JW, Thang HM, Kim HC. Socioeconomic inequality in compliance with precautions and health behavior changes during the COVID-19 outbreak: an analysis of the Korean Community Health Survey 2020. *Epidemiology and Health* 2022; **44**: e2022013.
5. Fujii R, Suzuki K, Niimi J. Public perceptions, individual characteristics, and preventive behaviors for COVID-19 in six countries: a cross-sectional study. *Environmental Health and Preventive Medicine* 2021; **26**: 29.
6. Agusto FB, Erovenko IV, Fulk A, *et al.* To isolate or not to isolate: the impact of changing behavior on COVID-19 transmission. *BMC Public Health* 2022; **22**: 138.
7. Cevik M, Baral SD, Crozier A, Cassell JA. Support for self-isolation is critical in Covid-19 response. *BMJ* 2021; **372**: n224.
8. Toon P. The ethics of self-isolation. *The British Journal of General Practice* 2022; **72**: 171.
9. Dang HH, Malesky E, Nguyen CV. Inequality and support for government responses to COVID-19. *PLoS One* 2022; **17**: e0272972. https://doi.org/10.1371/journal.pone.0272972.
10. Bodas M, Peleg K. Self-isolation compliance in the COVID-19 era influenced by compensation: findings from a recent survey in Israel. *Health Affairs* 2020; **39**: 936–41.
11. Potts W. SPI-B: Impact of financial and other targeted support on rates of self-isolation or quarantine. Published online Sep 16, 2020. Gov.UK. https://www.gov.uk/government/publications/spi-b-impact-of-financial-and-other-targeted-support-on-rates-of-self-isolation-or-quarantine-16-september-2020 (accessed Jan 24, 2024).
12. Spinhoven P, Cuijpers P, Hollon S. Cognitive-behavioural therapy and personalized treatment: an introduction to the special issue. *Behaviour Research and Therapy* 2020; **129**: 103595.
13. Why supported isolation is crucial to break community transmission. Find, test, Trace, isolate, support, mitigation measures. Independent SAGE. Published online Mar 22, 2021. https://www.independentsage.org/why-supported-isolation-is-crucial-to-break-community-transmission/ (accessed Jan 24, 2024).

14. Patel J, Fernandes G, Sridhar D. How can we improve self-isolation and quarantine for Covid-19? *BMJ* 2021; 372: n625.
15. Shridard D. Chapter 1: Spillover. In: Preventable: How a Pandemic Changed the World & How to Stop the Next One. Viking, New York, 2023: 45.
16. May Sidik S. How COVID has deepened inequality — in six stark graphics. *Nature*. Published online June 22, 2022. https://www.nature.com/immersive/d41586-022-01647-6/index.html (accessed Jan 24, 2024).
17. Reducing inequality benefits everyone — so why isn't it happening? *Nature* 2023; 620(7974):468.
18. De Vogli R. Neoliberalism, globalization and inequalities: consequences for health and quality of life. *Sociology of Health & Illness* 2008; 30: 647–8.
19. Saez E, Zucman G. Keeping business alive: the government will pay. Published online Mar 18, 2020. https://www.socialeurope.eu/keeping-business-alive-the-government-will-pay (accessed Jan 24, 2024).
20. Spagnolo. Gli anticorpi della solidarietà. Caritas Italiana. Published online Sept 14, 2022. https://www.caritas.it/rapporto-2020-su-poverta-ed-esclusione-sociale-in-italia/ (accessed Jan 24, 2024).
21. Lupia V. Pianista jazz Adriano Urso morto d'infarto. Seza lavoro durante la pandemia, faceva il rider. La Repubblica, Jan 13, 2021. https://roma.repubblica.it/cronaca/2021/01/13/news/adriano_urso_morto_rider_justeat_cordoglio_social_fratello_emanuele-282340658/
22. Riccardi K. Musicista rider morto di infarto, Emanuele Urso: 'Mio fratello Adriano, il pianista ucciso dal lockdown'. la Repubblica. https://roma.repubblica.it/cronaca/2021/01/15/news/emanuele_urso_adriano_jazz_lutto_intervista-282575526/?ref=fbpr&fbclid=IwAR1VxsRakD1SboCR0Pzy7lNsFgw-p8yszP1OJwi51lx8hnDizFgoBnhDLAY (accessed Jan 24, 2024).
23. De Vogli R. Blog | La crisi economica uccide. Ma l'austerità per i ricchi può fermarla. Il Fatto Quotidiano. Published online Mar 4, 2014. http://www.ilfattoquotidiano.it/2014/03/04/la-crisi-economica-uccide-ma-lausterita-per-i-ricchi-puo-fermarla/901522/ (accessed Jan 24, 2024).
24. Lecca T. Europa, Dopo la Spagna, anche il Belgio tassa i milionari. Today. Published online Nov 04, 2020. https://europa.today.it/attualita/spagna-belgio-tassa-milionari.html (accessed Jan 24, 2024).
25. Barone N. Pd: contributo di solidarietà sui redditi oltre gli 80mila euro. No di Italia Viva e M5S. Anche Conte si dissocia. Sala: non è buona idea. Il Sole 24 Ore. Published online Apr 11, 2020. https://www.ilsole24ore.com/art/pd-contributo-solidarieta-redditi-oltre-80mila-euro-ADI3nXJ?refresh_ce=1 (accessed Jan 24, 2024).
26. Sandbu M. Coronavirus: the moment for helicopter money. *Financial Times*. Published online Mar 20, 2020. https://www.ft.com/content/abd6bbd0-6a9f-11ea-800d-da70cff6e4d3.
27. Sandbu M. Coronavirus: the moment for helicopter money. March 20, 2020. https://www.ft.com/content/abd6bbd0-6a9f-11ea-800d-da70cff6e4d3
28. Al Daini A. What has become of the £375billion created by the Bank of England under quantitative easing? HuffPost. Published online Apr 18, 2015. https://www.huffingtonpost.co.uk/adnan-aldaini/quantitative-easing_b_6692038.html (accessed Jan 24, 2024).
29. Yanis Varoufakis: Capitalist nations bailed out banks while skimping on funds to vaccinate humanity. Democracy Now! Published online June 21, 2021. https://www.democracynow.org/2021/6/21/summit_for_vaccine_internationalism (accessed Jan 24, 2024).
30. Horti S. Biden ally Larry Summers, a former treasury secretary, said $2,000 stimulus checks would be a 'serious mistake' that could overheat the economy. Business Insider. https://www.businessinsider.com/2000-stimulus-checks-a-serious-mistake-biden-ally-larry-summers-2020-12 (accessed Jan 24, 2024).

31. da Costa PN. Wealth inequality is way worse than you think, and tax havens play a big role. Forbes. https://www.forbes.com/sites/pedrodacosta/2019/02/12/wealth-inequality-is-way-worse-than-you-think-and-tax-havens-play-a-big-role/ (accessed Jan 25, 2024).

32. Stefani S & De Vogli R. Coronavirus: Da una pandemia delle disuguaglianze a una politica economica della salute e del benessere. In-Mind. Published online 2020. https://it.in-mind.org/blog/post/coronavirus-da-una-pandemia-delle-disuguaglianze-a-una-politica-economica-della-salute-e (accessed Jan 24, 2024).

33. Shaxson N. Tackling tax havens: the billions attracted by tax havens do harm to sending and receiving nations alike. *Finance & Development* 2019; 56. https://doi.org/10.5089/9781498316040.022.A003.

34. The secret IRS files: trove of never-before-seen records reveal how the wealthiest avoid income tax. ProPublica. Published online June 8, 2021. https://www.pro-publica.org/article/the-secret-irs-files-trove-of-never-before-seen-records-reveal-how-the-wealthiest-avoid-income-tax (accessed Jan 24, 2024).

35. Sherman E. How these Fortune 500 companies (legally) paid $0 in taxes last year. *Fortune.* Published online Apr 11, 2019. https://fortune.com/2019/04/11/amazon-starbucks-corporate-tax-avoidance/ (accessed Jan 25, 2024).

36. Based on their wealth growth, 26 top billionaires paid an average income tax rate of just 4.8% over 6 recent years. Americans for Tax Fairness. Published online May 19, 2022. https://americansfortaxfairness.org/based-wealth-growth-26-top-billion-aires-paid-average-income-tax-rate-just-4-8-6-recent-years/ (accessed Jan 25, 2024).

37. Berkhout E, Galasso N, Lawson M et al. The inequality virus: Bringing to-gether a world torn apart by coronavirus through a fair, just and sustainable economy. Published online Jan 25, 2021. https://www.oxfam.org/en/research/inequality-virus (accessed Jan 24, 2024).

38. De Vogli R, Gimeno D, Mistry R. The policies–inequality feedback and health: the case of globalisation. *Journal of Epidemiology & Community Health* 2009; 63: 688–91.

39. D'Angelo A., Evasione, i paradisi offshore costano 427 miliardi di dollari. Fis-coOggi. Published online Dec 1, 2020. https://www.fiscooggi.it/rubrica/dal-mondo/articolo/evasione-paradisi-offshore-costano-427-miliardi-dollari?fbclid=IwAR04R19pr3PINV8IrwIg0zAEfLXnIAAPWz1J1xq76YeqrWjkdtHeoElsOwg (accessed Jan 24, 2024).

40. Sedik TS, Xu R. A vicious cycle: how pandemics lead to economic despair and social unrest. IMF. https://www.imf.org/en/Publications/WP/Issues/2020/10/16/A-Vicious-Cycle-How-Pandemics-Lead-to-Economic-Despair-and-Social-Unrest-49806 (accessed Jan 24, 2024).

41. World Bank. Poverty and Shared Prosperity 2022: Correcting Course. Wash-ington, DC: World Bank (accessed Jan 23, 2024).

42. Giles C. IMF proposes 'solidarity' tax on pandemic winners and wealthy. *Financial Times.* Published online Apr 7, 2021. https://www.ft.com/content/5dad2390-8a32-4908-8c96-6d23cd037c38?emailId=606d9db92999e6000430f59f&segmentId=3d08be62-315f-7330-5bbd-af33dc531acb (accessed Jan 24, 2024).

43. Kobe SL. Steve Biko's black theology of liberation from the perspective of Ubuntu. *The Ecumenical Review* 2022; 74: 589–99.

44. Palmisano L. Inside Helsinki | Come ha fatto la Finlandia a mantenere così basso il numero dei contagi, per ora. Linkiesta. Published online Nov 10, 2020. https://www.linkiesta.it/2020/11/finlandia-contagi-coronavirus/ (accessed Jan 24, 2024).

45. Tonon L. Perché in Italia il covid sembra uccidere di più. Internazionale. Pub-lished online Dec 24, 2020. Internazionale. https://www.internazionale.it/notizie/laura-tonon/2020/12/24/italia-covid-mortalita (accessed Jan 24, 2024).

46. Kuhn M and Bayer C. Intergenerational ties and case fatality rates: a cross-country analysis. CEPR. Published online Mar 20, 2020. https://cepr.org/voxeu/columns/intergenerational-ties-and-case-fatality-rates-cross-country-analysis (accessed Jan 24, 2024).
47. C Chen C, Frey C, and Presidente G. Culture and contagion: Individualism and compliance with COVID-19 policy. J Econ Behav Organ. 2021 Oct; 190: 191–200.
48. Collis A, Garimella K, Moehring A, *et al*. Global survey on COVID-19 beliefs, behaviours and norms. *Nature Human Behaviour* 2022; **6**: 1310–7.
49. Biddlestone M, Green R, Douglas KM. Cultural orientation, power, belief in conspiracy theories, and intentions to reduce the spread of COVID-19. *British Journal of Social Psychology* 2020; **59**: 663–73.
50. Wright L, Steptoe A, Fancourt D. Predictors of self-reported adherence to COVID-19 guidelines. A longitudinal observational study of 51,600 UK adults. *The Lancet Regional Health – Europe* 2021; **4**. https://doi.org/10.1016/j.lanepe.2021.100061.
51. Bollyky TJ, Hulland EN, Barber RM, *et al*. Pandemic preparedness and COVID-19: an exploratory analysis of infection and fatality rates, and contextual factors associated with preparedness in 177 countries, from Jan 1, 2020, to Sept 30, 2021. *The Lancet* 2022; **399**: 1489–512.
52. Williams S, Drury J, Michie S, Stokoe E. Covid-19: what we have learnt from behavioural science during the pandemic so far that can help prepare us for the future. *BMJ* 2021; **375**: n3028.
53. Roozenbeek J, Schneider CR, Dryhurst S, *et al*. Susceptibility to misinformation about COVID-19 around the world. *Royal Society Open Science* 2020; **7**: 201199.
54. Mo PKH, Wong ELY, Yeung NCY, *et al*. Differential associations among social support, health promoting behaviors, health-related quality of life and subjective well-being in older and younger persons: a structural equation modelling approach. *Health and Quality of Life Outcomes* 2022; **20**: 38.
55. An S, Schulz PJ, Kang H. Perceived COVID-19 susceptibility and preventive behaviors: moderating effects of social support in Italy and South Korea. *BMC Public Health* 2023; **23**: 13.
56. Sachs JD, Karim SSA, Aknin L, *et al*. The Lancet commission on lessons for the future from the COVID-19 pandemic. *The Lancet* 2022; **400**: 1224–80. https://doi.org/10.1016/S0140-6736(22)01585-9.
57. Radiotelevisione Itailana (RAI) 3. Puntata del 04/11/2022. Published online on Nov 4, 2022. https://www.rainews.it/tgr/rubriche/leonardo/video/2024/01/TGR-Leonardo-del-24012024-91bef19f-e35d-479b-b8b8-7002bee27fb2.html (accessed Jan 24, 2024).
58. Lazarus JV, Romero D, Kopka CJ, *et al*. A multinational Delphi consensus to end the COVID-19 public health threat. *Nature* 2022; **611**: 332–45.
59. Murray CJL. The public-health data systems we need. Project Syndicate. Published online July 7, 2021. https://www.project-syndicate.org/magazine/covid19-shows-need-to-overhaul-public-health-data-systems-by-christopher-j-l-murray-2021-07 (accessed Jan 24, 2024).
60. Maxmen A. Has COVID taught us anything about pandemic preparedness? *Nature* 2021; **596**: 332–5.
61. COVID minimizers rewriting pandemic's history. YouTube. People's Centers for Disease Control (CDC). Published online Mar 22, 2023. https://www.youtube.com/watch?v=W7loI39HT68 (accessed Jan 24, 2024).
62. Silvio Garattini. Prevenzione è rivoluzione. Per vivere meglio e più a lungo. Il Mulino, 2023.
63. Virchow R, Rather LJ. Collected essays on public health and epidemiology. Canton, MA: Science History Publications, 1985.

PART III

Preventing future pandemics

9

COVID-19

A human-made pandemic

"The pestilence is at once blight and revelation, it brings the hidden truth of a corrupt world to the surface."[1]

Albert Camus

"I remember when the poachers captured a pangolin and prepared to slit its throat, their eyes locked. One of them stared into the animal's eyes, and the pangolin met his gaze. I'll never forget it."[2] These are the first words of a National Geographic documentary broadcast a few years ago dedicated to this anteater, with a body almost entirely covered in scales. When it feels itself in danger, the pangolin curls up into a ball and its scales form a protective armor against predators. It is an effective defense against the claws of lions, tigers and leopards but not against humans.[3] Pangolins are endangered, as they are hunted for their meat and because of unfounded beliefs in the medicinal properties of their scales. In reality, there is no scientific evidence regarding their healing effectiveness, and China has fortunately removed them from the list of ingredients of traditional medicine. While this is a positive step, it might be too little, too late. The pangolin's plight is further exacerbated by rapid deforestation, endangering their habitat and survival. What captivates the most about pangolins are their eyes, often seeming to emit a tear-like liquid, possibly giving the impression of crying. They are among the world's most trafficked animals, with over a million of them poached in the last decade. Recently, pangolins gained international notoriety, not for their endangered status but as potential vectors in the origin of the coronavirus. While direct animal-to-human transmission cannot be ruled out, similar to previous pandemics such as SARS-CoV-1 and MERS, it's likely

DOI: 10.4324/9781003511977-13

that SARS-CoV-2 had an intermediate host.[4] Research suggests that the most probable intermediate host in the species jump of SARS-CoV-2 is this cute anteater.[5] The irony is tragic: already at risk of extinction, pangolins now are "blamed" for the onset of the worst global health crisis since World War II.

Perhaps the pangolin does indeed cry, but it is not the only wild animal "on trial" for the origin of the COVID-19 health disaster. There is another even more "guilty" suspect: the bat, well known already by researchers for being a primary global reservoir for coronaviruses.[6] There are other wild animals possibly implicated and the origin of SARS-CoV-2 is still a subject of scientific debate and controversy, yet the bat and the pangolin seem the most likely to have been involved in the species jump of the virus to humans.[7]

The Huanan horror market

Following the pandemic outbreak, the global community embarked on a quest not only to trace the species jump at the virus's origin but also to pinpoint the initial infections. This search led in various directions, with the most significant pointing to the Huanan market, a live animal and seafood market in Wuhan, Hubei.[8] This market, which was later shut down by Chinese authorities, used to sell a wide array of wild animals such as live wolf cubs, scorpions, squirrels, foxes, civets, salamanders, turtles and crocodiles. Often, these illegally captured creatures were slaughtered in front of customers, and parts of their bodies such as tails, bellies, tongues and intestines were on sale. While patient zero may remain elusive, swab tests have detected the virus in areas of the market where these animals were detained. Additional clues point to the significance of the Huanan market: the first confirmed COVID-19 death was a regular visitor to the market, and Wuhan doctors noted that many early patients hospitalized with an unprecedented form of pneumonia had links to this market. A significant proportion of the initial confirmed cases were either stall owners, employees or frequent visitors at the market.[9] As put in an article published in *Nature*, "when you analyze the evidence, it's clear that this all started at the market."[10] Furthermore, a geospatial analysis published in *Science* supports this conclusion, stating, "while there is insufficient evidence to determine the upstream events and the precise circumstances remain unclear, our analyses suggest that the emergence of SARS-CoV-2 was linked to the wildlife trade in China, with the Huanan market in Wuhan being the epicenter of the COVID-19 pandemic."[8]

In order to shed light on the topic, the WHO appointed a group of experts to explore the epidemiological roots at the origin of the virus.[11] Amidst controversies and allegations of a lack of transparency, the WHO team produced a report suggesting various hypotheses, ranked in terms of their likelihood. According to the ranking, the most likely hypothesis is a "natural" spillover through an intermediate host, while the idea that the coronavirus originated

in a lab has been described as "extremely unlikely."[12] This position is consistent with the lack of substantiated evidence supporting the hypothesis of
a lab leak.[13] Indeed, not only the WHO but the scientific community generally is more inclined toward the animal origin of the coronavirus.[14,15] Yet,
this narrative hasn't convinced everyone.[16,17] The debate over the origin of
SARS-CoV-2 has been mired in baseless attacks and conflicting viewpoints,
often influenced by strong biases and geopolitical interests.[18] While scientific
inquiry thrives on trials and errors, experimentation and correction, some
are keen to disregard facts and scientific findings, allowing confirmation biases to prevail. At the beginning of the pandemic, for example, former US
Secretary of State Mike Pompeo claimed without any proof that there was
"significant evidence" of the virus emerging from a Chinese lab.[19] Similarly,
a *Washington Times* editorial suggested that the virus might have originated
from a lab associated with China's biological warfare program.[20] These assertions gained enormous public traction, being widely disseminated by web-
sites such as ZeroHedge and media outlets like Fox News.[21]

Conspiracy theories aside, some respected scholars have maintained a justified caution regarding the origin of the virus.[22–24] A group of scientists, for
example, in a letter published in *Science*, argued that the possibility of an
accidental origin should not be prematurely dismissed a priori but taken seriously until sufficient data became available.[25] The *Lancet* COVID-19 Commission Task Force, chaired by renowned economist Jeffrey Sachs, took a
similar stance. As written in a *Lancet* article, "The proximal origins of SARS-
CoV-2 are still not known. Identifying these origins would provide greater
clarity into not only the causes of the current pandemic but also vulnerabili-
ties to future outbreaks and strategies to prevent them."[26] Sachs, however,
apart from accusing the US government institutions of a lack of transparency,[27] went so far as to state that he was "pretty convinced that the virus has
come out from an American biotechnology laboratory."[28] As explained in a
BMJ editorial, Sachs became increasingly skeptical of some narratives on the
origin of the virus and even decided to fold the *Lancet* commission because
of conflicts of interest and links to the Wuhan Institute of Virology of one
of its members. Moreover, he questioned the lack of scrutiny of both China
and the National Institutes of Health (NIH) in conducting virus research,
including "gain-of-function" studies, which look at what makes viruses more
transmissible and virulent.[24]

Sachs's position has been received with dismay by many scientists, including two world-renowned virologists who defined his claims as "wild speculation" and "shameful."[29] Robert Garry, a professor in the Department of
Microbiology and Immunology at Tulane University, dismissed Sachs and his
colleagues' conclusion as biased by misinterpretations of scientific data.[27] Determining the most plausible hypotheses in debates so fraught with controversies and accusations is very challenging, especially because the definitive

"smoking gun" evidence for SARS-CoV-2's origin has never been convincingly presented.[30] In such situations, Carl Sagan's famous adage, "extraordinary claims require equally extraordinary evidence,"[31] rings true, and although the majority of scientists view the "natural" origin as the most credible hypothesis,[32] it is important to remain open to various possible explanations. Doubts and skepticism are the building blocks of the scientific process.

Controversy on the natural origin of the virus hypothesis has also been generated by an episode that involved Kristian Andersen, a professor at the Scripps Research Institute in California and first author of one of the most significant contributions to the study of the natural hypothesis.[33] Although Andersen has been the target of shamelessly false accusations of bribery, in an email to Dr. Fauci in late January 2020, shortly after the coronavirus genome was first sequenced, he wrote: "the unusual features of the virus make up a really small part of the genome (<0.1%) so one has to look really closely at all the sequences to see that some of the features [potentially] look engineered." When asked to explain, he replied: "At the time, based on limited data and preliminary analyses, we observed features that appeared to potentially be unique to SARS-CoV-2. We had not yet seen these features in other related viruses from natural sources, and thus were exploring whether they had been engineered into the virus."[34] Is this proof of a cover-up, as depicted by advocates of the lab-leaked hypothesis? Or is it just an example of how a scientific inquiry evolves? A quote often misattributed to John Maynard Keynes says "when the facts change, I change my mind. What do you do, sir?"[35]

There is an important reason why most scientists believe that the natural origin of the virus is more likely. On top of the genetic analyses and epidemiological data from the Huanan market, there is overwhelming evidence that most previous health crises due to infectious diseases, such as SARS-CoV-1, MERS and Ebola, are zoonoses. They come from animals.[36,37] The number of global health crises created through these pathways is significant and well documented. How about lab leaks? Certainly, there have been examples of pathogens that escaped accidentally from laboratories, but how many of them caused large-scale outbreaks and global health crises? None.

Chinese shadows and the death of Li Wenliang

There are still significant uncertainties surrounding the origin of the virus. For example, the timing and identity of the first cases of SARS-CoV-2 are still under investigation. Some hypotheses maintain that the virus could have been circulating in one or more places outside China much before the outbreak in Wuhan.[38] One notable claim from Chinese authorities, for example, is that the pandemic started in Italy. Supporting this claim is a study by researchers from Italy's Cancer Institute, published in the institute's own journal and swiftly accepted the same day it was reviewed, suggesting the presence of anti-SARS-CoV-2 antibodies in asymptomatic patients as early as September 2019. Of course, these findings have been met with skepticism by the international scientific community, and there is no supporting evidence such as a corresponding increase in mortality during the same period.[39] Experts like virologist Gregory Towers of University College London dismissed them as implausible. As he put it, "when you eliminate the absurd, only Wuhan remains."[40]

While baseless conspiracy theories, false accusations and political weaponization of a challenging scientific topic can be easily debunked, there remain serious unanswered questions regarding China's handling of the early stages of the outbreak. One critical aspect still shrouded in mystery is the chain of events between the initial discovery of atypical pneumonia cases and the Chinese government's decision to act on January 23, 2020. Similar to what happened with the 2002 SARS-CoV-1 epidemic, the Chinese government initially did not inform the public about the emerging health threat. The story of Li Wenliang, the ophthalmologist who first raised the alarm about the coronavirus, exemplifies this. His warning, rather than spurring immediate infection control actions, led to his arrest for "causing alarm." However, the Chinese high court later reprimanded the police, allowing him to return to work at the Wuhan hospital, where he eventually contracted the virus and died on February 6, 2020. Li Wenliang is remembered for his courage and foresight and is regarded as a national hero in China.

What happened in the period between the first reported infections in mid-November 2019 and the initial virus control actions by Chinese authorities on January 23, 2020, remains a critical information gap.[41] A lingering question is, how many infections and deaths could have been avoided if China had acted more swiftly? Timeliness is crucial in pandemic management, but understanding the context of these delays is also essential. For instance, China's first official COVID-19 death was acknowledged in mid-January 2020, and the WHO declared a health emergency toward the end of January 2020. Despite these warnings, the Western world played down the threat for months. From mid-January to March 2020, political figures like Donald Trump and Boris Johnson publicly underestimated the virus's danger. Before turning into the most relentless critic of China, on January 24, 2020, Trump praised China's efforts and transparency, expressing optimism about the situation. As he put it, "China has been working very hard to contain the Coronavirus. The United States greatly appreciates their efforts and transparency. It will all work out well."[42] In late February 2020, even Anthony Fauci advised Americans not to excessively worry about the virus and to maintain their usual habits, citing a "still low" risk, although he acknowledged that this could change.[43]

Trump wasn't the only one to launch rambling attacks on China. A singular case comes from Veneto, where the governor of the region, in reference to the infections that exploded in China in the first months of the pandemic, stated: "it is a cultural fact. I think China paid a big price for this epidemic ... because ... we all saw them eating live mice or something like that."[44] A *New York Times* editorial in the early months of the pandemic connected the outbreak to China's cultural and political milieu, citing traditional beliefs about exotic meats and the government's tendency to suppress information, or "hitting the ambassador." While China has been the epicenter of several zoonoses, attributing the pandemic's origins solely to Chinese cultural and political practices grossly oversimplifies a complex issue. The real factors driving the emergence and spread of zoonotic diseases are structurally rooted in the interplay of environmental, economic and societal changes occurring in our increasingly globalized modern society.[45] As outlined in an article in *Infection, Genetics and Evolution*, the increasing interactions between humans and animals, driven by environmental and socioeconomic changes, are key to understanding these pandemics. Moreover, modern society's global exchanges and mobility act as amplifiers for these diseases, spreading them beyond their initial geographic locations.[46]

Pandemic risk amplifiers

The intense debate surrounding the origins of the pandemic, polarized between proponents of a lab leak and those asserting a natural species jump, has seemingly created a binary divide. However, focusing solely on these hypotheses may distract from understanding the broader, underlying causes of the increasing zoonotic problems. Genetic analyses might shed light on the virus's origins, but the deeper determinants – that facilitated the outbreak and spread of the virus – are rooted in global environmental, social and economic changes.[47] A report by the United Nations Environment Program (UNEP) and the International Livestock Research Institute (ILRI), titled "Preventing the Next Pandemic," highlights seven key factors that amplify pandemic risk:[48]

1 Increased trade, consumption and exploitation of wildlife
2 Deforestation
3 Excessive urbanization
4 Intensification of agriculture and industrialized animal production
5 Increased international travel and mobility
6 Overpopulation
7 Climate change

Let's examine each factor. The exponential growth in trade, consumption and exploitation of wildlife within the context of rapid economic growth and globalization has markedly increased the risk of pandemics. In the past 50 years, the frequency of pandemics has quadrupled compared to previous decades, and, as already mentioned, most of them originate from wild animals.[49] Markets like Huanan, which sell them, are particularly high-risk environments due to the diversity of species congregated in stressful, cramped conditions. These conditions not only cause immense suffering to these animals but also make them more prone to infectious diseases by weakening their immune systems. The crowded and unsanitary conditions in these markets further amplify the risk of disease transmission.[50] While this narrative might seem to support the idea of the virus's "natural" origin, as David Quammen notes in *Spillover* regarding the previous SARS pandemic, "we created the Coronavirus epidemic. It may have started with a bat in a cave [or a pangolin who knows where], but it was human activity that triggered it."[51] Indeed, the "natural" hypothesis of the virus's origin is not as natural as it seems.

The second major factor contributing to increased contact between wildlife and humans is the combination of deforestation and excessive urbanization. Deforestation, a well-known risk factor for exposure to various pathogens, has been linked to an increased risk of zoonotic diseases. A study in *Frontiers of Veterinary Science* found a strong correlation between global forest cover loss from 1990 to 2016 and heightened zoonotic outbreak risks in tropical regions.[52] The mechanism is straightforward: deforestation and conversion of forests to agricultural land create ideal conditions for pathogens through activities leading to high animal densities and forced interactions between species that wouldn't typically encounter one another. The transformation of rural environments and increased human presence have amplified pandemic risks by fostering environments conducive to diseases that are commonly transmitted by wild animals, such as bats.[53] In Australia, for instance, suburban expansion attracted infected bats from forests, facilitating the spread of the Hendra virus. The virus-carrying bats, adapting to urbanized areas, came into contact with horses, which subsequently had contact with humans.[54] Similarly, the species jump of the Nipah virus was linked to deforestation and the establishment of intensive pig farms that used fruit waste from bats. This created a synergistic condition for an outbreak of the virus. Bats are particularly adept at transmitting coronaviruses due to their ability to fly, their gregarious nature and their possession of a unique virus tolerance. Some have suggested eradicating all bats, which is not only ethically indefensible but also very counterproductive. Numerous scientific studies have demonstrated that the loss of biodiversity creates conditions that are conducive to the emergence of new pandemics. Therefore, engaging in such a reckless act would only further increase the risk of future health emergencies.[55]

During some of the most difficult months of the pandemic, a friend wrote to me: "Hi Roberto, how are you? It's been a while. I'd love to catch up, but first I must confess: I'm an anti-vaxxer. Will you still talk to me?" I replied: "Of course, I'll talk to you! Plus, aren't you vegan if I remember well? Ok, if everyone had adopted your diet, this pandemic may have probably never occurred!" The reason is simple: If deforestation is a major cause of zoonotic diseases, what causes deforestation? Worldwide, over two-thirds of forest loss occurs due to the conversion of primary forests into agricultural land, primarily for meat production. The meat industry and agriculture contribute to pandemic risk not only indirectly through deforestation but also through the transformation of animal farming practices.[56] Over the past 50 years, the rise of industrial farming has increased the likelihood of large animal populations to densely congregate, in a shift from the smaller, family-run farms of the past. Mega-farms and large-scale livestock production, with their overcrowded conditions, turn each animal into a potential breeding ground for viral mutations that could spark new pandemics.[57] The link between intensive agriculture and the emergence of new pathogens was highlighted in several research efforts, including the report titled "Is the Next Pandemic on Our Plate?"[58] The authors contend that the industrialization of animal farming has commodified animals, prioritizing profit at a great cost to the environment, health safety and animal welfare. Professor Robert Bragg from the Department of Microbial, Biochemical and Food Biotechnology at the University of the Free State warns, "There will be more pandemics, and some scientists believe this may just be a rehearsal for a much larger one."[50]

A systematic review published in the *Proceedings of the National Academy of Sciences (PNAS)*, which investigated how the intensification of animal agriculture escalates the risk of zoonotic diseases, concluded that the future emergence or re-emergence of such diseases will be intimately connected to changes in the agriculture-environment nexus.[59] A number of studies have examined how intensification of production increases the risk of epidemics, both directly through increased contact between wild and farmed animals, and indirectly through environmental impacts such as biodiversity loss, water use and climate change. Additionally, the intensification of animal agriculture exacerbates the spread of contagion due to factors such as high animal density, genetic similarities among farmed animals, heightened immunodeficiency and the transportation of live animals.[60]

Although intensive animal farming did not have a direct role in the origin and spread of SARS-CoV-2, this perspective may change when considering the interplay of multiple pandemic risk factors. As the author of the study "How a Pandemic Led to Another" argues, there is a link between the 2019 African swine flu outbreak, which devastated Chinese pig farms and halved pork production, and the COVID-19 pandemic. With China producing about half of the world's pigs, the swine flu crisis led to a significant decrease in pork supply, which seemingly triggered an increased demand for wild animal protein.[61,62] Some researchers have also suggested that the Chinese meat industry crisis, spurred by the mass culling of pigs due to African swine fever, might have been a contributing factor in the emergence of SARS-CoV-2.[63]

Robert Wallace, author of *Big Farms Make Big Flu*, argues that the origin of COVID-19 should be understood within the context of two areas significantly impacted by global economic production: forests and industrial farms. Following economic liberalization in China since the 1980s, there has been a rapid expansion in industrial livestock farming and the wild food sector, particularly in central and southern China, home to many bat populations. According to Wallace, increased interactions among livestock, wild animals, farmers and miners have facilitated the spread of various coronaviruses, including SARS-CoV-2. With the growing consumption of wild foods and agricultural production, many coronaviruses similar to SARS-CoV-2 infected animals or people in peri-urban areas before reaching the global travel network facilitated by globalization.[64] SARS-CoV-2 is just one of several pathogenic strains that have emerged or re-emerged in the 21st century. Diseases such as avian and swine flu, Ebola and Zika, while each having unique features, are all linked to changes in animal husbandry, logging and mining.[65] These increased dangers reflect changes in the economy and agriculture. In 1980, only 2.5% of Chinese livestock farms were industrial but now well over half are. Concurrently, Southeast Asia has seen the world's fastest deforestation rate in the past 40 years.

Spokespeople from WWF International, the United Nations Convention on Biological Diversity and the WHO's Department of Environment, Climate Change and Health see the coronavirus as a stark warning for humanity.[66] In their view, it should serve as a reminder to reassess our dysfunctional relationships with nature and animals. The fact that the pandemic originated in China, the world's largest producer of farmed animals with numerous large-scale animal farms, may or may not be a coincidence. However, these farms often feature billions of animals crowded in confined spaces, creating potential hotspots for disease emergence. Thankfully, the health crisis has spurred some legislative changes. For instance, new laws in China strengthened regulations on the management of wild animals bred in captivity, ensuring better control and oversight.[67] The infamous "wet" markets, known for selling and slaughtering bats and pangolins under dire sanitary conditions, are now subjected to stricter regulations. Yet, as the China policy specialist for Humane Society International noted, "There are glaring holes in the restrictions that still pose a zoonotic disease risk."[68] Stronger regulations are urgently needed, and they have to be adopted on a global scale to effectively mitigate pandemic risks. The WHO has urged a suspension of the sale of live wild-caught animals in food markets and recommended the implementation of enhanced hygiene standards. It has also advocated for the establishment of epidemiological surveillance systems to quickly detect new pathogen outbreaks.[69]

These measures represent critical steps in reducing the likelihood of future pandemics, emphasizing the need for a concerted global effort to reform practices that pose risks to both human health and biodiversity. Yet, they are not enough. A more thorough and comprehensive approach is required to address the underlying structural causes of major pandemic risk factors, such as deforestation, intensified animal agriculture, and the trade and exploitation of wild animals. These challenges stem from human and economic activities intrinsic to our current global development model. Over the past 50 years, humans have altered ecosystems more rapidly and extensively than in any previous historical period. The pace of these changes is unprecedented, driven by the escalating demand for animal proteins, a global increase in consumption and living standards and the growing need for food, water, wood and other natural resources.

Urbanization and population density are two additional factors significant in amplifying pandemic risks. While viruses responsible for recently emerging pandemics often originate from "animal assemblages," it's the "human assemblages" in densely populated areas that facilitate their global spread. The world's population has skyrocketed from about 1 billion in the early 19th century to over 8 billion today, with projections indicating another billion by 2050 if current trends continue. Furthermore, by 2050, two-thirds of the global population will reside in urban areas or megacities. This exponential growth in people and crowded cities, combined with the increased mobility due to travel and trade fostered by economic and social globalization, created unprecedented challenges for global health. In 2018, over 4 billion people traveled by plane, a stark increase from just 310 million in 1970.

After the repeal of isolation rules and the self-monitoring of COVID-19 data in Italy, Francesco Vaia, the Director of Prevention at the Italian Ministry of Health, expressed triumphantly that the decree marked "the end of the pandemic" and that there would be no more "obligations, sanctions, and restrictions."[70] This is very optimistic. Without changes in our model of economic development and lifestyle, which leads to environmentally destructive practices like deforestation and wildlife exploitation, the risk of facing future viruses such as SARS-CoV-3, SARS-CoV-4, and beyond remains dangerously high.[71]

Ecological crisis: sister to the pandemic one?

Among the numerous factors contributing to heightened pandemic risk, climate change stands out as one of the most critical. A study featured in *Nature Climate Change* analyzed the impact of ten climate risks sensitive to greenhouse gas (GHG) emissions on known pathogenic diseases. The findings revealed that approximately 58% (218 out of 375) of infectious diseases that have emerged globally were intensified by climate risks.[72] This underscores the critical need to tackle the climate crisis as a measure to mitigate future pandemic risks. Research from the University of Cambridge has further highlighted the role of the climate emergency, in conjunction with other factors, in exacerbating conditions that could trigger new pandemics. The study showed that over the last century, rising temperatures and related extreme weather events have led to a significant increase in bat populations in China's Yunnan province, adjacent to Myanmar and Laos. Intriguingly, this is the same region where genetic studies suggest SARS-CoV-2 may have originated. The study emphasized that around 40 bat species, carrying approximately 100 different types of coronaviruses, have migrated to Yunnan over the past century, and climate change has transformed Yunnan into an ideal habitat for these wild animals.[73]

The effects of the COVID-19 pandemic on society have sometimes been portrayed as a kind of appetizer to what the planet will face as the worst effects of climate change unfold. Indeed, both crises share some similarities: they are the result of human interference with ecosystems and are driven by common factors like exponential growth in living standards, consumption and population, as well as deforestation and industrialized animal farming. Deforestation and intensification of animal farming are not only pandemic risk factors but also major contributors to greenhouse gas (GHG) emissions globally, accounting for about a fifth and a third of them, respectively.[74–76] The climate crisis and the pandemic have another aspect in common: they are global crises that cannot be be resolved through nationalistic and unilateral approaches. Yet, there are also crucial differences. The climate crisis unlike COVID-19 could lead to an irreversible collapse of modern civilization.[77] The Lancet Countdown 2021 report labeled climate change the most significant global health threat of the century,[78] showing that rising global temperatures and related ecological changes have increased the likelihood of extreme weather events, resulting already in significant adverse health outcomes.[79,80] Indeed, the ecological crisis poses a serious threat to our future survival.[81] In *Collapse: How Societies Choose to Fail or Survive*, Jared Diamond outlined several factors that have led to the collapse of past civilizations, such as deforestation, habitat destruction, soil erosion and overpopulation. He also highlighted environmental issues like climate change, energy shortages and the overuse of Earth's photosynthetic capacity. His analysis showed that many civilizations have collapsed due to these factors, but ours is uniquely threatened by most of them. Moreover, for the first time in history, the risk of collapse is not confined to specific regions of the world but is global. As Diamond noted, "globalization makes it impossible for modern societies to collapse in isolation."[82] As the environmental adage says, "there is no planet B."

A recent study on the effects of global population growth on deforestation assessed the likelihood of averting a catastrophic collapse at around 10%.[83] Another slightly less dire analysis from the *PNAS* study suggested a 1 in 20 chance of "catastrophic or existential outcomes" from climate change. The authors pointed out: "it's like taking a flight with a one in twenty chance that the plane … will crash"[84] and added, "we would never get on a plane with a one in twenty chance of crashing but why then are we willing to send our children and grandchildren?"[85]

These grim predictions outlined by climate scientists may seem surreal, yet they represent a concrete danger. Some authors argue that our planet risks facing conditions similar to those experienced at the end of the Permian era, known as "the mother of all extinctions," when a significant portion of marine and terrestrial species vanished. This mass extinction event was preceded by a rapid increase in global temperatures due to the release of massive amounts of GHG. The worst projections of a world warmer by 6°C by the end of the century raise serious questions about its habitability. Such a scenario would likely bring frequent and more devastating hurricanes, heatwaves and other catastrophic natural disasters. Large swaths of the Earth could become arid deserts, and many major cities and nations might find themselves submerged, even as drinking water became scarce. The likelihood of frequent droughts, floods, famines and epidemics would increase significantly in this scenario. Irreversible climate change could lead to the displacement of hundreds of millions of people, creating climate refugees on an unprecedented scale. Crop failures could severely impact global food security, threatening our ability to sustain ourselves. Beyond environmental and health crises, social tensions could escalate. Global shocks might spark civil conflicts and wars as nations compete for dwindling natural resources, as underlined by Gwynne Dyer in his book *Climate Wars: The Fight for Survival as the World Overheats*.[86]

One of the most concerning aspects is the uncertainty about whether we can still avert the so-called ecological "point of no return" or climate tipping points, thresholds beyond which abrupt, dangerous and often irreversible changes occur. To reduce the risk of overcoming them, scientists suggested keeping the global average temperature increase below 1.5°C above preindustrial levels. This entails maintaining atmospheric GHG levels below 350 ppm and reducing carbon dioxide emissions by about 90% by 2050 compared to 1990 levels (Figure 9.1). It's a very ambitious goal. However, some research seems to suggest that even achieving this target may not prevent the crossing of several critical thresholds. These include the collapse of the Greenland and West Antarctic ice sheets, the demise of tropical coral reefs at low latitudes and the sudden thawing of permafrost in the northern regions of the planet.[87] Some research estimates suggest that we might have already surpassed this critical juncture, making it potentially too late to reverse course.[88] Research using mathematical models to envision a scenario where GHG ceased entirely in 2020 suggests that even if we stopped emitting these gases today, the world would continue to warm. This continued warming is due to positive feedback loops, such as the thawing of permafrost, which release additional GHG into the atmosphere. The IPCC's 2022 report corroborates this grim outlook, noting that increasingly extreme weather and climate conditions have already caused irreversible impacts, as both natural and human systems have been pushed beyond their adaptive capacity.[89] *The Guardian* described this report as the "darkest warning ever," indicating that the window for ensuring a livable future for our species is rapidly closing.[90] Additionally, the 'nine planetary boundaries' model, developed by Johan Rockström, professor in Earth System Science at the University of Potsdam, together with

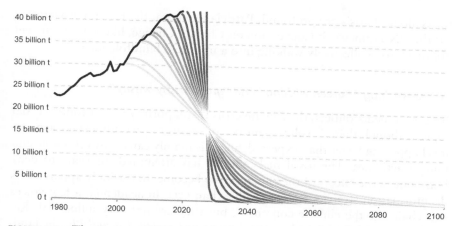

FIGURE 9.1 The (im)possible undertaking: carbon dioxide reductions needed to keep global temperature rise below 1.5°C

Source: Robbie Andrew, based on the Global Carbon Project – processed by Our World in Data. IPCC SR15 – "CO_2 mitigation curves to meet a 1.5C target" [dataset]. Robbie Andrew, based on the Global Carbon Project [original data]. Retrieved February 14, 2024 from https://ourworldindata.org/grapher/co2-mitigation-15c

Note: Annual emissions of carbon dioxide are shown under various mitigation scenarios to keep the global average temperature rise below 1.5°C. Scenarios are based on the carbon dioxide reductions necessary if mitigation had started – with global emissions peaking and quickly reducing – in the given year. Carbon budgets are based on a >66% chance of staying below 1.5°C from the IPCC's SR15 Report.

a team of 28 researchers, shows that we have already crossed six of the boundaries: climate change, biodiversity loss, land exploitation, overexploitation of water resources, chemical pollution and biogeochemical flows. This trajectory seemingly sets us on the path toward the sixth mass extinction.[91] Bill McGuire, Professor Emeritus of Geophysics and Climate Hazards at University College London and author of *Hothouse Earth*, argued that the "point of no return" has already been passed. According to his analyses, children born in 2020 will inherit a world far more hostile than the one known by their grandparents.[92]

Fortunately, a segment of the scientific community offers a less dark outlook. According to a notable analysis, the latest cycle of climate model simulations suggests that if GHG emissions ceased immediately, there could be a decrease in global temperatures, with no resumption of warming in the foreseeable future.[93] This hopeful scenario is echoed by articles published in *Nature* and *Science*, as well as organizations like the United Nations and the IPCC.[94–96] Clearly, there are significant uncertainties, and definitive evidence about future scenarios will only become available in the future. Despite such uncertainties, the risks humanity faces by delaying action against the ecological crisis are profound. Patricia Espinosa, the Executive Secretary for the UN Framework Convention on Climate Change, likened our current approach to "collectively walking into a minefield blindfolded."[97]

"Greenwashing," "green wishing" and "green wishy-washy"

In certain media outlets, the climate crisis is still portrayed as a controversial topic, although there is solid scientific consensus on two important aspects: it is happening faster than expected, and it is mainly caused by economic and human activities. The fossil fuel industry has attempted for years to deny both, but as the effects of the climate crisis become increasingly apparent, its disinformation strategy is less credible than ever. In academia, a few voices still challenge the climate consensus, but they are not very influential. Recently, an article published in *The European Physical Journal Plus* in January 2022, which claimed that the climate crisis was not evident, was later retracted due to the editors' "concerns regarding data selection, analysis, and conclusions."[98] Although the editors did not mention it explicitly, it appears to be a typical case of "cherry picking," or the deliberate exclusion of data or facts that do not confirm one's hypothesis and the selection of those few data or facts that do confirm it. Of course, research that criticizes the scientific consensus on a topic can be very important precisely because, in some cases, exceptions that do not confirm a hypothesis can teach important lessons and even open up new interpretations of the hypothesis studied. A significant portion of studies that have challenged the climate science consensus, however, have not improved our understanding of the phenomenon. They have only distorted and manipulated reality and, more importantly, delayed policy action that could increase our chances to survive in the future.

In recent years, talks and policy proposals on global commitments to fight climate change have increased exponentially. Although empirical analyses by James Hansen and colleagues estimated that the aim of keeping the global average temperature below 1.5°C above preindustrial levels, as per the Paris Agreement, will inevitably be missed because of the recent acceleration of global warming,[99,100] in recent years there has been a mobilization of efforts to address the climate crisis. In spite of the growing institutional attention and public awareness, political action has been totally inadequate, characterized by what, during a conference organized by the Human Rights Centre at the University of Padova, I described as "greenwashing, green wishing or green wishy-washy." Greenwashing refers to the practice of making misleading or fake claims about the environmental benefits of a policy. Companies or governments may engage in greenwashing to present themselves as more environmentally responsible than they are, without making significant changes to their practices. Green wishing implies that climate policies might be about making optimistic or hopeful statements without substantial actions or strategies to address the root causes of environmental problems. In this context, policies celebrated as key changes toward sustainability might appear environmentally friendly, but their effectiveness is limited. Green wishy-washy suggests a lack of decisiveness or commitment to environmental policies.

Recent years have produced an unprecedented number of new policies and initiatives on the environment. However, these commendable efforts to avoid global climate collapse have barely scratched the surface of the problem. The practicality of even the most achievable ecological goals is challenged by current political and economic impasse. In the last 15 years alone, approximately 30% of all CO2 emissions since the start of the Industrial Revolution have been released, amounting to over 1.5 trillion tons. The concentration of GHG in the atmosphere has already surpassed 385 ppm and continues to rise. More than half a century of international meetings, academic discussions, policy proposals and IPCC reports have not successfully altered this ecological trend. While the wealthiest nations, led by the United States, fall short in environmental sustainability efforts, most developing countries prioritize their developmental goals over ecological concerns. Even if adhered to, the emission reduction commitments made by governments, are projected to result in insufficient decreases in emissions.[101]

This dire situation emphasizes the urgent need for decisive action. The first step is to acknowledge that climate change is more than just an ecological crisis. It's a systemic failure that encompasses philosophical, political, economic and psychological dimensions of modern society and its culture. Like the threat of new pandemics, the climate change crisis is a manifestation of "deep fractures" in our societal fabric, where economic considerations are still prioritized over ecological and human goals. Underlying issues such as deforestation, agricultural intensification, wildlife trade, travel, overconsumption and overpopulation are driven by a global economic model that prioritizes profit and markets above all else.[102, 103] As suggested by Johan Rockström and colleagues, humanity must reorganize itself, by redirecting economic incentives and capital toward environmentally beneficial solutions. This reorientation could include adopting a circular bioeconomy, enhancing resource efficiency and striving for zero waste.[91] An article in *The Lancet* also emphasized the need to realign society's priorities to prevent breaching ecosystem limits.[104] These are reasonable suggestions; however, they overlook an important aspect that can be summarized by slightly modifying a well-known slogan by former American President Bill Clinton: "It's the economy and power, baby!"

References

1. Marmot M. Why did England have Europe's worst Covid figures? The answer starts with austerity. *The Guardian*. Published online Aug 10, 2020. https://www.theguardian.com/commentisfree/2020/aug/10/england-worst-covid-figures-austerity-inequality (accessed Jan 24, 2024).

2. The tragic tale of a pangolin, the world's most trafficked animal | short film showcase. YouTube. National Geographic. Published online Feb 20, 2017. https://www.youtube.com/watch?v=XMx13JZ5FZU (accessed Jan 24, 2024).

3. Trentin R., Il pangolino, minacciato di estinzione per colpa dell'uomo. Il Bo Live UniPD. Published online Sept 6, 2018. http://ilbolive.unipd.it/it/news/pangolino-minacciato-estinzione-colpa-delluomo (accessed Jan 24, 2024).

4. Burki T. The origin of SARS-CoV-2. *The Lancet Infectious Diseases* 2020; 20: 1018–9.

5. Cyranoski D. Did pangolins spread the China coronavirus to people? *Nature* Published online Feb 7, 2020. https://doi.org/10.1038/d41586-020-00364-2

6. Karlsson EA, Duong V. The continuing search for the origins of SARS-CoV-2. *Cell* 2021; **184**: 4373–4.

7. Turcios-Casco MA, Cazzolla Gatti R. Do not blame bats and pangolins! Global consequences for wildlife conservation after the SARS-CoV-2 pandemic. *Biodivers Conserv* 2020; **29**: 3829–33.

8. Worobey M, Levy JI, Malpica Serrano L, *et al.* The Huanan seafood wholesale market in Wuhan was the early epicenter of the COVID-19 pandemic. *Science* 2022; 377: 951–9.

9. Boseley S. Origin story: what do we know now about where coronavirus came from? *The Guardian*. Published online Dec 12, 2020. https://www.theguardian.com/world/2020/dec/12/where-did-coronavirus-come-from-covid (accessed Jan 24, 2024).

10. Maxmen A. Wuhan market was epicentre of pandemic's start, studies suggest. *Nature* 2022; 603: 15–6.

11. Zarocostas J. WHO team begins COVID-19 origin investigation. *The Lancet* 2021; 397: 459.

12. World Health Organization. WHO-convened global study of origins of SARS-CoV-2: China part. Joint report. 2021.

13. Why many scientists say it's unlikely that SARS-CoV-2 originated from a 'lab leak'. Sccience. https://www.science.org/content/article/why-many-scientists-say-unlikely-sars-cov-2-originated-lab-leak (accessed Jan 25, 2024).

14. Andersen KG, Rambaut A, Lipkin WI, Holmes EC, Garry RF. The proximal origin of SARS-CoV-2. *Nature Medicine* 2020; **26**: 450–2.

15. Cohen J. Evidence suggests pandemic came from nature, not a lab, panel says. Science. Published online Oct 10, 2022. https://www.science.org/content/article/evidence-suggests-pandemic-came-nature-not-lab-panel-says (accessed Jan 25, 2024).

16. Segreto R, Deigin Y, McCairn K, *et al.* Should we discount the laboratory origin of COVID-19? *Environmental Chemistry Letters* 2021; **19**: 2743–57.

17. Maxmen A. Divisive COVID 'lab leak' debate prompts dire warnings from researchers. *Nature* 2021; **594**: 15–6.

18. Rasmussen AL. On the origins of SARS-CoV-2. *Nature Medicine* 2021; **27**: 9.

19. Pompeo says 'significant' evidence that new coronavirus emerged from Chinese lab. Reuters. Published online May 4, 2020. https://www.reuters.com/article/idUSKBN22G049/ (accessed Jan 24, 2024).

20. Gertz B. Coronavirus link to China biowarfare program possible, analyst says. *The Washington Times*. https://www.washingtontimes.com/news/2020/jan/26/coronavirus-link-to-china-biowarfare-program-possi/ (accessed Jan 24, 2024).

21. Dreyfuss B. Trump has no secret intel on the coronavirus's origins. *The Nation*. Published online May 22, 2020. https://www.thenation.com/article/world/trump-china-coronavirus-bush-iraq/ (accessed Jan 24, 2024).

22. BMJP Group. Lab leaks? ... and other stories. *BMJ* 2021; 373: n811.

23. Maxmen A, Mallapaty S. The COVID lab-leak hypothesis: what scientists do and don't know. *Nature* 2021; 594: 313–5.

24. Thacker PD. Covid-19: Lancet investigation into origin of pandemic shuts down over bias risk. *BMJ* 2021; 375: n2414.

25. Bloom JD, Chan YA, Baric RS, *et al*. Investigate the origins of COVID-19. *Science* 2021; 372: 694.

26. Sachs JD, Karim SSA, Aknin L, *et al*. The Lancet commission on lessons for the future from the COVID-19 pandemic. *The Lancet* 2022; 400: 1224–80.

27. Harrison NL, Sachs JD. A call for an independent inquiry into the origin of the SARS-CoV-2 virus. *Proceedings of the National Academy of Sciences* 2022; 119: e2202769119.

28. Boyd C. Covid leaked from AMERICAN – not Chinese – lab, top US professor says. Mail Online. Published online July 4, 2022. https://www.dailymail.co.uk/health/article-10980715/Covid-leaked-AMERICAN-lab-claims-professor-Jeffrey-Sachs.html (accessed Jan 25, 2024).

29. Kilander G. Lancet report claiming Covid could have come from US lab prompts anger. *The Independent*. Published online Oct 4, 2022. https://www.independent.co.uk/news/world/americas/covid-report-lancet-us-lab-b2168248.html (accessed Jan 25, 2024).

30. Thorp H. Continued discussion on the origin of COVID-19. Science. Published online May 13, 2021. https://www.science.org/content/blog-post/continued-discussion-origin-covid-19 (accessed Jan 25, 2024).

31. McMahon S. Do extraordinary claims require extraordinary evidence? The proper role of Sagan's dictum in astrobiology. In: Smith KC, Mariscal C, eds. Social and conceptual issues in astrobiology. Oxford University Press, 2020: 117–129.

32. Pekar JE, Magee A, Parker E, *et al*. SARS-CoV-2 emergence very likely resulted from at least two zoonotic events. Zenodo. Published online Feb 26, 2022. https://doi.org/10.5281/zenodo.6291628

33. Cohen J., Politicians, scientists spar over alleged NIH cover-up using COVID-19 origin paper. Science. July, 2023. https://www.science.org/content/article/politicians-scientists-spar-over-alleged-nih-cover-up-using-covid-19-origin-paper (accessed Jan 25, 2024).

34. Gorman J, Zimmer C. Scientist opens up about his early email to Fauci on virus origins. *The New York Times*. Published online June 14, 2021. https://www.nytimes.com/2021/06/14/science/covid-lab-leak-fauci-kristian-andersen.html (accessed Jan 25, 2024).

35. Ineichen A. Letter: Keynes changed his mind, even if the quote isn't his. *Financial Times*. Published online Sep 6, 2022. https://www.ft.com/content/76e6fae7-f273-49e6-8238-288d9e4991c7 (accessed Jan 25, 2024).

36. Dharmarajan G, Li R, Chanda E, *et al*. The animal origin of major human infectious diseases: what can past epidemics teach us about preventing the next pandemic? *Zoonoses* 2022; 2: 989.

37. Song Z, Xu Y, Bao L, *et al*. From SARS to MERS, thrusting coronaviruses into the spotlight. *Viruses* 2019; 11: 59.

38. Wu Z, Jin Q, Wu G, *et al*. SARS-CoV-2's origin should be investigated world-wide for pandemic prevention. *The Lancet* 2021; 398: 1299–303.

39. Chang L, Zhao L, Xiao Y, *et al*. Serosurvey for SARS-CoV-2 among blood donors in Wuhan, China from September to December 2019. *Protein & Cell* 2023; 14: 28–36.

40. Cohen J. Where did the pandemic start? Anywhere but here, argue papers by Chinese scientists echoing party line. Science. Published online on Aug 18, 2022. https://www.science.org/content/article/pandemic-start-anywhere-but-here-argue-papers-chinese-scientists-echoing-party-line (accessed Jan 25, 2024).

41. Il Fatto Quotidiano. Coronavirus, media: 'Primo caso d'infezione accertato in Cina risale al 17 novembre e non all'8 dicembre'. *Il Fatto Quotidiano*. Published

online March 13, 2020. https://www.ilfattoquotidiano.it/2020/03/13/coronavirus-media-primo-caso-dinfezione-accertato-in-cina-risale-al-17-novembre-e-non-all8-dicembre/5736081/ (accessed Jan 25, 2024).

42. Trump: U.S. appreciates China's 'efforts and transparency' on coronavirus. Reuters. Published online Jan 24, 2020. https://www.reuters.com/article/idUSKBN1ZN2IK/ (accessed Jan 25, 2024).

43. Farley R. Trump misquotes Fauci on coronavirus threat. FactCheck.org. Fact Check. Published online April 29, 2020. https://www.factcheck.org/2020/04/trump-misquotes-fauci-on-coronavirus-threat/ (accessed Jan 25, 2024).

44. Wollner A. Coronavirus, frasi choc di Zaia sui cinesi: "Li abbiamo visti tutti mangiare i topi vivi". TrevisoToday. Published online Feb 28, 2020. https://www.trevisotoday.it/video/zaia-cinesi-topi-vivi-treviso-28-febbraio-2020.html (accessed Jan 25, 2024).

45. Yi-Zheng Lian. Opinion | Why did the coronavirus outbreak start in China? *The New York Times*. Published online Feb 20, 2020. https://www.nytimes.com/2020/02/20/opinion/sunday/coronavirus-china-cause.html (accessed Jan 25, 2024).

46. Frutos R, Serra-Cobo J, Chen T, Devaux CA. COVID-19: time to exonerate the pangolin from the transmission of SARS-CoV-2 to humans. *Infection, Genetics and Evolution* 2020; 84: 104493.

47. Frutos R, Lopez Roig M, Serra-Cobo J, Devaux CA. COVID-19: the conjunction of events leading to the coronavirus pandemic and lessons to learn for future threats. *Frontiers in Medicine (Lausanne)* 2020; 7: 223.

48. Preventing the next pandemic. United Nations Environment Programme and International Livestock Research Institute. Published online Feb 7, 2020. https://www.ilri.org/preventing-next-pandemic (accessed Jan 25, 2024).

49. Jones KE, Patel NG, Levy MA, et al. Global trends in emerging infectious diseases. *Nature* 2008; 451: 990–3.

50. Dalton J. Meat-eating creates risk of new pandemic that 'would make Covid look like a dress rehearsal'. *The Independent*. Published online Jan 30, 2021. https://www.independent.co.uk/climate-change/news/meat-coronavirus-pandemic-science-animals-b1794996.html (accessed Jan 25, 2024).

51. Quammen D. Spillover: animal infections and the next human pandemic. New York, NY: WW Norton & Co, 2013.

52. Morand S, Lajaunie C. Outbreaks of vector-borne and zoonotic diseases are associated with changes in forest cover and oil palm expansion at global scale. *Frontiers in Veterinary Science* 2021; 8. https://www.frontiersin.org/articles/10.3389/fvets.2021.661063 (accessed Jan 25, 2024).

53. Afelt A, Frutos R, Devaux C. Bats, coronaviruses, and deforestation: toward the emergence of novel infectious diseases? *Frontiers in Microbiology* 2018; 9. https://www.frontiersin.org/articles/10.3389/fmicb.2018.00702 (accessed Jan 25, 2024).

54. Scillitani L. Aids, Hendra, Nipah, Ebola, Lyme, Sars, Mers, Covid.... Scienza in rete. Published online March 18, 2020. https://www.scienzainrete.it/articolo/aids-hendra-nipah-ebola-lyme-sars-mers-covid%E2%80%A6/laura-scillitani/2020-03-18 (accessed Jan 25, 2024).

55. Lawler OK, Allan HL, Baxter PWJ, et al. The COVID-19 pandemic is intricately linked to biodiversity loss and ecosystem health. *The Lancet Planetary Health* 2021; 5: e840–50.

56. Ritchie H, Roser M. Drivers of deforestation. *Our World in Data*. Published online Jan 15, 2024. https://ourworldindata.org/drivers-of-deforestation (accessed Jan 25, 2024).

57. Wallace RG. Big farms make big flu: dispatches on infectious disease, agribusiness, and the nature of science. New York, NY: Monthly Review Press, 2016.

58. Is the next pandemic on our plate? Compassion in World Farming. Published online May 6, 2020. https://www.ciwf.org.uk/news/2020/05/is-the-next-pandemic-on-our-plate (accessed Jan 25, 2024).

59. Jones BA, Grace D, Kock R, *et al.* Zoonosis emergence linked to agricultural intensification and environmental change. *Proceedings of the National Academy of Sciences* 2013; **110**: 8399–404.

60. Espinosa R, Tago D, Treich N. Infectious diseases and meat production. *Environmental and Resource Economics* 2020; **76**: 1019–44.

61. Grover N. Deadly pig disease could have led to Covid spillover to humans, analysis suggests. *The Guardian.* Published online March 10, 2021. https://www.theguardian.com/environment/2021/mar/10/deadly-pig-disease-could-have-led-to-covid-spillover-to-humans-analysis-suggests (accessed Jan 25, 2024).

62. Xia W, Hughes J, Robertson D, Jiang X. How one pandemic led to another: ASFV, the disruption contributing to Sars-Cov-2 emergence in Wuhan. Published online Feb 25, 2021. https://doi.org/10.20944/preprints202102.0590.v1

63. Lytras S, Xia W, Hughes J, Jiang X, Robertson DL. The animal origin of SARS-CoV-2. *Science* 2021; **373**: 968–70.

64. Robert Wallace. Resilience. Planet farm. Published online March 22, 2021. https://www.resilience.org/stories/2021-03-22/planet-farm/ (accessed Jan 25, 2024).

65. Ramankutty N, Mehrabi Z, Waha K, *et al.* Trends in global agricultural land use: implications for environmental health and food security. *Annual Review of Plant Biology* 2018; **69**: 789–815.

66. White paper on a GEF COVID-19 response strategy. Global Environment Facility. Published online Nov 17, 2020. https://www.thegef.org/council-meeting-documents/white-paper-gef-covid-19-response-strategy (accessed Jan 25, 2024).

67. Arieff A. How Covid-19 is changing the wet markets of China. City Monitor. Published online Sept 21, 2020. https://citymonitor.ai/government/public-health/how-covid-19-is-changing-the-wet-markets-of-china (accessed Jan 25, 2024).

68. Guarascio F, Guarascio F. Exclusive: China out of UN's wildlife survey for pandemic controls. Reuters. Published online April 13, 2023. https://www.reuters.com/world/china/china-out-uns-wildlife-survey-pandemic-controls-source-2023-04-13/ (accessed Feb 9, 2024).

69. Boseley S. Calls for global ban on wild animal markets amid coronavirus outbreak. *The Guardian.* Published online Jan 24, 2020. https://www.theguardian.com/science/2020/jan/24/calls-for-global-ban-wild-animal-markets-amid-coronavirus-outbreak (accessed Jan 25, 2024).

70. Covid. Via l'isolamento per chi contrae il virus. Schillaci: "Abrogato l'ultimo divieto reale". Quotidiano Sanità. https://www.quotidianosanita.it/governo-e-parlamento/articolo.php?articolo_id=116100 (accessed Jan 25, 2024).

71. Valigia Blu. Gli Stati di tutto il mondo stanno trattando i sintomi ma non le cause ecosistemiche della pandemia'. Valigia Blu. Published online July 8, 2020. https://www.valigiablu.it/onu-pandemie-cause-zoonosi/ (accessed Jan 25, 2024).

72. Mora C, McKenzie T, Gaw IM, *et al.* Over half of known human pathogenic diseases can be aggravated by climate change. *Nature Climate Change* 2022; **12**: 869–75.

73. Beyer RM, Manica A, Mora C. Shifts in global bat diversity suggest a possible role of climate change in the emergence of SARS-CoV-1 and SARS-CoV-2. *Science of the Total Environment* 2021; **767**: 145413.

74. Palmer C, Pearson N and Kyriacou G. What is the role of deforestation in climate change and how can 'Reducing Emissions from Deforestation and Degradation' (REDD+) help? Grantham Research Institute on Climate Change and the Environment. Published online on Feb 10, 2023. https://www.lse.ac.uk/granthaminstitute/explainers/whats-redd-and-will-it-help-tackle-climate-change/ (accessed Jan 25, 2024).

75. Pearson TRH, Brown S, Murray L, Sidman G. Greenhouse gas emissions from tropical forest degradation: an underestimated source. *Carbon Balance and Management* 2017; **12**: 3.
76. Lynch J, Cain M, Frame D, Pierrehumbert R. Agriculture's contribution to climate change and role in mitigation is distinct from predominantly fossil CO_2-emitting sectors. *Frontiers in Sustainable Food Systems* 2021; **4**. https://www.frontiersin.org/articles/10.3389/fsufs.2020.518039.
77. Willcock S, Cooper GS, Addy J, Dearing JA. Earlier collapse of Anthropocene ecosystems driven by multiple faster and noisier drivers. *Nature Sustainability* 2023; **6**: 1331–42.
78. Romanello M, Mc Gushin A, Di Napoli C, et al. The 2021 report of the Lancet Countdown on Health and Climate Change: code red for a healthy future. *The Lancet* 2021; **398**(10311):1619–1162. https://www.thelancet.com/article/S0140-6736(21)01787-6/fulltext.
79. NOAA. Global climate summary for July 2022 | Climate.gov. http://www.climate.gov/news-features/understanding-climate/global-climate-summary-july-2022 (accessed Jan 25, 2024).
80. How is climate linked to extreme weather? Met Office. https://www.metoffice.gov.uk/weather/climate/climate-and-extreme-weather (accessed Jan 25, 2024).
81. Kemp L, Xu C, Depledge J, et al. Climate endgame: exploring catastrophic climate change scenarios. *Proceedings of the National Academy of Sciences* 2022; **119**: e2108146119.
82. Diamond JM. Collapse: how societies choose to fail or succeed, Ed. with a new afterword. New York, NY: Penguin Books, 2011.
83. Bologna M, Aquino G. Deforestation and world population sustainability: a quantitative analysis. *Scientific Reports* 2020; **10**: 7631.
84. Xu Y Ramanatha V. Well below 2°C: mitigation strategies for avoiding dangerous to catastrophic climate changes. PNAS, 2017; **114**(39): 10315–10323P. https://www.pnas.org/doi/10.1073/pnas.1618481114 (accessed Jan 25, 2024).
85. Monroe R. New climate risk classification created to account for potential 'existential' threats. Scripps Institution of Oceanography. Published online Sept 14. https://scripps.ucsd.edu/news/new-climate-risk-classification-created-account-potential-existential-threats (accessed Jan 25, 2024).
86. Dyer G. Climate wars: the fight for survival as the world overheats. Oxford: Oneworld Publications, 2010.
87. McKay A, Jesse A, Abrams J, et al. Exceeding 1.5°C global warming could trigger multiple climate tipping points. Science, 2022; **377**(6611): 1–10. https://www.science.org/doi/10.1126/science.abn7950 (accessed Jan 25, 2024).
88. Randers J, Goluke U. An earth system model shows self-sustained thawing of permafrost even if all man-made GHG emissions stop in 2020. *Scientific Reports* 2020; **10**: 18456.
89. Pörtner H-O, Roberts DC, Tignor MMB, et al., editors. Climate change 2022: impacts, adaptation and vulnerability: contribution of working group II to the sixth assessment report of the Intergovernmental Panel on Climate Change. 2022. Cambridge University Press, Cambridge, UK and New York.
90. Harvey F. IPCC issues 'bleakest warning yet' on impacts of climate breakdown | Climate crisis. *The Guardian*. Published online on Feb 28, 2022. https://www.theguardian.com/environment/2022/feb/28/ipcc-issues-bleakest-warning-yet-impacts-climate-breakdown (accessed Jan 25, 2024).
91. Richardson, K., Steffen, W., Lucht, W., et al. Earth beyond six of nine planetary boundaries. *Science Advances* 2023; **9**:37. https://www.science.org/doi/epdf/10.1126/sciadv.adh2458

92. McKie R. 'Soon the world will be unrecognisable': is it still possible to prevent total climate meltdown? *The Observer*. Published online July 30, 2022. https://www.theguardian.com/environment/2022/jul/30/total-climate-meltdown-inevitable-heatwaves-global-catastrophe (accessed Jan 25, 2024).
93. Dunne D. Is the climate crisis pushing the world towards a 'point of no return'? *The Independent*. Published online Nov 12, 2020. https://www.independent.co.uk/climate-change/news/climate-change-crisis-tipping-point-world-warm-b1721822.html (accessed Jan 25, 2024).
94. Glacier shrinkage is past the point of no return. *Nature* 2018; 555: 562–2.
95. Avasthi A. Climate's point of no return. Science. Published online March 17, 2005. https://www.science.org/content/article/climates-point-no-return (accessed Jan 25, 2024).
96. Earthtalk. Have we passed the point of no return on climate change? *Scientific American*. https://www.scientificamerican.com/article/have-we-passed-the-point-of-no-return-on-climate-change/ (accessed Jan 25, 2024).
97. Harvey F. CO_2 emissions: nations' pledges 'far away' from Paris target, says UN. *The Guardian*. Published online Feb 26, 2021. https://www.theguardian.com/environment/2021/feb/26/co2-emissions-nations-pledges-far-away-from-paris-target-says-un (accessed Jan 25, 2024).
98. Alimonti G, Mariani L, Prodi F, Ricci RA. Retracted article: a critical assessment of extreme events trends in times of global warming. *The European Physical Journal - Plus* 2022; **137**: 112.
99. Hansen J, Kharecha P, Loeb N, *et al.* How we know that global warming is accelerating and that the goal of the Paris Agreement is dead. Columbia University. Published online Nov 10, 2023. https://mailchi.mp/caa/how-we-know-that-global-warming-is-accelerating-and-that-the-goal-of-the-paris-agreement-is-dead (accessed Jan 25, 2024).
100. Harvey C. Open secret at climate talks: the top temperature goal is mostly gone. Politico. Published online March 12, 2023. https://www.politico.com/news/2023/12/03/cop28-global-temperature-goal-00129766 (accessed Jan 25, 2024).
101. "Climate commitments not on track to meet Paris Agreement goals" as NDC synthesis report is Published. UNFCCC. Published online on Feb 26, 2021. https://unfccc.int/news/climate-commitments-not-on-track-to-meet-paris-agreement-goals-as-ndc-synthesis-report-is-published (accessed Jan 25, 2024).
102. Tonissen P. IPBES #PandemicsReport: escaping the 'era of pandemics'. IPBES Secretariat. Published online Oct 19, 2020. https://www.ipbes.net/pandemics (accessed Jan 25, 2024).
103. De Vogli R. Progress or collapse: the crises of market greed. London, New York: Routledge, 2013.
104. Mair S. Neoliberal economics, planetary health, and the COVID-19 pandemic: A Marxist ecofeminist analysis. *The Lancet Planetary Health* 2020; 4: e588–96.

10

THE ECONOMIC FABRIC OF ZOONOSES

Once upon a time there was a planet where life was "nasty, brutal and short"[1] and the average lifespan didn't exceed 30 years. Poverty and hunger were widespread, and health was precarious, often threatened by lethal infectious diseases. The Black Death, for instance, wiped out nearly a third of Europe's population between 1347 and 1352.[2] For nearly 200,000 years, Homo sapiens grappled with early death and fatal diseases. Whether we were happier at the time is unknown and unknowable. However, what is certain is that over the last two centuries, longevity has significantly increased, with global life expectancy now exceeding 70 years. (Figure 10.1) While longevity isn't everything, how old are you? Are you more than 30 years of age? Then count all the extra years you have lived thanks to being born in the modern era. If you are under 30, however, count the years you would have left if you had been born in an earlier historical period. To paraphrase a famous phrase by Schopenhauer, "longevity is not everything, but without it, health is nothing."[3]

The changes generated after the Industrial Revolution caused enormous human suffering and injustices, and yet they marked a historical turning point. Without these transformations, maybe our lives would likely have remained "nasty, brutal and short." The societal changes associated with this historical event enabled improvements in nutrition, sanitation and medical care, granting access to goods, services and technologies that have enhanced not just our lifespan but also our quality of life. Such advancements are the result of large-scale improvements in socioeconomic conditions, fundamental to the material, nutritional, hygienic, health and technological success of our society. Of course, for the farmers whose lands were expropriated during the "enclosures," then forced to emigrate and work in the nascent English textile industries, the Industrial Revolution

DOI: 10.4324/9781003511977-14

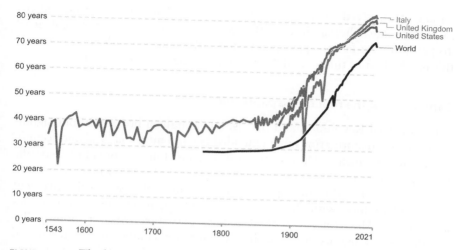

FIGURE 10.1   The longevity revolution: life expectancy at birth in the world, Italy, the United Kingdom and the United States (1543–2021)

Sources: UN WPP (2022); HMD (2023); Zijdeman et al. (2015); Riley (2005) – with minor processing by Our World in Data. "Life expectancy at birth – Various sources – period tables" [dataset]. Human Mortality Database, "Human Mortality Database"; United Nations, "World Population Prospects 2022"; United Nations, "World Population Prospects"; Zijdeman et al., "Life Expectancy at birth 2"; James C. Riley, "Estimates of Regional and Global Life Expectancy, 1800–2001" [original data]. Retrieved February 14, 2024 from https://ourworldindata.org/grapher/life-expectancy?country=OWID_WRL~ITA~GBR~USA

was a horrible and tragic event. The situation was even worse for child slave workers in the first English mills and mines, who were to unspeakable risks, very long working hours and unthinkable hygiene conditions, as well as premature death.[4]

Even today, due to the gross maldistribution of power and economic resources within and across societies, grotesque inequalities remain, where hunger and poverty continue to cause premature mortality associated with preventable diseases. At the same time, dramatic improvements in global living standards are undeniable. Longevity has increased more in the last century than in the previous two millennia.

Even critics of this model of economic progress acknowledge its remarkable achievements. Economic development has improved the health of billions globally, reducing infectious diseases and infant mortality everywhere including in less affluent countries. We now have healthcare and medications that make diseases curable and disabilities more tolerable. We are healthier, freer, taller and more educated than ever before. Many enjoy luxuries once unimaginable: comfortable homes, automobiles, smartphones, laptops and travel opportunities. Despite the dire ecological troubles we face, we live in an era of unprecedented possibilities, a period that can be considered the most fortunate in human history. But, we also face unprecedented challenges. To paraphrase a famous passage in Charles Dickens's *A Tale of Two Cities*, this is "the best of times" and "the worst of times" at the same time.

Capital sins at the root of the pandemic

The Industrial Revolution and the rise of capitalism brought about significant social transformations that extended beyond mere material and technological advancements. These changes were rooted in the spread of a specific ideology – a set of ideas aimed at defining the ideal organization of a social system. Central to this ideology is utilitarianism, a philosophical movement equating happiness with pleasure or consumption, also known in economics as "utility." This concept marked a sharp departure from previous philosophical and religious views of life, which never emphasized material and economic success as a path to achieving happiness. Before this era, in spite of cultural and philosophical differences, the pursuit of wealth and consumer excess was seen almost as a form of mental pathology. The advent of utilitarianism has radically changed this perspective, and economic prosperity became the primary goal of life, especially in Western nations, but also globally.

With the rapid and unprecedented improvements in material conditions in recent centuries, it might be reasonable to expect a cultural transition toward what many philosophers, psychologists and even economists define as the "true" goal of progress: human actualization or personal fulfillment. But this has not happened. On the contrary, material wealth has remained the comet star of our model of human progress, and in recent times it became even more important as a life goal. Surveys from various US university campuses indicate a growing emphasis on financial success as a main life aspiration among students. This trend is not limited to American college students but reflects a global shift, propelled by cultural globalization and the geopolitical, media and economic influence of the United States. The frenetic march toward higher economic status and material success has occurred at both the personal and societal level. Despite obvious differences and inequalities, the prototypical individual in modern society expects to constantly advance his or her own career, wealth and power. Nations do the same collectively, for example by striving toward ever-increasing GDP. Dominant and high-income nations, which have achieved privileged economic conditions, continue to enrich themselves and compete to improve their economy, while those with low and middle incomes aspire to reach the same standards of living as the richer countries.

There is a term that can be used to describe the cultural inclination to prioritize economic activities over all other forms of human endeavor: economism.[5] Its etymology can be traced back to various thinkers, but Karl Polanyi was notably influential in shaping this concept. In his seminal work, *The Great Transformation: The Political and Economic Origins of Our Time*, Polanyi argued that in modern capitalist societies, "it is not the economy that is embedded in social relations, but it is social relations that are embedded in the economic system."[6] This has led to a progressive commodification of people and interpersonal exchanges, often referred to as "social or human capital," in which their value is determined by the needs of the economy. Under this economistic perspective, nature and animals are also viewed as "natural capital," merely resources for exchange in the market. The value of occupations is similarly distorted; jobs that are very beneficial to society and contribute to the public welfare (e.g. school teachers, nurses) tend to be undervalued or poorly paid. Conversely, some highly paid job roles, particularly in speculative financial markets, that not only fail to produce any public good but can cause significant harm to society, known as "bullshit jobs,"[7] are objects of respect and even admiration.

The increasing dominance of economic principles in all sectors of society, including education and politics, can be observed in additional ways. Universities, traditionally bastions of public knowledge and learning, have undergone a gradual shift toward privatization. They are increasingly being viewed and operated as businesses competing in the educational market. This change reflects a broader trend by which economic values and motivations are permeating almost every facet of modern life. One striking example of this trend is the uniquely superior status of economics among all the social sciences.[8] Have you ever wondered why, among numerous social sciences (e.g., philosophy, sociology, psychology, anthropology, international relations, political science), only economics is awarded a Nobel Prize?

An even more significant symptom of the dysfunctional impact of economism is the intrusion of economic motives into politics. Over the past five decades, democratic processes have been increasingly swayed by the financial clout of wealthy individuals and large corporations. Economic inequality and the escalating costs of political campaigns have further entrenched this trend. The wealthier segments of society contribute significantly to political funding, making it challenging for less affluent candidates to compete. This financial influence extends beyond national borders, with markets and international financial institutions acquiring significant power to sway political decisions even abroad. The democratic principle of voting is thus increasingly overshadowed by market and profit motives. Former European Budget Commissioner Gunther Oettinger's comment following a referendum in Italy encapsulates this sentiment: "the markets will teach the Italians to vote for the right thing."[9] As British political philosopher John Gray explains in the book *False Dawn: The Delusions of Global Capitalism*, governments are increasingly at the mercy of the political demands of speculative capital, and this has made redistributive and social policies almost impracticable. The growing internationalization of finance has offered wealthier investors the ability to influence the political decisions of governments: from their computers, by deciding whether or not to transfer large quantities of investments across borders, they can carry out real-time referenda on the policies of national governments. As US Senator Mark Hanna once observed, "There are two important things in politics. The first is money and I don't remember the second."[10]

The critique of modern society's relentless pursuit of economic growth, especially in the context of climate change, highlights a paradoxical problem. Robert Costanza, in his book *Addicted to Growth*, argues that modern society's addiction to economic expansion is so profound that it is even hampering our collective ability to respond effectively even to existential threats like climate change.[11] The global economy, which aims for infinite growth and is predominantly driven by market forces, lacks the capacity to steer societal efforts toward democratically planned, sustainable goals. Utilitarianism was perhaps justified for alleviating widespread poverty in times of material scarcity but is now obsolete and even destructive. As John Kenneth Galbraith observed, "furnishing an empty room is one thing. Continuing to pile furniture until the foundation begins to buckle is another."[12] Modern progress seems, in fact, driven by what can be called "futilitarianism," or a collective psychological tendency characterized by the inability to distinguish what is useful (that in Italian means "utile") from what is futile. Some sociologists argue that the pursuit of well-being primarily through financial success is a form of "cultural fraud." Consumerism, ironically defined as the idea of "spending money we don't have, to buy things we don't need, to create impressions on people we don't care about," is not only disastrous on an ecological level but also harmful psychologically. American economist William Baumol observed that a capitalist economy thrives on GDP growth, which is promoted by consumer spending. Therefore, it must be driven by the perpetual dissatisfaction of our desires. If our wants are completely satisfied, the economy is destined to go into crisis.[13] Just like a zero-sum game, the economy is happy when we are not.

Some economists find criticism of utilitarianism and capitalism unfair, arguing that humanity owes a clear debt of gratitude to this model of development, which has generated such exceptional results in terms of material well-being and life expectancy. What seems to escape proponents of this argument, however, is the realization that the exponential growth in our living standards cannot continue indefinitely. The feast of material success of humanity, based on the exponential growth of the satisfaction of ever-increasing new wants, which began with the Industrial Revolution, will sooner or later be interrupted by the reaching of the limits of the ecosystem.

Those who have studied the problem in depth already understood this a long time ago. In the essay "Civilized Man's Eight Capital Sins," Konrad Lorenz observed that while natural organisms have homeostatic regulatory mechanisms with "negative feedback," our model of development is structured in exactly the opposite way: like a tumor cell, it is based on "positive feedback," or infinite growth, without self-regulation. As the scientist explains, "The neoplastic cell is distinguished from the normal one by having lost the genetic information necessary to make it a useful member of the community of interests represented by the body."[14]

The neoliberal variant of capitalism

In discussing the "development model," or the overarching strategies and philosophies that guide economic progress across different nations, it's important to note that this is not a uniform approach; different countries adopt various political-economic methods and reforms. However, in recent decades, amidst rapid increases in consumption, industrial production and population growth, there has been a convergence toward a particular form of global economic development. This shift is characterized by growing internationalization and the rise of a specific variant of capitalism, commonly referred to as "neoliberalism." Social scientists who have investigated neoliberal reforms and their effects on society have often been 'unwelcome' and even the target of stigmatising labels. Historian Philipp Mirowsky, author of *The Political Movement That Dared Not to Speak Its Name*, for example, claims that colleagues' responses to his work on the history of neoliberalism have taken, roughly, two major paths. The first rests on the argument that neoliberalism is nothing more than a "fevered delusion of his addled brain." The second says that if neoliberalism does indeed exist, "it is far too uneven and inconsistent to count as a serious analytical category."[15] Indeed, the idea that modern society has been transformed into a self-regulating global market and most countries simultaneously decided to adopt the same neoliberal policies almost sounds like a conspiracy theory, a kind of plot. Some of the critics, who admit that the ideology of neoliberalism does exist, think, however, that its study has largely been undertaken by its detractors to vent their criticism and ideological dissent. As Thomas Biebricher notes, neoliberalism "has now become a dirty word."[16]

Despite the controversies, the sheer volume of scientific work on the subject refutes the idea that neoliberalism is a mere figment of the imagination of some academics, or a reservoir of their frustrations. Sometimes called the "Washington consensus," "laissez-faire capitalism," "hyper-capitalism," "turbo-capitalism," "shock therapy" (in Eastern Europe) or "structural adjustment policies" (in developing countries), neoliberalism broadly refers, as David Harvey noted, to "a theory of political economic practices which proposes that human well-being can best be improved by liberating individual entrepreneurial freedoms and capacities within an institutional framework characterized by strong protection of private property, free markets and free trade."[17] In the global health courses I have taught at various universities, to help my students remember the key policy components of "neoliberal globalisation", I suggest that they memorise five terms ending in "-ation":[18]

- (Financial) deregul-ation
- Privatiz-ation (of state-owned enterprises)
- Liberaliz-ation (of trade)
- Flexibiliz-ation (of the labor market)
- Stabiliz-ation (of the state budget), or austerity

Neoliberalism derives primarily from the ideas of economists of the Mont Pelerin Society such as Friedrich Von Hayek and Milton Friedman, who, after the end of the Second World War, developed its main cornerstones. However, it is only thanks to the political rise of Ronald Reagan in the United States and Margaret Thatcher in the United Kingdom that these policies have gained global political dominance. In the previous post-war period, national and international policies were primarily inspired by the ideas of English economist John Maynard Keynes. Keynes placed particular emphasis on full employment and a type of capitalism capable of limiting or even reducing economic inequities. In the 1980s, however, the world was subjected to a neoliberal turning point that cornered Keynesianism. This radical shift was facilitated by a series of historical events and economic crises, as well as political pressure and funding from powerful stakeholders frustrated by the post-war Keynesian policies. In effect, in the most privileged circles of society, the reforms of the post-war period (1945–1980) were experienced as a kind of "financial repression" that required a political reaction, sometimes described as a "revolution in reverse."[19]

According to some critical and disenchanted scholars, neoliberalism is nothing other than the ideology underlying a "class war," – that is, the one launched (even if never declared) by the most powerful sectors of society, the best, over the middle class and the poor, the rest. Undoubtedly the advent of neoliberalism, first in the United States and the United Kingdom, then around the world, has offered the ultra-rich enormous opportunities to increase their wealth, power, political control and dominance. At the national level, countries that had at least attempted to adopt economic policies partly inspired by the Universal Declaration of Human Rights – aimed, for example, at guaranteeing work and universal access to essential goods and services for all – abandoned these aspirations to adopt neoliberal measures of deregulation, privatization and liberalization. Globally, neoliberal reforms such as the removal of capital controls and financialization have generated rapid movements of money, speculation and new opportunities for large-scale financial investments internationally. These policies have resulted in rapid growth in the power and wealth of the financial industry and facilitated the spread of tax havens. Tax cuts for the super-rich, tax havens and the creation of a world market where commercial and financial flows are promoted without too much state interference have generated a rapid increase in economic inequalities and a disproportionate concentration of political power in the wealthier classes. We now live in an age of grotesque socio-economic inequality. According to a study by Oxfam, the eight richest individuals in the world have as much wealth as the 3.6 billion people who make up the poorest half of the world.[20]

According to a neoliberal understanding of social processes, inequality is not an issue. On the contrary, this narrative supports the idea that the enrichment of society should take place through "the trickle-down approach," which postulates that it is possible to improve the living standards of the middle and lower classes through policies capable of generating wealth among the richer social classes, which will ultimately benefit everyone through a "cascade" effect. But what often trickles down is not wealth, but the toxic effects of financial crises fuelled by inequality and excessive speculation by the ultra-rich. A further neoliberal assumption is the assertion that "economic liberation" and the well-being of society can be ensured only if state interventions are reduced to a minimum. According to this school of thought, the free market, with rare exceptions, does not require strong regulations because it regulates itself. Ronald Reagan famously joked about this concept when he said, "Do you know what the nine most feared words in the English language are? I'm here from the government, I'm here to help. This narrative carefully avoids admitting that without some government interventions, poverty takes away liberty.[21] Like all theories, however, neoliberalism has often been applied inconsistently in the real world and political practice. Despite the theoretical opposition to the state and the ideal of an unlimited free market, neoliberal policies have at times been paired with strong state interventions on behalf of private powers, as in the case of the bailouts of large companies and aid to too-big-to-fail banks after the 2008 global financial crisis. In some cases, such as in Chile during the dictatorship of Augusto Pinochet, neoliberalism was imposed on the basis of highly repressive politics. In spite of the obvious conceptual contradictions, many neoliberals find some form of authoritarianism totally compatible with their preferred policy doctrines. As observed in an article entitled "Preventing the Abuses of Democracy," one of the founders of neoliberal thought, Friedrich von Hayek, expressed a preference for "a liberal dictator" (such as Pinochet) over "a democratic government lacking liberalism" (such as that of Salvador Allende).[22]

Neoliberalism has become the dominant economic policy worldwide not only under the pressure of the most powerful classes and conservative political leaders such as Reagan and Thatcher but also thanks to the interventions of international financial agencies, such as the International Monetary Fund (IMF), the World Bank and the World Trade Organization (WTO), or the former General Agreement on Tariffs and Trade (GATT). In theory, these institutions were supposed to act as 'lenders of last resort' to countries in economic crisis. In practice, they have promoted neoliberal policies around the world by granting loans only after 'conditionalities' have been met. Indebted developing countries and, more recently, European nations hit by economic crises have been obliged to adopt "structural adjustment" reforms, which involve deregulating, liberalizing and privatizing as quickly as possible. According to some officials of international financial institutions and mainstream economists, these "one size fits all" policies are the only way forward to achieve what could be conceived of as "economic salvation" in response to recessions. *New York Times* journalist Thomas Friedman equated these reforms with a kind of "straitjacket" that countries must wear in order to prosper economically.[23] Despite the rhetoric, the results of these policies have not lived up to expectations even from an economic standpoint. As Prof. Dani Rodrik eloquently remarked, "Neoliberalism is not just a morally bankrupt ideology … it's also bad economics."[24]

The liberalization of viruses

Neoliberal reforms have not only failed to deliver optimal economic outcomes such as financial stability; they have also generated deleterious effects in terms of environmental and animal health, thus fueling the danger of ecological disaster and new pandemics. Few authors have ventured to study the links between neoliberal policies and the amplifiers of pandemic risk.[25] As already argued, the neoliberal ideology has influenced the management of the COVID-19 pandemic by favoring, for example, a "laissez-faire" approach to the virus, the privatization of healthcare in the years preceding the health crisis and policies that fostered unequal access to COVID-19 vaccines. On top of these processes, however, neoliberal policies have also played an important role in favoring the origin and spread of pandemics. Perhaps, the most significant effect concerns the impact of trade liberalization policies in encouraging the spread of large-scale industrial agriculture and intensive animal farming. According to neoliberal theories, the deregulation of the agricultural market and the removal of restrictions that limit trade in the international food market are absolutely necessary to allow countries to prosper economically and reduce poverty. In addition, this economic ideology requires the elimination of agricultural subsidies to allow economic competition to push small farmers unable to produce surpluses to sell on the global market or go out of business. For the neoclassical economist, this is a fair price to pay to promote economic "progress." According to neoliberal theory, to combat food insecurity, the poorest nations in the world should exploit their countryside and industrialize agriculture as much as possible. The key word in this approach is "efficiency": we must always produce more in the shortest time possible. This often translates into a gradual vertical integration of smaller agricultural farms into larger agri-food companies.[26] It's the same logic used by the US Secretary of Agriculture Earl Butz, when he said, "get big or get out."[27]

Although the rise and consolidation of food chains and the concomitant decline of local food systems and small farms were phenomena first observed in the United States at the onset of the so-called neoliberal revolution, agricultural deregulation ended up becoming a worldwide phenomenon even before then. From the 1980s onward, the IMF, World Bank and WTO have urged developing countries to abandon domestic agriculture and turn to cash crops for export. Globalization and the interaction between global and local food systems have forced poor and middle-income farmers to compete with multinationals and agribusinesses like Tyson, transnational food manufacturers like Nestlé, global fast-food companies like McDonald's and global supermarkets like Walmart.[28] These policies and the removal of economic support for small farmers, instead of favoring free markets, have in fact generated food oligopolies[29] – a largely predictable outcome. In a market without rules, the winners of a commercial competition find it advantageous and rational to suppress the very same competition that made them winners. Large multinational food corporations (which exploit tax havens and have revenues as large as the GDP of entire countries) control ample segments of the "farm-to-table" food production system. With the gradual decline of less well-off economic actors, pushed out of business or "swallowed up" by mergers and acquisitions ("corporate cannibalism"), free market policies have produced the perfect antithesis of the free market: an economy where a few actors exercise great control over products, prices, producers and market conditions. The dominance of food multinationals has also indirectly generated changes in food consumption from a diet based on fruit and vegetables and other fresh foods grown and sold by local suppliers to a modern diet based on ultra-processed products. The consequences for public health are clear: obesity has tripled worldwide, and chronic diseases such as type II diabetes have become so prevalent that they affect more than half a billion people and are expected to double within a few decades.[30]

In addition to changing diets worldwide, neoliberal trade liberalization reforms have influenced another major risk factor for pandemics: deforestation. A 2020 study appearing in the *Journal of the Association of the Environment and Resource Economists* analyzed the historical association between regional trade liberalization agreements and deforestation, using data from 189 countries. The results show a large and statistically significant increase in deforestation in the three years following the enactment of a regional (free) trade agreement.[31] Free trade agreements destroy forests, and this increases the risk of new pathogens. As Andreas Malm emphasizes in his book 'Corona, Climate, Chronic Emergency', "if it were not for the economy ... which attacks nature, invades it, tears it apart, tears it to pieces, destroys it with a zeal that borders on the desire for extermination, these things [pandemics] would not happen."[32] These pathogens, trapped in the forests, would not reach us if we were not the ones who made them reach the cities. Often, free trade agreements have involved an increase in the conversion of agricultural land to animal husbandry. The expansion and consolidation of the meat sector, in particular, have inevitably increased the opportunities for the spread of new emerging infectious diseases. This is not only because of its effects on deforestation but also because of the conditions in which animals are raised. While it has certainly brought benefits in terms of efficiency, prices and speed of food production, as Rob Wallace observed, "the industrialization of food production has caused the industrialization of the creation of new pathogens."[33]

Trade liberalization policies are often associated with financial deregulation reforms, which are additional potential risk factors for deforestation. These policies are linked to investment in the extraction industry and phenomena such as land grabbing of agricultural land from small landowners in favor of agribusiness. A report by the University College London highlighted the agri-financial links between financial practices such as maximizing the productivity of agricultural land and realizing capital gains on the one hand and changes in land use and the adoption of intensive agricultural practices on the other, to the detriment of biodiversity and ecological protection.[34] The impoverishment of local communities caused by land grabbing also seems to facilitate another pandemic risk factor, the exploitation and trade of wild animals. Populations dispossessed of their land and rural agricultural activities have found themselves forced to find employment in sectors such as the trade in wild fauna (often captured in the forests and sold in city markets). As Rob Wallace points out, although pandemics often originate in places like the Wuhan market or farms that engage in intensive animal farming, to fully understand the origins of pandemics we should "follow the money." As he put it, "if we pay attention to entities that finance deforestation and highly pathogenic methods of agriculture, we should consider international financial centers such as London, Hong Kong and New York City as viral epicenters and then proceed to rename viruses and their variants to reflect their political-economic origins (e.g., 'NAFTA swine flu' and 'neoliberal Ebola')."[35]

Trade and financial liberalization reforms create new opportunities for the global propagation of pathogens also through their contribution to increasing commercial and tourist travel, as well as migration and job relocation. Globalization and the flexibilization of labor markets on a world scale have made viruses that once remained isolated in the forests of remote developing countries now connected to large cities, thanks to the phenomenal network of international trade, commerce, work and travel. International policies that have favored the rapid movement of capital, consumer goods and workers have also generated a series of conditions facilitating the rapid increase in climate conditions that facilitate the outbreak of new pandemics. It has been estimated that more than a quarter of GHG emissions are related to the international trade of goods and services.[36]

As the report 'The Climate Cost of Free Trade' points out, free trade agreements not only promote an export-led industrial agricultural model, but also influence environmental and energy policies and urbanisation, which have a significant impact on climate change.[37] In a chapter of the book entitled *Disappearing Peasantries? Rural Labour in Africa, Asia and Latin America* Deborah Bryceson explains that small farmers have been subjected to a "swim or drown" economic strategy.[38] Those whose land has been expropriated for extraction or industrial agriculture projects in particular have been left with little option apart from migrating to urban slums of megacities or overcrowded shantytowns. This may have caused not only further opportunities for virus transmission, but also a significant burden on their mental health. A recent meta-analysis conducted on over half a million people in 45 countries revealed that people who live in cities, especially the most crowded and chaotic ones, are much more likely to be depressed than those who live in rural areas.[39]

Of course, there are conflicting opinions about the effects of neoliberal policies. According to some authors, the benefits of trade liberalization, such as greater efficiency and new technologies, have increased the ability of countries to implement environmental regulations and protect ecosystems.[40,41] This argument, however, is at odds with data trends on deforestation and annual carbon emissions over time. Even some institutions that promoted trade and financial liberalization policies, such as the World Bank and IMF, have admitted that their own "structural adjustment" programs, which resulted in the approval of hundreds of fossil fuel extraction projects, have produced billions of tons of carbon dioxide emissions in developing countries.[42,43] A review published by the World Bank's Environment Department concluded that despite some positive effects, including technology transfer after trade liberalization and more efficient use of scarce natural resources after the removal of subsidies, there were significant negative environmental impacts of structural adjustment policies.[44] It is also important to underline that privatization and cuts in public sector spending, an essential component of the neoliberal policy agenda, go hand in hand with reforms that push for less stringent regulations in international forestry policy.[45]

Even if neoliberalism is presented as a neutral, scientific theory, in reality there is nothing neutral about its consequences: it favors private investors' right to profit over the public right to a healthy environment. For example, during the negotiations of the United Nations Climate Conference in Paris (COP21), an internal European Union (EU) document revealed that European governments instructed their representatives to "oppose any discussion on measures to combat climate change which could be a restriction on international trade."[46]

Neoliberalism is largely incompatible with ecological sustainability not only in everyday political practice but also on a theoretical level. As Robert Nadeau, author of *The Wealth of Nature: How Mainstream Economics Failed the Environment*, noted, neoclassical economics predicts that markets, over time, tend toward stability, not sustainability.[47] Neoclassical economic theory not only promotes a greater role for the private sector in the management of public goods but also advocates for voluntary commitments to self-preservation in opposition to national and international regulations. Neoliberal skepticism toward the development of legally binding environmental standards and science-based quantitative targets and sanctions arises from the assumption that government regulations are essentially distorting the magic working of free markets. Conceiving of natural resources as mere exchange goods to be traded and bartered in a fiercely competitive and unregulated market means that they will be protected only when the price is what "consumers" are willing to pay.[48] If measures to avoid an ecological collapse are too costly, they will be avoided. Clearly, as long as the dominant economic development paradigm remains based on neoliberal principles, the term "sustainable development" will remain an oxymoron.

Free markets "made in China"

In Western media, China is often at the center of controversies not only for its alleged culpability in triggering the COVID-19 pandemic and adopting the zero-COVID strategy, but also for being one of the major contributors to the climate change crisis. According to an editorial in the *Wall Street Journal*, one of the media outlets that has contributed to spreading climate denialism, China is "the worst polluter [in the world]."[49] Even in the opinion of a *Time* columnist, China is the worst country in the world in terms of pollution.[50] The American Enterprise Institute, a neoliberal think tank that, has propagated false climate news, proposed "coercing" China (and India) to adopt policies capable of addressing climate change.[51] The role played by China in terms of pollution and climate change is certainly an important problem for the future of humanity. If we still hope to avoid the worst effects of the ecological crisis, Chinese environmental policies must be radically changed. But is China really the worst polluter in the world?

To understand who has contributed the most to global climate change, it is crucial to verify which countries, historically or since the Industrial Revolution, have emitted the most GHG into the atmosphere per capita (Figure 10.2). Those who try to point to China as the world's main polluter have engaged in a typical exercise of "cherry picking": focusing all attention on one element of reality (the country's total greenhouse gas emissions) while deliberately ignoring other very important aspects (such as the country's population size and historical emissions).

It is also important to note that recent reductions in GHG in richer countries are partly caused by the effects of outsourcing (a reform often

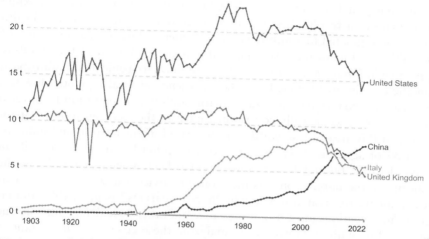

FIGURE 10.2 Confronting historical pollution: per capita carbon dioxide emissions in the United States, China, Italy and the United Kingdom (1903–2022)

Source: Global Carbon Budget (2023); Population based on various sources (2023) – with major processing by Our World in Data. "Per capita CO_2 emissions – GCB" [dataset]. Global Carbon Project, "Global Carbon Budget"; Various sources, "Population" [original data]. Retrieved February 14, 2024 from https://ourworldindata.org/grapher/co-emissions-per-capita?tab=chart&time=1903.latest&country=ITA~USA~GBR~CHN

Note: In carbon dioxide emission from fossil fuel and industry, fossil emissions measure the quantity of carbon dioxide emitted from the burning of fossil fuels and directly from industrial processes such as cement and steel production, while fossil carbon dioxide includes emissions from coal, oil, gas, flaring, cement, steel and other industrial processes. Fossil emissions do not include land use change, deforestation, soils or vegetation.

adopted in connection with trade liberalization policies) of their production to developing countries including China.[52,53] Historical GHG in Western countries are far higher than China's; moreover, this model of economic development was not conceived and promoted by China but by the most powerful Western countries together with the international financial institutions they dominate. Those who have called for the dismantling of regulations and global laws to protect the environment and ecosystems for more than half a century, have only one place to look for the main culprit of the climate catastrophe: their mirror. All countries in the world share responsibility for increasing the ecological and pandemic risk through the exponential growth of consumption, population and economy. However, some countries that have polluted more and pushed for this development model to become globalized are more responsible than others.

Obviously, it is essential that the Chinese also do their part in tackling the climate catastrophe. It is no coincidence that a good portion of health crises has originated in South Asia, and southern China was ground zero of the COVID-19 pandemic. As explained in a critical review of the literature appearing in *Environmental Research*, in addition to tropical and subtropical climatic conditions that facilitate the emergence of viral zoonotic diseases, increasingly broader regional trade, deforestation and migration from rural to urban areas, what really contributed most to the emergence of new pandemics in this area of the world were the rapid intensification and industrialization of agriculture. Global meat consumption has increased rapidly in recent decades, but in China this increase has been much faster and now the majority of the population eats meat once or twice a day.[54] The outrage at how animals are treated in Chinese "horror markets" is justifiable, and effective interventions must be adopted to avoid other "accidents" like the one happened in Wuhan. However, in analyzing these crises, it is important to also address the structural reasons that pushed many former farmers to hunt wild animals and sell them in wet markets, including economic policies, free trade treaties that favor land grabbing and the expropriation of the land of small farmers.[55]

The rapid industrialization and liberalization of Chinese agriculture is an event that generates a certain interpretative confusion, especially in the West. China is often conceived of as a socialist or communist society, although since the 1970s, despite obvious differences from Western countries, it has adopted "free market" policies, generating what some authors have defined as a "Chinese version of neoliberalism."[56] Although it has often disobeyed neoliberal precepts in various sectors of its economy, China has adopted liberalizing reforms especially in the agricultural sector.[57,58] "Chinese neoliberalism," in addition to causing a rapid increase in economic inequalities (the Gini coefficient increased from 0.309 in 1981 to 0.465 in 2019), has generated a revolution in agriculture. The sector, previously based on subsistence activities, has gradually become increasingly dominated by intensive animal farming. As already observed, the rapid industrialization of agriculture has pushed many small farmers to seek new ways of survival and to become suppliers and traders of wild animals. These transformations have also contributed to generating gatherings in urban environments, facilitating the rapid transmission of viruses. Before the advent of SARS-CoV-2, there was a rapid increase in strains of new influenzas, including H5N1, H6N1, H7N9 and H9N2, as well as SARS-CoV-1 and an explosion of cases of African swine fever.[59,60]

Many intellectuals, even the most perspicacious, seem to minimize the role of structural factors at the origin of pandemics, but there are also voices that have studied the economic and political determinants of environmental and animal health.[61,62] A United Nations Environment Programme (UNEP) report published in 2022 indicated a series of recommendations to mitigate the risk of new zoonoses. In addition to the usual warnings about respecting nature and animals by adhering to the One Health strategy and reducing meat consumption, the authors of the report recommended developing "new and better economic systems measures of progress," as well as giving up endless economic growth as a fundamental value of society.[63] According to some, the UN has now become a purely symbolic, toothless, powerless organisation: perhaps, but even if this is the case, we should still be developing alternatives to this model of development, which is like a train driven towards a precipice by some autistic drivers. And make no mistake: among the UN's staunchest opponents are those who have their foot firmly on the accelerator.

Neoliberal unrealism: the viral utopia of global "disorder"

In July 2022, during one of the hottest summers on record, a catastrophe struck the Italian Alps. The freezing point repeatedly exceeded 4,500 meters, leading a significant portion of the Marmolada glacier to collapse. This tragic event resulted in the death of 11 climbers, a particularly poignant incident for me, as I have climbed "the queen of the Dolomites" three times. The path leading to the top of the mountain is part of a magnificent natural landscape, but in recent years it has been transformed, mirroring the widespread changes affecting all the Italian Alps' glaciers.

Following the disaster, the Trento prosecutor's office launched an investigation into possible manslaughter charges. The central question was, who if anyone, should have closed access to the Marmolada glacier? In the wake of the tragedy, there were calls for new laws, stricter rules and enhanced monitoring of Alpine glaciers. Some journalists sought the perspective of renowned mountaineer Reinhold Messner, perhaps to confirm their views on who was to blame. Messner silenced them all. He argued that natural mountain phenomena like collapses or avalanches cannot be equated with mechanical failures like a cable car accident. Holding institutions responsible for such natural events, he insisted, made no sense and could even spell the end of traditional mountaineering. According to Messner, mountaineers must understand that their survival depends on their skills, choices and, to some extent, chance. As he put it, "those who do mountaineering must know that their life depends on their abilities, on the choices they will be called upon to make and, to a not entirely alienable extent, on chance. For those who don't realise this or don't think it's worth it (which makes perfect sense …), there are amusement parks."

A few weeks after the Marmolada disaster, the Trento prosecutor's office ended the investigation, finding no criminal responsibility. Amidst national grief, a prominent Italian science communicator suggested that we all share some guilt for this tragedy. His point centered on the idea that our lifestyle choices, consumer habits and environmentally harmful behaviors contributed to the climate crisis, which in turn accelerated the glacier melting that led to the Marmolada disaster. While there's some merit to this perspective, it over-simplifies the issue by echoing (even if inadvertently, in this case) a neoliberal viewpoint: the premise that the ecological crisis is an individual problem re-quiring individual solutions. However, there are deeper and broader factors influencing our behavior and the ecological crisis. The root causes of the ecological crisis aren't merely personal lifestyle choices but rather stem from the political and economic decisions shaping our model of progress globally. While individuals are not helpless puppets of corporate and economic forces, they are undoubtedly affected by them. It's these systemic forces influencing our behavior that need to be addressed if we are to confront the ecological crisis. Yet, there are some who would rather abolish mountaineering, which is becoming too dangerous due to climate change, instead of neoliberalism, which produces climate change and makes it too dangerous.

Claiming that the ecological crisis is "Homo sapiens' fault" means shoot-ing into the mix and putting corporate lobbyists on the same level as those who have opposed policies that allow fossil fuel industries to obtain trillions of dollars in state contributions. Saying "it's Homo sapiens' fault" means putting activists and scientists who for half a century have been warning humanity about the ecological risks of this development model on the same level as those who have instead promoted and financed "climate denialism." Among the figures most active in disseminating fake news on the climate are big oil companies such as Exxon Mobil,[64] neoliberal foundations such as the American Enterprise Institute, foundations funded by tycoons such as the Koch Brothers[65] and newspapers such as the *Wall Street Journal*.[66] Say-ing "it's Homo sapiens' fault" means ignoring the efforts of those who have fought against climate misinformation, such as the contributions of Naomi Oreskes, author of *Merchants of Doubt: How a Handful of Scientists Ob-scured the Truth on Issues from Tobacco Smoke to Global Warming*,[67] and James Hoggan, author of *Climate Cover Up: the Crusade to Deny Climate Change*.[68] Saying "it's Homo sapiens' fault" means putting Greenpeace and Fridays for Future activists on the same level with those politicians who for decades have hindered the advancement of laws to protect the environment. A tragicomic example is former US Congressman John Shimkus, who said we shouldn't worry about the planet being destroyed because God promised Noah it wouldn't happen again after the great flood.[69]

No, we are not all equally responsible for the ecological crisis and the Marmolada disaster. Those who have supported this model of development and those who have stood in the way of curbing its environmental impact are a very different category of contributors to climate change. Modern so-ciety may have made us all neoliberals, but some are more neoliberal than others. Nearly 80 years ago, Karl Polanyi explained that "allowing the market mechanism to be the sole director of the destiny of the human being and his natural environment … entails the demolition of society." They are prophetic words, however ignored or poorly digested by mainstream politicians, economists and journalists who accuse all those who question this development model of "utopianism" and "extremism."

The ideology beyond all ideologies

One may wonder why, despite the pandemic risks and the ecological disasters it seemingly contributes to, neoliberalism has not been supplanted by an alternative economic model. The primary justification for its perceived inevitability hinges on the belief that all other political-economic systems have failed. As Margaret Thatcher famously stated, "There is no alternative. There's nothing else to try."[70] Proponents of neoliberalism argue that its dominance is backed by historical events such as the fall of the Berlin Wall and the collapse of the Soviet Union, which they see as evidence of the failure of planned economies. Martin Wolf of the *Financial Times* reflected this view, suggesting that a sophisticated market economy is superior to any alternative and those dreaming of different models are envisioning a utopian society that never has and never will exist. This perspective, in a sense, similar to that of Francis Fukuyama, a professor at Johns Hopkins University, who posited that the success of "liberal democracies" represents an "End of History," or a culmination of ideological evolution and the "ultimate form of human government." This triumph of neoliberal thought is also often uncritically echoed by the media industry, which is increasingly influenced by the private interests of the wealthiest and most powerful social classes. Echoing this sentiment, Thomas Friedman of the *New York Times* asserted that the "historical debate" over economic systems is over, with free-market capitalism as the only viable political model.

In political and even academic debates, the term "ideology" is frequently associated with totalitarian regimes or used pejoratively, often being confused with "dogmatism." However, as Thomas Piketty highlights in *Capital and Ideology*, often the most ideological thinkers are those who believe they are pragmatists, especially if, in their post-ideological claim, they hide a series of prejudices and assumptions that come from an ideology of which they are not aware. In a way, it is an even deeper ideology precisely because it makes individuals believe that it is not.[71] This supposedly "pragmatic political posture" is well represented by the position of modern center-left parties who espouse the so-called third way,[72] or what, in the opinion of many, would be a political "renewal" of socialism on the basis of new modern "realities." In effect, this represents a political shift toward increasingly indistinct positions, where neoliberalism becomes the universally accepted political reality across both right-wing and left-wing parties. When Margaret was asked to define her greatest achievement, she replied: "Tony Blair and New Labour. We forced our opponents to change their minds."[73] Thatcher made neoliberalism the dominant political ideology, from the right to the left and, and the claim of non-ideological pragmatism by neoliberal advocates is a prime example of delusion. Every economic-political doctrine carries underlying values and priorities. There's nothing ideology-free about the philosophical underpinnings and political choices that shape the distribution of power and wealth in a society. As John Maynard Keynes pointed out, "the ideas of economists and political philosophers, both right and wrong, are more powerful than is commonly believed. In reality the world is governed by little else. Practical men, who think themselves completely free from all intellectual influence, are generally the slaves of some defunct economist."[74]

The uncritical support for economism and the imprisonment of the collective imagination within the mental cage of the "no alternatives" slogan represent the greatest hegemonic-cultural "success" of neoliberal ideology. Far from being the only possible alternative, neoliberalism is just one of the many ideological options available. There are and always will be countless alternatives for how to organize society, and the choices are made on the basis of the values considered most important. Although supporters of neoliberalism are convinced that the doctrine they support is the only one that works there is no need to do too much research to identify realistic alternatives. These alternatives are far beyond "communism," that has nothing to do with the authoritarian regime adopted in the former Soviet Union, which recalls the famous Russian joke that goes, "under capitalism man exploits man, and under communism it is exactly the opposite." Political-economic approaches capable of offering concrete suggestions on how to build a different development model, one that is economically stable, more socially compassionate, less unequal and less destructive from an environmental point of view, are already available. Andrew Simms, in his book *Canceling the Apocalypse*,[75] presented the idea of a possible society called "Goodland", where well-being is more important than economic growth, where there is a national plan for good living and where cities are green and produce healthy food. In Goodland, Simms explain, "most fossil fuels have been phased out, health and education services are free and child and elderly care is subsidized by the state." It is a nation where "the constitution was written by the citizens, there are laws that establish the protection of ecosystems and the president donates a large part of his salary to the poor." Goodland has a "dynamic local banking system that goes out of its way to help small businesses," "trade is largely dominated by cooperatives" and "the working week is much shorter than in other countries." Goodland may sound like a utopia, an impossible idea? Yet, Simms explains, that all these virtuous examples exist or have existed in various countries around the world. Of course, the challenge is to put them all together and apply them globally.

It remains to be seen whether the eventual construction of Goodland would allow us to avert the imminent environmental destruction under way. There is no guarantee, given the latest overwhelming evidence on the speed of the climate crisis. However, the belief that there are no alternatives is rooted in a selective historical amnesia that rests on a fallacious and Panglossian vision of the world, seen as "the best of all possible worlds." In fact, the world presented in this narrative is deeply utopian. Mark Fisher has defined this one-dimensional thinking that sees capitalism as the only option as "capitalist realism,"[76] but what has anesthetized the political imagination of humanity is an even more radical idea: the belief that the only acceptable alternative among all forms of capitalism is neoliberalism. This narrow mindset makes not only socialism but also postwar Keynesian capitalism impractical and idealistic. Furthermore, one can also object to the term "realism," given that our model of development seems to be based on a complete detachment from reality resembling a mild form of psychosis. Whatever its supporters say, this economic approach is not "realistic" precisely because, in the long term, it is destined to crash into its own ecological contradictions. Assuming that this is truly "the best of all possible worlds," it would in any case remain an impossible one. This ideology should not be called "capitalist realism" but "neoliberal unrealism."

Economics: science or religion?

In the book *The Tragic Science: How Economists Cause Harm Even as They Aspire to Do Good,*[77] George De Martino tells how many economists, despite having good intentions, show a sense of presumption that often leads them to "do without knowing" and cause irreparable damage to society. This attitude derives not only from the power given to the discipline by rampant economism but also from the limits and idiosyncrasies of education in the subject. Indeed, there is no better place than economics programs in universities to study the limits of the one-dimensionality of neoliberal thought. As described in the book *Econocracy: The Perils of Leaving Economics to the Experts*, an analysis of 174 economics degree programs in as many universities has shown that the pedagogical approach to teaching economics reflects a total disconnect from reality and ordinary people. In particular, the authors highlighted an excessive use of abstract theory and an obsessive search for mathematical purity to the detriment of real-world empirical analysis and a lack of attention to historical factors and to the role of social class and power, and a heavy reliance on memorizing concepts through multiple-choice tests. The authors of the study also noted the almost total absence of tasks requiring critical evaluation or independent judgment in the evaluation of academic success.[78]

Although the study of economics is characterized by a very high degree of heterogeneity, uncertainty and complexity, economic disciplines are often equated with exact sciences such as physics and mathematics. For mainstream economists like the former president of Harvard University, former chief economist of the World Bank, and economic advisor to two US presidents (Clinton and Obama) Lawrence Summers, "the laws of economics are like the law of engineering. One set of laws works everywhere."[79] By "economics," in reality, Summers is referring to a single economic narrative, neoclassical economics, an approach strongly influenced by neoliberal theoretical assumptions. As Summers revealed, "Despite economists' reputation for never being able to agree on anything, there is a striking degree of unanimity in the[ir] advice … The three '-ations' – privatization, stabilization, and liberalization – must all be completed as soon as possible."[80] In reality, there is no unanimity and this position involves marginalizing knowledge that comes from other schools of thought. The marginalization of alternatives is corroborated by the fact that only 17 out of 174 economics programs analyzed in the study cited before teach perspectives and approaches different from the traditional neoclassical model. The same study found that university programs in economics tend to only marginally address key historical events such as the 2008 financial crisis, as well as societal trends such as increasing economic inequality, money creation and climate change.[78]

Although most economists present themselves as champions of freedom of thought and independence of judgment, their uncritical adherence to only one main disciplinary approach, neoclassical economics, causes them to act as a "herd of independent minds." Pondering whether mainstream economics possesses some qualities that could be found in a religion may sound exaggerated, but there is no shortage of academic contributions studying this parallelism. This is a topic investigated, for example, by Robert Nelson, author of *Economics as Religion*,[81] Harvey Cox in the book *The Market as God*[82] or John Rapley, author of the editorial "How Economics Became a Religion."[83] In investigating the analogies between economics and religion, some have tried to examine the potential myths. In addition to the contribution *America's Free Market Myths*[84] by Joseph Shaanan, in the book *Economyths: 11 Ways Economics Gets It Wrong*,[85] the mathematician and writer David Orrell focused his attention on some of the completely unrealistic aspirations shared by mainstream economists. One of the most powerful, deeply rooted and widespread myths is the illusion of having infinite growth on a finite planet,[86] which is clearly a mathematical and physical impossibility.

Another myth widely spread in the world of mainstream economics is the idea that markets do not require too much state intervention or regulation because they regulate themselves. The idea comes from the so-called efficient markets hypothesis of an economist called Eugene Fama, who argued that because a free market collects all the information available to economic actors, the prices it produces can never be wrong. The naïvety of the hypothesis is astonishing. In the real world, market failures are often the rule, not the exception. As carefully and brilliantly explained by Ha Joon Chang in *Bad Samaritans: The Myth of Free Trade and the Secret History of Capitalism*, markets work best when they are carefully supported and regulated by government interventions, not when they are left free.[87]

A third myth of modern economics and political practice is the proposition conceiving of human beings as rational, efficient, individualistic beings, mostly motivated by material profit. This is obviously a biased and limited vision of human behavior, which is also influenced by emotions, relationships, irrationality and psychological conditions that lie below consciousness. According to Noam Chomsky, the most dangerous system of convenient myths of modern industrial civilization is the hypothesis that "individual material gain" is the driving force behind our actions, together with the speculation that "private vices yield public benefits." As Chomsky argued, "a society that is based on this principle will destroy itself in time" and added, "At this stage of history, either one of two things is possible: either the general population will take control of its own destiny and will concern itself with community-interests, guided by values of solidarity and sympathy and concern for others; or, alternatively, there will be no destiny for anyone to control."[88]

Comparing economics to a religion with its own myths is perhaps unfair to economists who have provided important insights on society and public policies. Economics is not necessarily "the dismal science"[89] but can be a fascinating discipline offering a wide range of approaches and tools to understand society and behaviors.[90] There are many brilliant economists who have provided invaluable contributions to making the world a better place.[91,92] Yet, the idea of comparing economics to an exact science with no reasonable alternatives to the dominant neoclassical approach is consistent with a dogma. Fortunately, many economists have challenged the neoliberal and neoclassical paradigms that have long dominated and still dominate economic curricula. Forward-thinking economists are exploring new ways to make economics contribute to developing sustainable, healthy and equitable societies. For example, by increasing the cost of carbon-intensive activities, thereby creating economic incentives for environmentally friendly practices and innovation in low-carbon technologies and renewable energies, economics can make a difference in attempting to tackle the climate catastrophe.[93]

These are small but important changes that need to be escalated in different areas and societal sectors.

Our chances of survival increasingly depend on our ability to bring about a paradigm shift capable of prioritizing the health of human relation with the health of the environment and other animals. A new development model capable of incorporating such principles is not simply the most important antidote against new pandemics; it is the humanitarian immune response we need to avoid societal collapse and the risk of extinction. Critics of this mode of economic development or visionaries of alternatives are accused of lacking realism, but the true utopians are those who believe in continuing with this "normality." Fooling ourselves into thinking that the "magic" of markets and technologies will avert the looming ecocatastrophes is a sign of being disconnected from reality, akin to a specific version of autism.[94] We need a "real-world economics," that encompasses alternatives to neoliberalism and embraces new approaches to progress that balance economic priorities with values of well-being, cooperation, solidarity, empathy and creativity. To effectively address the ecological crisis, it is necessary to reorganize societal priorities, recalibrating the position and importance of the economy as just one component within a larger system.[95]

References

1. Norton MI, Anik L, Aknin LB, Dunn EW. Is life nasty, brutish, and short? Philosophies of life and well-being. *Social Psychological and Personality Science* 2011; 2: 570–5.
2. Glatter KA, Finkelman P. History of the plague: an ancient pandemic for the age of COVID-19. *The American Journal of Medicine* 2021; **134**: 176–81.
3. Zhang J, Prettner K, Chen S, Bloom DE. Beyond GDP: using healthy lifetime income to trace well-being over time with estimates for 193 countries. *Social Science & Medicine* 2023; **320**: 115674.
4. Humphries J. Childhood and child labour in the British industrial revolution. *The Economic History Review* 2013; **66**: 395–418.
5. Kwak J, Johnson S. Economism: bad economics and the rise of inequality, 1st ed. New York, NY: Pantheon Books, 2017.
6. Polanyi K, Stiglitz JE, Block FL. The great transformation: the political and economic origins of our time, 2nd ed. Beacon Paperback [reprinted]. Boston, Mass: Beacon Press, 2010.
7. Heller N. The bullshit-job boom. *The New Yorker*. Published online June 7, 2018. https://www.newyorker.com/books/under-review/the-bullshit-job-boom (accessed Jan 25, 2024).
8. Fourcade M, Ollion E, Algan Y. The superiority of economists. *Journal of Economic Perspectives* 2015; **29**: 89–114.
9. Anderson E. Oettinger apologizes after Italy remarks spark storm. Politico. Published online May 29, 2018. https://www.politico.eu/article/oettinger-italy-markets-will-give-signal-not-to-vote-for-populists/ (accessed Jan 25, 2024).
10. Bartlett B. Money and politics. Forbes. Published online Jul 11, 2012. https://www.forbes.com/2009/06/11/terry-mcauliffe-virginia-primaries-opinions-columnists-fundraising.html (accessed Jan 25, 2024).

11. Costanza R. Addicted to growth: societal therapy for a sustainable wellbeing future. London, New York: Routledge, Taylor & Routledge Group, 2023.
12. Dale E. Are we living too high on the hog? *New York Times*. Published online June 1, 1958. https://archive.nytimes.com/www.nytimes.com/books/99/05/16/specials/galbraith-affluent.html?scp=32&sq=current%2520economic%2520events&st=cse (accessed Feb 9, 2024).
13. Baumol WJ. Introduction: The engine of free-market growth. The Free-Market Innovation Machine: Analyzing the Growth Miracle of Capitalism. Princeton: Princeton University Press, 2002:1.
14. Lorenz K, Latzke M. Civilized man's eight deadly sins. Methuen, 1973.
15. Mirowski P. The political movement that dared not speak its own name: the neoliberal thought collective under erasure. *Institute for New Economic Thinking Working Paper Series No. 23, SSRN Electronic Journal* 2014. https://doi.org/10.2139/ssrn.2682892
16. Biebricher T. The political theory of neoliberalism. Stanford, Calif.: Stanford University Press, 2018.
17. Harvey D. A brief history of neoliberalism, 1. Publ. in Paperback, reprint (twice). Oxford: Oxford University Press, 2011.
18. De Vogli R. Progress or collapse: the crises of market greed. London, New York: Routledge, 2013.
19. Lehmann C. Neoliberalism, the revolution in reverse. *The Baffler* 2014; 104–17.
20. Just 8 men own same wealth as half the world. Oxfam International. Published online Jan 16, 2017. https://www.oxfamamerica.org/press/just-8-men-own-same-wealth-as-half-the-world/ (accessed Jan 25, 2024).
21. The president's news conference. Ronald Reagan. Ronald Reagan Presidential Library & Museum. Pulished online Aug 12, 1986. https://www.reaganlibrary.gov/archives/speech/presidents-news-conference-23 (accessed Feb 9, 2024).
22. Farrant A, McPhail E, Berger S. Preventing the 'abuses' of democracy: Hayek, the 'military usurper' and transitional dictatorship in Chile? *American Journal of Economics and Sociology* 2012; 71: 513–38.
23. Friedman TL. The Lexus and the olive tree: understanding globalization, first Picador edition. New York: Picador, 2012.
24. Rodrik D. The fatal flaw of neoliberalism: it's bad economics. *The Guardian*. Published online Nov 14, 2017. https://www.theguardian.com/news/2017/nov/14/the-fatal-flaw-of-neoliberalism-its-bad-economics (accessed Jan 25, 2024).
25. Saad-Filho A. The age of crisis: neoliberalism, the collapse of democracy, and the pandemic. Cham, Switzerland: Palgrave Macmillan, 2021. https://doi.org/10.1007/978-3-030-81608-7
26. The economics of food and corporate consolidation. FoodPrint. Published online Oct 11, 2018. https://foodprint.org/issues/the-economics-of-food-and-corporate-consolidation/ (accessed Jan 25, 2024).
27. Carlson M. Earl Butz. *The Guardian*. Published online Feb 4, 2008. https://www.theguardian.com/world/2008/feb/04/usa.obituaries (accessed Jan 25, 2024).
28. McMichael P. Political economy of the global food and agriculture system. In: Amir K, Laila K, eds. Rethinking food and agriculture. Burlington: Woodhead Publishing, 2021: 53–75.
29. Food barons 2022. ETC Group. Crisis Profiteering, Digitalization and Shifting Power. Published online Sept 7, 2022. https://www.etcgroup.org/content/food-barons-2022 (accessed Jan 25, 2024).
30. Global, regional, and national burden of diabetes from 1990 to 2021, with projections of prevalence to 2050: a systematic analysis for the Global Burden of Disease 2021 Diabetes Collaborators. *The Lancet* 2023;402(10397):203-234. https://www.thelancet.com/journals/lancet/article/PIIS0140-6736(23)01301-6/fulltext.

31. Abman R, Lundberg C. Does free trade increase deforestation? The effects of regional trade agreements. *Journal of the Association of Environmental and Resource Economists* 2020; 7: 35–72.

32. Malm A. On the political ecology of zoonotic spillover. In: Corona, climate, chronic emergency: war communism in the twenty-first century. London, New York: Verso, 2020.

33. Robert Wallace. Resilience. Planet farm. Resilience. Published online Mar 22, 2021. https://www.resilience.org/stories/2021-03-22/planet-farm/ (accessed Jan 25, 2024).

34. UCL. From financial risk to financial harm: exploring the agri-finance nexus and drivers of biodiversity. UCL Institute for Innovation and Public Purpose. Published online Mar 24, 2022. https://www.ucl.ac.uk/bartlett/public-purpose/publications/2022/mar/financial-risk-financial-harm-exploring-agri-finance-nexus-and-drivers (accessed Jan 26, 2024).

35. Whalen E. The unemployed epidemiologist who predicted the pandemic. The Nation. Published online Aug 30, 2021. https://www.thenation.com/article/society/rob-wallace-profile/ (accessed Jan 26, 2024).

36. Peters GP, Minx JC, Weber CL, Edenhofer O. Growth in emission transfers via international trade from 1990 to 2008. *Proceedings of the National Academy of Sciences* 2011; **108**: 8903–8.

37. Lilliston B. The climate cost of free trade. IATP. Institute for Agriculture & Trade Policy. Published online Sep 6, 2016. https://www.iatp.org/documents/climate-cost-free-trade (accessed Jan 26, 2024).

38. Bryceson D, Kay C, Mooij J, eds. Disappearing peasantries? Rural labour in Africa, Asia and Latin America, reprint. Warwickshire: ITDG Publishing, 2005.

39. Xu C, Miao L, Turner D, DeRubeis R. Urbanicity and depression: a global meta-analysis. *Journal of Affective Disorders* 2023; **340**: 299–311.

40. Bhagwati JN. In defense of globalization: with a new afterword. Oxford: Oxford University Press, 2007.

41. Antweiler W, Copeland BR, Taylor MS. Is free trade good for the environment? *American Economic Review* 2001; **91**: 877–908.

42. World development report 1992. World Bank. Oxford University Press, 1992. https://elibrary.worldbank.org/doi/abs/10.1596/0-1952-0876-5 (accessed Jan 26, 2024).

43. Schreuder Y. The corporate greenhouse: climate change policy in a globalizing world. London, New York, NY: Zed, 2009.

44. Gueorguieva A, Bolt K. A critical review of the literature on structural adjustment and the environment. World Bank. Published online Apr, 2003. http://hdl.handle.net/10986/18396 (accessed Jan 26, 2024).

45. Kessler JJ, Van Dorp M. Structural adjustment and the environment: the need for an analytical methodology. *Ecological Economics* 1998; **27**: 267–81.

46. Hilary J. There is no EU solution to climate change as long as TTIP exists. The Independent. Published online Dec 7, 2015. https://www.independent.co.uk/voices/there-is-no-eu-solution-to-climate-change-as-long-as-ttip-exists-a6763641.html (accessed Jan 26, 2024).

47. Nadeau RL. The wealth of nature: how mainstream economics has failed the environment. Columbia University Press, 2003. https://doi.org/10.7312/nade12798

48. Humphreys D. Discourse as ideology: neoliberalism and the limits of international forest policy. *Forest Policy and Economics* 2009; **11**: 319–25.

49. Browne A. China is the world's worst polluter. Don't expect it to be a climate crusader. Publisher online on June 6, 2017. *Wall Street Journal.* https://www.wsj.com/articles/dont-count-on-china-as-next-climate-crusader-1496741425.

50. Plucinska J. Could China, the World's Biggest Carbon Emitter, Ever Go Green? Time. Published online June 23, 2015. https://time.com/3918728/china-green-coal-carbon-emissions-pollution/ (accessed Jan 26, 2024).
51. Zhang L. Coercing China on climate change? American Enterprise Institute. Published online Feb 5, 2020. https://www.aei.org/foreign-and-defense-policy/asia/coercing-china-on-climate-change/ (accessed Jan 26, 2024).
52. You've heard of outsourced jobs, but outsourced pollution? It's real, and tough to tally up. *New York Times.* https://www.nytimes.com/2018/09/04/climate/outsourcing-carbon-emissions.html (accessed Jan 26, 2024).
53. Plumer B. How rich countries 'outsource' their CO_2 emissions to poorer ones. Vox. Published online Apr 18, 2017. https://www.vox.com/energy-and-environment/2017/4/18/15331040/emissions-outsourcing-carbon-leakage (accessed Jan 26, 2024).
54. Goldstein JE, Budiman I, Canny A, Dwipartidrisa D. Pandemics and the human-wildlife interface in Asia: land use change as a driver of zoonotic viral outbreaks. *Environmental Research Letters* 2022; 17: 063009.
55. Wallace R, Liebman A, Chaves LF, Wallace R. COVID-19 and circuits of capital. Monthly Review. Published online May 1, 2020. https://monthlyreview.org/2020/05/01/covid-19-and-circuits-of-capital/ (accessed Jan 26, 2024).
56. Weber I. Origins of China's contested relation with neoliberalism: economics, the world bank, and Milton Friedman at the dawn of reform. *Global Perspectives* 2020; 1: 12271.
57. Duckett J. Neoliberalism, authoritarian politics and social policy in China. *Development and Change* 2020; 51: 523–39.
58. Harvey D. Neoliberalism 'with Chinese characteristics'. In: Harvey D, ed. A brief history of neoliberalism. Oxford University Press, 2005: 1–147 .
59. Wallace R. Are influences in southern China byproducts of the region's globalizing historical present? In: Influenza and public health learning from past pandemics. London: Earthscan Press, 2010.
60. Wallace RG, Kock R, Bergmann L, *et al.* Did neoliberalizing West African forests produce a new niche for Ebola? *International Journal of Health Services* 2016; 46: 149–65.
61. Wallace R. Neoliberal Ebola: the agroeconomic origins of the Ebola outbreak. CounterPunch. Published online July 29, 2015. https://www.counterpunch.org/2015/07/29/neoliberal-ebola-the-agroeconomic-origins-of-the-ebola-outbreak/ (accessed Jan 26, 2024).
62. Kentikelenis A, King L, McKee M, Stuckler D. The International Monetary Fund and the Ebola outbreak. *The Lancet Global Health* 2015; 3: e69–70.
63. UN Environmental Prigramme. COVID-19, a warning: addressing environmental threats and the risk of future pandemics in Asia and the Pacific. UNCP. Published online Oct 25, 2022. http://www.unep.org/resources/report/covid-19-warning-addressing-environmental-threats-and-risk-future-pandemics-asia (accessed Jan 26, 2024).
64. Supran G, Oreskes N. Rhetoric and frame analysis of ExxonMobil's climate change communications. *One Earth* 2021; 4: 696–719.
65. Leonard C. Opinion | David Koch was the ultimate climate change denier. *The New York Times.* Published online Aug 23, 2019. https://www.nytimes.com/2019/08/23/opinion/sunday/david-koch-climate-change.html (accessed Jan 26, 2024).
66. Nuccitelli D. The Wall Street Journal keeps peddling Big Oil propaganda. The Guardian. Published online June 11, 2018. https://www.theguardian.com/environment/climate-consensus-97-per-cent/2018/jun/11/the-wall-street-journal-keeps-peddling-big-oil-propaganda (accessed Jan 26, 2024).

67. Oreskes N, Conway EM. Merchants of doubt: how a handful of scientists obscured the truth on issues from tobacco smoke to global warming, Paperback. ed. London: Bloomsbury, 2012.

68. Hoggan J, Littlemore R. Climate cover-up: the crusade to deny global warming. Vancouver, Berkeley: Greystone Books, D & M Publishers Inc, 2009.

69. What's the harm? Let's ask congressman John Shimkus. YouTube. 2009 https://www.youtube.com/watch?v=U5yNZ1U37sE (accessed Jan 26, 2024).

70. Berlinski C. 'There is no alternative': why Margaret Thatcher matters, Paperback 1. publ. New York, NY: Basic Books, 2011.

71. Piketty T, Goldhammer A. Capital and ideology. Cambridge, Mass.: Harvard University Press, 2020.

72. Giddens A. The third way: the renewal of social democracy, Reprint. Cambridge: Polity Press, 2008.

73. CentreRight: Margaret Thatcher's greatest achievement: New Labour. Conservative Home. https://conservativehome.blogs.com/centreright/2008/04/making-history.html (accessed Jan 26, 2024).

74. Keynes JM. The general theory of employment interest and money 1936. Kessinger Publishing, 2010.

75. Simms A. Cancel the apocalypse: the new path to prosperity. Little, Brown Book Group, 2014.

76. Fisher M. Capitalist realism: is there no alternative? Winchester, UK Washington: Zero Books, 2009.

77. DeMartino G. The tragic science: how economists cause harm (even as they aspire to do good). Chicago, London: University of Chicago Press, 2022.

78. Earle J, Moran C, Ward-Perkins Z. The econocracy: the perils of leaving economics to the experts. Manchester: Manchester University Press, 2017.

79. Selwyn B. Ha-Joon Chang has exposed the fallacies of neoliberalism. Developing Economics. Published online Nov 27, 2022. https://developingeconomics.org/2022/11/27/ha-joon-chang-has-exposed-the-fallacies-of-neoliberalism/ (accessed Jan 26, 2024).

80. Summer L. Comment. In: Chapter 7: Fisher S. Russia and the Soviet Union Then and Now (pp. 252-3). In Blanchard O, Froot K, Sachs J, eds. The transition in Eastern Europe, volume 1, country studies. Chicago: University of Chicago Press, 1994 https://www.nber.org/system/files/chapters/c6021/c6021.pdf

81. Nelson RH. Economics as religion: from Samuelson to Chicago and beyond. University Park, PA: Pennsylvania State University Press, 2001.

82. Cox H. The market as God. Cambridge, Mass.: Harvard University Press, 2016.

83. Rapley J. How economics became a religion. *The Guardian*. Published online July 11, 2017. https://www.theguardian.com/news/2017/jul/11/how-economics-became-a-religion (accessed Jan 26, 2024).

84. Shaanan J. America's free market myths. Cham: Springer International Publishing, 2017. https://doi.org/10.1007/978-3-319-50636-4

85. Orrell D. Economyths: 11 ways economics gets it wrong, revised and expanded edition. Duxford: Icon Books Ltd, 2017.

86. Terzi A. Growth for good: reshaping capitalism to save humanity from climate catastrophe. Cambridge, Mass.: Harvard University Press, 2022.

87. Chang H. Bad Samaritans: the myth of free trade and the secret history of capitalism, Paperback edition. New York: Bloomsbury Publishing, 2019.

88. Achbar M. Manufacturing Consent: Noam Chomsky and the Media. The Companion Book to the Award-Winning Film by Peter Wintonick and Mark Achbar. Montreal: Institute for Policy Alternatives, 1994:221.

89. Marglin SA. The dismal science: how thinking like an economist undermines community, First Harvard University Press Paperback edition. Cambridge, Mass.: Harvard University Press, 2010.

90. Mearmen A, Berger S and Guizzo D. What is Heterodox Economics? Conversations with Leading Economists 2019. Routledge. London and New York.
91. Chang H. Economics: the user's guide; a Pelican introduction, 1. London: Pelican, 2014.
92. Wolf M. The crisis of democratic capitalism. London: Allen Lane, 2023.
93. Clark D, Grantham Research Institute. Why do economists describe climate change as a 'market failure'? *The Guardian*. Published online May 21, 2012. https://www.theguardian.com/environment/2012/may/21/economists-climate-change-market-failure (accessed Feb 11, 2024).
94. Fullbrook E, ed. Real world economics: a post-autistic economics reader. Anthem Press, 2006. https://doi.org/10.2307/j.ctt1gxp77q
95. Schoenmaker D, Stegeman H. Can the market economy deal with sustainability? *Economist (Leiden)* 2023; **171**: 25–49.

11

HUMANITARIAN IMMUNE RESPONSES

Ever since Charles Darwin explained that we are just another animal trying to survive and reproduce on the planet, a part of our collective consciousness has struggled to deny this humbling fact. Although science tells us that we share about 99% of our DNA with chimpanzees, we Homo sapiens like to think of ourselves as something unique, something special.[1] Even in the way we have chosen to define "zoonoses," as animal infections transmissible to humans, our sense of unrealistic superiority shines through. Are they not just another example of animal to animal infections?

There is nothing wrong with feeling special. Psychologists say that cultivating positive illusions is a healthy attitude.[2] An optimistic prejudice may even help us face life's difficulties, and, as the dominant species, we have overcome many of them. However, as we continue to evolve, we may have acquired a sense of overestimation of our own power, resulting in a dangerous unawareness of our limitations. This inflated collective self-esteem has created some myths in the representation of who we are and what our evolutionary superiority represents. The idea of being creatures deserving of a special place in the universe has combined with the undue presumption that we can perpetually progress economically by disposing of the environment and other animals as we please. This could become the most serious cognitive-evolutionary error we have ever made. We haven't fully realized it yet, but our health now depends more than ever on the health of the environment and other animals, not on their exploitation and destruction. If we fail to ensure a healthy future for them, ours will not be ensured either.

DOI: 10.4324/9781003511977-15

Homo hubris

In an article that appeared in *Nature* a few months after the outbreak of the health crisis, anthropologist Martha Lincoln hypothesized that the pandemic could be conceived of as a natural experiment capable of testing the effects of human hubris.[3] In Greek mythology, the term "hubris" refers to a sense of superiority or manifestation of arrogance destined to generate a "nemesis," or punishment, imparted by the blindfolded goddess, Justice. The author of the editorial was mainly referring to the poor management of the pandemic by governments led by political figures such as Donald Trump, Boris Johnson and Jair Bolsonaro. However, the most important test of human arrogance that the pandemic could impart does not concern political leaders who have been shown to be particularly inept in dealing with the virus. It has to do with the collective decision-making process that, on a historical level, generated this model of human "progress." Many have interpreted the pandemic as "nature's revenge" or, as Pope Francis explained, "the response to man's mistreatment of nature and animals."[4] But this is not the case. Nature and animals have not plotted any revenge against us. We did everything ourselves.

In the search for scapegoats to blame for the origin of the health crisis, we have been looking everywhere, a lab, a bat, a pangolin, carefully avoiding our own mirror. This attempt to misdirect our responsibility for the environmental disasters we create is the main obstacle to our healthy future. There is a toxic pride in the philosophy of a development model based on an anthropocentric and narcissistic vision of the world that presupposes the systematic destruction of nature as a foundation of our well-being. On the surface, this propensity would appear to be destructive only to the environment and other animals, but, like a boomerang, it is proving to be the most powerful cause of human self-harm in slow motion in history. As Canadian astrophysicists Hubert Reeves made clear, "we're at war with nature. If we win, we're lost."[5]

The roots of our pervasive sense of superiority can be perhaps traced to a self-aggrandizing mindset that has underpinned many of our evolutionary achievements. The last few centuries of progress and discovery have injected our collective ego with an intoxicating sense of confidence in our abilities to evolve. Economic, scientific and technological advances have contributed to the inflation of our self-esteem and have persuaded us to think we can overcome any limit. A particularly perilous aspect of this mindset is the belief that human creativity, science and technology can solve any challenges we face. Intoxicated by the feeling of being able to do as we please with the planet and other animals, we show off a sense of superiority that is not only cognitive but also ethical. Religion has significantly contributed to this attitude. Convincing ourselves to believe that we are created in the image and likeness of various deities seems to be one of the most popular and recurring explanations to justify our sense of moral exceptionalism. However, a careful look at history reveals a less flattering picture. Our evolutionary journey and historical successes are a succession of wars, conquests, genocides and domination. Our collective might and ostentatious success have come at the cost of the relentless destruction of the environment and the prolonged and unspeakable suffering of other animals. We are the dominant species on the planet certainly not because of our moral superiority but only because we have been the most capable, brutal and systematic "serial ecological killers" in history. Now, however, we have become so effective at killing that we risk killing ourselves.

The disconnect from the real world promoted by our economic system, a topic already addressed previously, has certainly contributed to this toxic pride, but we have not become who we are only because of capitalism or its more recent neoliberal variant. The myth of the "noble savage," has been a source of controversies and historical constructions often fueled by political agenda.[6] However, criticising modernity and contemporary economics deserves a nuanced approach. Even today, a significant proportion of the population believes that modernity is characterized by a general moral decline, but evidence shows that our contemporaries' assessment of morality has remained largely unchanged.[7] Moreover, the modern era has brought significant advances in civil progress and respect for human rights and even some appreciable improvements in sustainability. Despite these desirable changes, the speed, scale and globalization of recent economic and consumption trends (together with the demographic explosion) that have characterized human development over the last half-century raised the bar of the process of ecological destruction. There is ample proof that such trends have pushed the ecosystems beyond their limits and that the climate crisis could soon become catastrophic. As underlined in an article published in the *Proceedings of the National Academy of Sciences,* higher temperature scenarios have the potential to create systemic risk and a cascade of effects on different sectors of society that can generate what the authors defined as a "climate endgame."[8]

"Climate endgame" is a very strong expression, especially for scientists. Yet, there seems not to be a corresponding sense of urgency in our policies, decision-making processes and economic activities. Our "overdeveloped nations"[9] are too absorbed in a "Promethean march" toward ever-increasing status and new material expectations. While this search for more will never satisfy us, it will certainly destroy Earth's ecologies. Perhaps, the global climb toward the acquisition of material success (which, however, has not been shared by large sections of the population), urbanization and industrialization have transformed us into a species incapable of relating to the natural world.

It is so easy to forget that the ecosystem is the fundamental basis upon which our very existence depends. Enveloped in a suburban lifestyle, unaware of how quickly resources like food, water and oil are being consumed, we have stopped perceiving ourselves as part of the natural system. We behave like aliens who think they live on a planet full of infinite resources, mostly unaware of the damage inflicted on the environment. Having nurtured the conviction of being an exceptional species has maybe blinded us into overestimating the probability that "everything will be fine." Our culture is permeated with the obsession of optimism, positive vibes and other positive psychology clichés, but perhaps, as the philosopher Benjamin Fondane explained in his book Existential Monday, modern society could benefit from a little more pessimism? We certainly do not need more pessimism. Yet, according to the philosopher, modern man, driven by the positivism of science and psychology, now feels a bit like a god. This unrealistic representation of ourselves may be a precursor to the sense of collective invincibility that, is typical of civilizations that, after reaching a peak of success and progress, face decline and then collapse. Most of the empires in history that disappeared practically overnight believed themselves to be exceptional and invulnerable just before they fell.

In 1972, a group of scientists known as the Club of Rome embarked on a critical mission to assess the potential risks facing modern civilization in its blind pursuit of unchecked economic expansion. Their analysis pointed to some alarming future trends: a looming decline in food production, industrial output, and population growth. While some critics questioned their predictions, recent data trends confirm that we are indeed heading in a troubling direction. These ominous forecasts don't necessarily spell the end of humanity; however, they do predict significant global impacts in the future, including economic disruptions, reduced food availability and a decline in living standards.[10] We stand at a critical juncture, teetering on the brink of a momentous shift. At the very least, as highlighted in the 2022 Global Report of the Lancet Countdown, we must break free from our addiction to gas, oil and coal.[11] This would involve transforming agricultural practices, reimagining economic structures and challenging the deep-seated anthropocentrism that places humans at the universe's center. Tackling this crisis requires bold and transformative steps. We must look beyond the narrow confines of GDP as a measure of progress,[12] invest heavily in renewable energy sources and adopt energy-saving practices. This would require not just emission reductions but also additional measures like carbon sequestration. Energy efficiency in electricity production, agriculture, forest management, transport and construction along with significant investments in wind and solar power are also crucial. These are not mere adjustments but challenges that may require a transitional period of economic de-growth and changes in our lifestyle. Relying on the hope that "normalcy" can be restored through simple fixes, miracle cures or breakthrough technologies is a dangerously flawed approach. It's akin to leaning on a flimsy cardboard wall for support. The solution isn't about implementing a few laws here and there; it's about fundamentally altering humanity's trajectory. Our approach to progress has been characterized by industrialized exploitation of natural and animal resources, driven by an insatiable desire to increase our power, lifespan, expectations, comfort and material wealth. But the rules of human progress have changed: the exploitation and destruction of nature and other animals, as we are now doing, are the driving force behind our collective ecological suicide.

Collateral sustainability, healthy "de-growth"

When, in the days of the first lockdown in Italy, various media outlets published videos and photos of clear skies and clean waters in the canals of Venice, many pondered whether the pandemic, despite its tragic nature, might have inadvertently brought some unexpected environmental benefits. Indeed, there is some truth to these observations. Satellite maps from that period revealed a significant drop in pollution levels across cities, a direct consequence of reduced industrial activity and transportation. While the early videos of dolphins in Venice's Grand Canal turned out to be fabrications, they were later genuinely sighted in the waters near Punta della Dogana.[13] Nature, at the time, seemed to be reclaiming its own spaces.

The pandemic has generated some additional unintended "blessings in disguise" beyond environmental improvements. For example, there has been a reduction in mortality from some causes of death such as road accidents, and people's lifestyles have changed not always for the worse. Many individuals found themselves investing more time in their own passions, enhancing their social relationships and improving the overall quality of their lives. While for some, lockdowns were akin to a personal hell, for others, they provided a rare opportunity for self-reflection. Some people may have reconsidered what truly mattered in life, distinguishing the ephemeral from the essential. The pandemic, in its own harsh way, has highlighted the fragility of our existence and the intricate interdependence we share with our environment. It also underscored the need for a collective reassessment of our life goals and values, both as individuals and as a society, in pursuit of a more meaningful and sustainable future.

The impact of social distancing during the pandemic has been a mixed bag. On the one hand, it has led to increased feelings of loneliness and isolation for many. On the other, it has provided a unique opportunity for introspection and meditation, a chance to engage with thoughts and ideas often sidelined in the frenetic, work-obsessed rush of modern everyday life. Blaise Pascal's observation, "all our miseries arise mostly from our inability to sit quietly alone in a room,"[14] resonates deeply. While this is somewhat of an overstatement, it helps to illustrate the limited scope for self-reflection in modern life. The dramatic and tragic moments of the crisis, such as the heart-wrenching images of Italian Army vehicles transporting coffins in Bergamo, did more than evoke pain and sorrow. They also offered a stark opportunity to contemplate the meaning of death, a topic frequently ignored or denied in a world increasingly focused on materialistic and status-driven pursuits. Stephen Jenkinson, author of *Die Wise*, has explored this issue, and identified two maladies prevalent in modern culture: a phobia of death and an illiteracy of pain. According to Jenkinson, instead of avoiding thoughts of death and attempting to exorcise its inevitability, we should bravely confront it and even stare at it. The transience of life does not need to be seen as a curse but as a catalyst that enhances the beauty and value of each moment.[15] Realizing that our days are numbered, or that we are living "on borrowed time," makes each of them precious, because any moment could be our last. This realization prompts us to ask, are we spending our time on activities that are truly meaningful, that align with our deepest passions and values? The thought of death and the recognition of our vulnerability to pain can indeed teach us to value life more, to treat each day as a gift not to be squandered. It can also guide us to focus on what really makes a difference, encouraging us to live more authentically, passionately and with a greater appreciation for the fragile, fleeting nature of our existence. In this way, the pandemic, with all its hardships, could serve as a philosophical teacher, inspiring a deeper understanding and appreciation of life itself.

The pandemic has not only put us face to face with the ephemeral finiteness of our lives through a sharp, albeit temporary, slowdown in an unsustainable lifestyle. It has also pushed us to question the values on which modern civilization is structured, re-evaluating ideals such as gratitude, kindness and simplicity as well as the importance of feeling in tune and part of nature. Research analyzing social media behavior during the first lockdowns in Lombardy, Italy, and Wuhan, China, shed light on this shift, revealing not only a decrease in stress levels but also a heightened focus on leisure and free time.[16] Furthermore, a study that analyzed Google Trends data in 20 European countries noted a significant increase in interest in environmental issues since the onset of the health crisis.[17] Interestingly and paradoxically, the pandemic has also had an unexpected effect on the global effort to combat climate change. In the years most impacted by the health crisis, there was the fastest annual decline in carbon dioxide emissions in history.[18] Decades of environmental activism, international climate change treaties, IPCC reports, Earth Day celebrations, recycling, calls to save species, battles against plastic in the oceans, collective switching off of household lights and other virtuous green initiatives, while important, had failed to reverse the global rise in GHG emissions – but the SARS-CoV-2 virus had. (Figure 11.1)

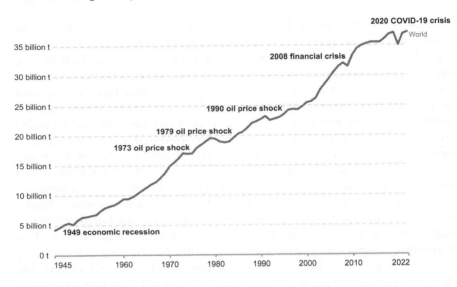

FIGURE 11.1 It takes a crisis: annual carbon dioxide emissions in the world and major economic recessions (1945–2022)

Source: Global Carbon Budget (2023) – with major processing by Our World in Data. "Annual CO₂ emissions – GCB" [dataset]. Global Carbon Project, "Global Carbon Budget" [original data]. Retrieved February 14, 2024 from https://ourworldindata.org/grapher/annual-co2-emissions-per-country?time=1920.latest&country=~OWID_WRL

Additional historical circumstances characterized by significant reductions in carbon dioxide worldwide are periods of economic crisis, such as the global financial crisis of 2008, the two oil crises of the 1970s and other similar events. Although these data can be interpreted in various ways, they suggest that, at least until now, only recessions, or reductions in GDP, have led to significant reductions in carbon dioxide emissions globally.[19] The idea of adopting a regime of economic de-growth is viewed with extreme skepticism if not derision by most politicians and economists and by a good part of the public. Yet, it could perhaps be the only hope to attempt to reduce our environmental impact collectively. Critics may point to countries like Sweden and states like California as examples of areas where GDP growth appears to be compatible with falling CO₂ emissions.[20] These cases are pointed to as models for how technological innovation, regulatory changes and shifts in consumption patterns can lead to more sustainable forms of growth. However, as already mentioned, a significant portion of the emissions decrease in affluent countries is tied to the outsourcing of polluting activities to less economically privileged nations.

The structural forces influencing historical trends in GHG emissions are often downplayed in favour of conceptualising the ecological crisis as a problem of individual behaviour and choices. Indeed, adopting more sustainable lifestyles can make a difference. We can fight climate change not only by advocating for a new economy but also through our everyday individual actions. These forces are not only contextual but partly personal. To paraphrase a famous phrase, the ecological problem is not just about neoliberalism itself but also about neoliberalism within ourselves. If we genuinely aspire to prevent ecological collapse through individual choices, however, it's imperative to identify the most effective pro-ecological behaviors. Science provides guidance in this endeavor. A study published in *Environmental Research Letters* a few years ago categorized ecological behaviors based on their potential to reduce annual carbon dioxide emissions.[21] The most important behaviors are the following:

1 Reducing car usage
2 Limiting air travel
3 Opting for renewable energy sources
4 Selecting energy-efficient vehicles
5 Transitioning to electric cars or forgoing car ownership
6 Adopting a vegetarian diet
7 Using cold water for laundry
8 Engaging in recycling
9 Replacing incandescent bulbs with LEDs

This study's results, however, also showed that, when combined, these eco-friendly actions collectively contribute less than one-fifth (9.1 tons of carbon dioxide reduction per year) of the impact achievable through a single impactful individual choice: having one fewer child, which can reduce carbon dioxide emissions by a staggering 58.6 tons annually. This is especially relevant for high-income individuals in high-income nations whose lifestyle generates a far higher impact on the ecosystem.

The urgency of making profound shifts in our notions of "growth," "success" and "progress" is often underestimated, and efforts to promote a collectively sober lifestyle are sometimes dismissed as unrealistic. Worse, these efforts are often opposed because they are perceived as limitations on individual freedoms and the right to ever greater wealth and status. Some even mockingly refer to the approach that calls for abandoning the idea of promoting unlimited GDP as "unhappy de-growth." This reflects a lack of understanding of the issue: either we plan a transition that may involve reducing economic activities or the limits of the ecosystem will cause a reduction of GDP anyway.

Fortunately, pro-ecological changes do not necessarily mean large sacrifices to our well-being. On the contrary, de-growth-related transformations can even improve health and quality of life, producing what economists might define as "positive externalities." Despite epidemiological evidence indicating that periods of reduced GDP per capita can lead to adverse health outcomes, numerous analyses also show that economic recessions can paradoxically coincide with increased life expectancy and reduced mortality. The relationship between GDP per capita and two indicators of health and happiness (life expectancy and life satisfaction) shows that at lower levels of GDP there's a strong correlation: as GDP increases, life expectancy and life satisfaction also tend to rise. However, the strength of this relationship significantly diminishes beyond a certain GDP threshold, suggesting that beyond a certain level of economic wealth, further increases in GDP do not necessarily lead to proportionate increases in health and happiness (Figures 11.2A and 11.2B). Moreover, data show that there are countries that have demonstrated remarkable achievements in life expectancy and life satisfaction with relatively low carbon emissions, suggesting that it's possible to promote longevity and wellbeing without creating major negative impacts on climate change.

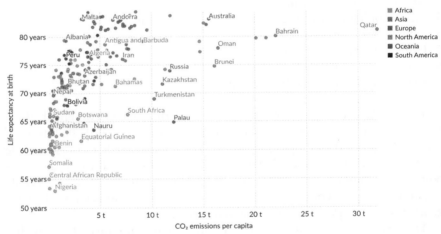

FIGURE 11.2A Long lives, low carbon: life expectancy at birth and carbon dioxide emissions per capita across countries (2019)

Sources: UN, World Population Prospects (2022) – processed by Our World in Data. "Life expectancy at birth – alls, period, estimates" [dataset]. UN, World Population Prospects (2022) [original data]. Data compiled from multiple sources by World Bank – processed by Our World in Data. "CO_2 emissions per capita" [dataset]. Data compiled from multiple sources by World Bank [original data]. Retrieved February 14, 2024 from https://ourworldindata.org/grapher/life-expectancy-at-birth-vs-co-emissions-per-capita?xScale=linear

Note: Average life expectancy, measured in years across both sexes, is a metric that summarizes death rates across all age groups in one particular year. For a given year, it represents the average lifespan for a hypothetical group of people if they experienced the same age-specific death rates throughout their lives as the age-specific death rates seen in that particular year.

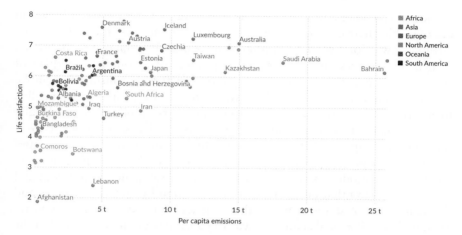

FIGURE 11.2B   Happy lives, low carbon: life satisfaction and carbon dioxide emissions per capita across countries (2022)

Sources: World Happiness Report (2023) – processed by Our World in Data. Global Carbon Budget (2023); Population based on various sources (2023) – with major processing by Our World in Data. Retrieved May 31, 2024 from https://ourworldindata.org/grapher/life-satisfaction-vs-co-emissions-per-capita?xScale=linear

Note: Average life satisfaction measured from survey responses to the 'Cantril Ladder' question in the Gallup World Poll. The survey question asks respondents to think of a ladder, with the best possible life for them being a 10, and the worst possible life being a 0.

In modern societies, an increasingly significant number of people are aware of the "cultural fraud" of pursuing well-being through material wealth and status symbols.[22] A significant portion of the population has rejected the illusion of improving life satisfaction by focusing all their energies on their career and social status, and is devoting more of their time to socially and personally fulfilling activities. Ecological behaviors are also changing with the rapid growth of recycling, energy saving, pro-environmental practices and conservation.[23] Veganism is becoming more and more popular in some countries.[24] Such behavioral transformations mark important steps forward, but can they alone be enough to avert the impending climate disaster? Unfortunately, the answer is no. The belief that the ecological crisis can be addressed through individual sacrifices is delusional. In an editorial published in *The Guardian*, titled "Neoliberalism Has Conned Us into Fighting Climate Change as Individuals," Martin Lukacs investigated this idea.[25] Lukacs highlighted that, despite earnest individual efforts to live more sustainable lives, the overarching influence of the economy, fossil fuel companies and other large-scale industrial activities renders our individual efforts relatively inconsequential.

Certainly, there is a need for individual changes such as consuming less, changing diet and adopting a pro-ecological lifestyle. However, the significance of individual choices can only become significant when the economic system offers viable environmental options for everyone, not just the privileged or virtuous few. Moreover, it's essential to recognize that behaviors, often seen as personal choices, are, in fact the by-product of a complex interplay of social, environmental, economic and political factors. For instance, if public transport is not widely accessible at affordable prices, people are compelled to resort to alternative means of travel, often cars. Similarly, when locally sourced organic food is prohibitively expensive, citizens may opt for fossil fuel-intensive supermarket chains. Downshifting and voluntary simplicity[26] are important pro-environmental personal choices. However, if advertising and economic production continuously encourage rampant consumerism and create the illusion that personal worth is measured by material displays and the acquisition of status symbols, their impact on the climate crisis will remain limited.[27] Personal changes toward a sober lifestyle are laudable, but the sacrifices of a minority of virtuous and healthy consumers cannot do much without a systematic and sustained effort to change the economic and political forces that drive the conditions facilitating environmental destruction and anti-ecological behaviors.

Far beyond "One Health"

Although the desire to "go back to normal" has tempted us to completely forget about the COVID-19 crisis and its paradoxical effects on carbon emissions, repeated warnings have been raised to prepare to face the possibility of new zoonoses.[28] In an editorial published by the World Economic Forum, approximately 20 scientists shared their insights regarding the root causes of emerging health crises and the necessary measures to prevent them. Their collective opinion resounds with a unanimous call for global interventions, as they firmly believe that "prevention is better than reaction." According to these experts, the costs associated with preparing for future pandemics are significantly lower than the toll we would pay when managing a new pandemic akin to COVID-19. The Global Preparedness Monitoring Board echoed this sentiment, stressing the importance of collective action for "global health security" through substantial investments in public health and preparedness. Additionally, experts within the G20 group have underscored the significance of investing in "global commons," while cautioning that "the time until the next pandemic may be shorter than many expect."[29]

Despite clear warnings from scientists and environmentalists, the societal, economic and political factors contributing to pandemics and ecological crises often receive inadequate attention in science, policy and practice. The lack of decisive actions against global deforestation, the risks posed by intensive animal farming and the inadequate regulations curbing the commercial exploitation of wildlife are notable examples. While there is emphasis on developing pandemic plans and pharmaceutical interventions post-outbreak, proactive measures to prevent zoonoses seem to lag behind, not yet treated as a priority. This inertia or reluctance to address the underlying causes of pandemics effectively means acquiescing to a future where the "new normal" includes recurrent health crises and a global ecological catastrophe.[30]

How can we prevent all this? For many scientists and politicians, the answer lies in the "One Health" approach, now used like salt and pepper – you can find it almost everywhere. Undoubtedly, the need to safeguard the health of animals and the environment in order to protect human health is a worthy idea. While it is widely accepted as a valuable concept, concrete actions and reforms are lacking. Sometimes, however, we read concrete proposals: according to the authors of a study that appeared in *Science Advances*, based on the opinions of global public health experts, "primary prevention of pandemics" interventions should include laws to stop deforestation, better management of the wildlife trade and improved surveillance of zoonotic pathogens. At the end of a plenary presentation entitled "COVID-19 and the Ecological Crisis: What Do They Have in Common?" at the 19th conference of the European Society for Health and Medical Sociology,[31] an attendee asked me why I had never used the term "One Health" during my presentation. I replied that I favoured the approach named "Structural One Health," which addresses the root causes of pandemics and the ecological crisis, not just the proximal factors. To understand and intervene in these crises, it is not enough to act on the environmental determinants of pandemics. It is also necessary to address the economic and political factors that influence them.[32,33] Without tackling the structures of power and economic interests that influence human behavior, animal health and the environment, calls for One Health will remain empty slogans.

To understand the limitations of the One Health approach it is sufficient to discuss the idea of curbing global deforestation without acting on the economic-political forces that fuel it. According to analysis by the University of Maryland and the online monitoring platform Global Forest Watch, the last 20 years have seen forest loss well above the historical average.[34] Although various countries have adopted measures to combat this phenomenon, national policies are not enough, nor are the current regulations at the global level. The fundamental problem is that there are not sufficient financial incentives to stop deforestation. A case in point is the environmental policy of Jair Bolsonaro's government, which has made Brazil the world's biggest deforester. This is a perfect example of how a single developing country, left alone or unincentivized to conserve its forests, can turn into an ecological damnation for all. As highlighted in an editorial in *NEJM*, the efforts of governments and institutions to confront climate change and respect international agreements need to consider the "cumulative historical contribution" that each country has made, as well as its capacity to respond. The authors say it explicitly: "countries that have disproportionately created the environmental crisis must do more to support low- and middle-income countries to build cleaner, healthier and more resilient societies."[35] Research published in *Nature Sustainability* showed that although poor people and poor countries are more vulnerable to the effects of climate change, they are the least responsible. On average, each citizen is responsible for 6 tons of CO_2 per year, while an individual belonging to the top 1% in terms of wealth is responsible for about 101 tons. Data on the global inequality of individual greenhouse gas emissions between 1990 and 2019 highlighted that the poorest half of the world population has been responsible for 16% of overall emissions growth, while the richest 1% generated 23% of emissions growth. Empirical evidence has also highlighted that in more recent decades, per capita emissions have increased for the richest 1%, while they have decreased among low- and middle-income populations in rich countries.[36]

In addition to vigorous economic policies to stop deforestation, interventions are urgently needed in the food industry sector, which is responsible for a significant portion of global GHG emissions worldwide.[37] As noted by scholars in a letter published in *The Lancet*, the growth of the industrial livestock sector is a significant obstacle in the fight against global warming. The suggested reconfiguration of the agricultural sector includes a shift away from increasing livestock production to reducing meat consumption and encouraging the intake of more environmentally friendly and health-beneficial foods such as legumes, grains, fruits, vegetables, nuts and seeds.[38] The EAT-Lancet Commission on Healthy Diets from Sustainable Food Systems further emphasized the need for a radical dietary and agricultural revolution. The Commission did not advocate for a vegan diet but recommended a flexitarian approach, allowing for moderate consumption of fish, meat and dairy. According to the authors of the report, this flexible diet, would be sufficient to balance environmental sustainability with health benefits.[39] Importantly, any global strategy to transform diets must consider the issue of malnutrition, particularly in poorer countries where over 800 million people suffer from undernourishment and more than 2 billion have micronutrient deficiencies.[40] The challenge is to enhance global food systems in a way that addresses the dual burden of undernutrition and obesity, ensuring access to nutritious and sustainable diets for all.

As emphasized by Ronald Vargas, an official from the Food and Agriculture Organization (FAO), it is necessary to develop a new agricultural system, as an alternative to the industrial model. In his opinion, the conventional approach of substituting human labor with agricultural machinery, chemicals and fossil fuels is unsustainable. Instead, Vargas advocates for investing in small-scale farming, which he deems the most promising solution for combating hunger and malnutrition while minimizing the ecological impact of agriculture. Contrary to the widespread belief that large industrial agricultural corporations are the primary food producers and indispensable to global food security, small farms are vital. Approximately 90% of the world's farms are operated by individuals or families, contributing to around 80% of the world's food supply.[41]

Agroecology emerges as a compelling alternative to industrialized agriculture. This approach encompasses a variety of agricultural techniques aimed at minimizing environmental impact and promoting sustainability. Advocacy for agroecology suggests that it could not only help prevent further pandemics by protecting forests and promoting biodiversity but also replace large-scale animal agriculture with methods that are more sustainable and animal-friendly. Emphasizing the role of indigenous people and small landowners, the move toward agroecology involves valuing their contributions and reversing the adverse effects modern agriculture has had on these communities.[42] Despite the efforts of organizations like the Landless Workers' Movement in Brazil and La Via Campesina, the transition to a more sustainable and equitable agricultural system faces significant challenges: the power of large multinational food companies and a political economic system that favor them at the expense of sustainable farmers.

As underlined by an editorial in the *World Economic Forum* and an article I co-authored together with other members of the Alliance for Sustainability and Prosperity (ASAP) in the online journal *Solutions*, the world needs a new governance system capable of tackling the systemic causes of climate and zoonotic crises.[43,44] Urgent investments are needed in sustainable infrastructure such as renewable energy, energy efficiency, public transport, watershed protection measures, green public spaces, clean technology, drastic changes in agriculture with radical reduction of factory farming and a ban on eating and trading wild animals. A study published in the journal *Energy Strategy Review* says that switching to electricity from renewable sources for cars, trucks and trains will only be possible by reducing the population's levels of consumerism.[45] But a review by LUT University and 14 other leading international universities suggests that creating a renewable energy system on a global, regional and national scale is realistic. As the authors explain, "the entire demand of the energy system can be met on the basis of renewable energy."[46] The key pillars of this new energy system are solar and wind energy, energy storage, sector coupling and electrification of all energy and industry sectors, to be added to gas sequestration and "natural solutions" like restoring ecosystems such as wetlands.[47]

Progress or collapse: between the impossible and the unthinkable

The concurrent crises of new pandemics and climate change have prompted calls for profound shifts in economic development and norms guiding human progress. High-profile figures, including the Secretary-General of the United

Nations and the director of the World Economic Forum, have recognized the need for systemic change, advocating for a departure from the systems that precipitated these crises and calling for a "great reset" of capitalism. However, despite such acknowledgments and rhetoric, there has been little substantive change. So far, the solutions retained as "politically acceptable" or proposed within the mainstream mindset of "sustainable development" have failed to address the root causes of these crises.

A genuine social transformation away from ecological collapse would necessitate a comprehensive revolution across economic, political, cultural, philosophical and behavioral dimensions. This would include reconfiguring the economic system to recognize the intrinsic value of nature and restructuring global economic policy to move beyond treating natural resources as mere commodities for generating wealth. Markets would need to be recalibrated to create strong incentives for consuming sustainable goods and services, reversing the prevalent logic of short-term profit maximization. In addition to economic reforms, it would be necessary to develop innovative mechanisms of transnational cooperation between affluent and less wealthy nations, fostering a finance sector oriented toward sustainable well-being instead of speculative activities based on toxic financial products. Other interventions, such as promoting the circular economy and new modalities of commerce that reduce environmental and animal impacts, would also be essential.[43]

Creating a wish list of desired policies and societal transformations for a more equitable, happy and sustainable world is important. Yet, the implementation of such transformative proposals requires addressing those strong economic interests and powerful private institutions that oppose them. A report by the Climate Accountability Institute revealed that about 100 companies, including Saudi Aramco, Gazprom, Chevron, ExxonMobil, National Iranian Oil, Royal Dutch Shell and British Petroleum, are responsible for more than two-thirds of global emissions from fossil fuels and cement since the Industrial Revolution.[48,49] Moreover, despite the urgent need for climate action and widespread protests from activists and environmental groups, the fossil fuel industry continues to receive substantial government subsidies, totaling nearly 6 trillion dollars in 2020. To put things in perspective, global GDP in the same year was just under 85 trillion dollars.[50] Despite all the emphasis surrounding the goal of achieving zero carbon emissions by 2050, as shown in the report titled "Banking on Climate Chaos 2023," large banks continue to heavily invest in fossil fuels. In the seven years following the adoption of the Paris Agreement, these banks collectively invested a staggering 5.5 trillion dollars.[51] Fossil fuel financing is dominated by a handful of institutions, or the "dirty thirty," which include large investment banks that were rescued with taxpayer-funded government bailouts after the 2008 global economic collapse.

In protection of these powerful economic and political interests, there is a political stalemate at the global level, perpetuated by a deeply entrenched ideology and *modus operandi*. While addressing climate change necessitates a significant paradigm shift, the entrenched economic policies and power dynamics rooted in half a century of neoliberalism are proving to be formidable obstacles. The ideologies of neoliberalism and economism, which prioritize privatization, market deregulation and limited state intervention, have created a socioeconomic environment where the interests of the wealthy and powerful outweigh the welfare, well-being and environmental sustainability of the general public. The mainstream economic policies have contributed to an imbalanced power distribution between social classes and the erosion of democratic processes, making it challenging to implement the significant policy changes required for an effective ecological transition. This includes transforming essential sectors such as railway activities, public services and energy networks, where the pursuit of private profit often takes precedence over the promotion of the common good. While the current crisis require reforms that increase democratic control over markets and the private sector, including the transformation and conversion of industries such as fossil fuel companies, neoliberalism drives politics in the opposite direction. Deregulation, which is hailed as a virtue in neoliberal economics, undermines governments' ability to implement reforms that could turn fossil fuel companies into true proponents of sustainability.

At a time when averting ecological catastrophe requires large-scale government policies akin to those seen during times of war, austerity measures and budget stabilizations limit the necessary investments in renewable energy infrastructure and welfare policies that could provide wider access to resources like solar panels. Moreover, governments have become culturally and politically subservient to private powers, leading to a crisis of ungovernability.

While Western nations like to portray themselves as "democratic," this is only true in the realm of politics. Nonetheless, it is crucial to recognize that genuine democracy cannot be fully achieved without democratizing the economy. As philosopher John Dewey noted nearly a century ago, "politics is the shadow cast over society by big business interests," and if it remains so, "an attenuation of the shadow will not change the substance." The neoliberal political project has systematically defended the interests of private power while eroding the capacity for democratic planning and collective well-being. The power of wealthy elites and large multinational corporations still outweighs societal and common interests, resulting in a democracy dominated by nearly identical options. Without economic democracy, politics will continue to resemble Thomas Friedman's metaphor of a "free" choice between "Pepsi and Coke."[52]

Economic democratization is a concept rooted in the idea of redistributing power and decision-making authority within economic systems. It involves expanding the influence and control of workers and communities over private companies and other economic institutions. This shift aims to move away from traditional hierarchical structures where decision-making is concentrated in the hands of a few executives or shareholders, towards a more participatory and inclusive model. Richard Wolff, author of *Democracy at Work: A Cure for Capitalism*,[53] explored this concept extensively. In his book, he advocates for worker cooperatives and other forms of employee ownership where workers have a direct say in company decisions, such as production processes, investment strategies, and distribution of profits. Economic democratization extends beyond the workplace to include broader social transformations. It encompasses initiatives aimed at decentralizing economic power and fostering community control over resources. This can involve policies such as community land trusts, participatory budgeting, and municipal ownership of utilities.

Addressing the ecological crisis would require more than just new reforms and policies; it would also demand a cultural transformation embracing values of cooperation, equity, civic dignity and solidarity on a planetary scale. Only with a shift in this underlying philosophy, economic interests and power structures can the changes necessary to address the existential threat of the ecological crisis possibly be attempted. It is no less than an epochal, epic task.

Whether it's possible to address the impending ecological crisis within the framework of capitalism is uncertain. What is certain, however, is that neoliberalism has failed. The emphasis on markets as self-regulating, the pursuit of infinite economic growth and the dominance of the profit motive in all societal sectors, hallmarks of neoliberal thought, are fundamentally at odds with the goals of environmental sustainability. Overcoming these dogmatic economic principles does not mean depriving ourselves of free markets and free trade, but rather questioning the root precepts of capitalism. Is this a realistic goal? According to libertarian eco-socialist Murray Bookchin, "capitalism can no more be persuaded to limit growth than a human being can be persuaded to stop breathing."[54] Capitalism appears deeply entrenched not only in perpetual growth and profit-seeking, but also in a myopic perspective that prioritizes short-term gains over long-term sustainability and ecological stewardship. As Jørgen Randers, Professor of Climate Strategy at the Norwegian Business School, observes, "the tyranny of the short term seems to prevail because it is convenient to postpone global climate action." This focus on short-term benefits is not merely incidental but intrinsic to capitalist economics, where the pursuit of immediate profit frequently outweighs considerations of environmental health. In other words, the economic logic of capitalism makes it more advantageous to "let the world go to hell" than to undertake costly actions that might mitigate or prevent environmental and health crises.[55] Similarly, in the prevention of new pandemics, capitalist, profit-making, market-oriented solutions seem incompatible with the large-scale policy efforts required to address their risk factors. Agribusinesses may prioritize maximizing short-term gains from intensive animal farming, despite the long-term risks posed by the emergence of dangerous pathogens. For these companies, it may be more profitable to let the world have another pandemic, than to invest in costly technologies to prevent it.

The incompatibility between ecological sustainability and capitalist, profit-making, market-oriented policies was shown very clearly during the COP28 meeting in Dubai, attended by more than 2,400 individuals somehow tied to the fossil fuel industry.[56] The outcome of the meeting has been cherished by the mainstream media as a "historic agreement" consisting of the decision to "transition away from fossil fuels."[57] But beyond the rhetoric and the hype, the text of the agreement did not include any concrete steps to phase out fossil fuels and insufficient efforts to phase in a new energy system.[58] Moreover, in an international order shaped by national competition, geopolitical tensions and economic interests, expecting fossil fuel industries and nations whose wealth heavily relies on these natural resources to put themselves out of business for the global common good is naïve at best. Unless we devise a new global economic order with large-scale cooperation and emergency ecological policies, it is unreasonable to expect a transition away from fossil fuels. Our global collective ecological suicide makes perfect economic sense.

Although another world economic order has never been so necessary, at least for now there seems to be no signs of radical changes in the economic-political paradigm on the horizon. Capitalism is widespread in the vast majority of nations, and the prospects of its imminent demise are, for the moment, statistically insignificant. As Fredric Jameson's famous quote observes, "it seems to be easier for us today to imagine the thoroughgoing deterioration of the earth and of nature than the breakdown of late capitalism."[59] Despite the perceived improbability of a radical systemic overhaul, the call to oppose this system of power and economic interests that pushes us all toward collapse underscores a widespread sense of civic duty. This transcends political and ideological preferences, uniting individuals around the human imperative of existence. While the task may be daunting and the path unclear, striving for a more just, sustainable and healthy world requires passion, commitment, creativity and collective action. The journey toward "another possible world" involves exploring and promoting alternatives, advocating for policy changes, fostering cultural shifts and building movements that prioritize new values and a new philosophy of life.

Outcasts at the end of the world

On August 30, 2021, the American magazine *The Nation* dedicated its front page to the person whom the editor of the article named as "the unemployed epidemiologist who predicted the pandemic."[60] It concerns Robert Wallace, an evolutionary biologist who studied the root causes of emerging pandemics. In one of his books, *Big Farms Make Big Flu*, published in 2007, he virtually predicted the COVID-19 crisis: "a pandemic could now be almost inevitable. In what would be a catastrophic failure on the part of governments and health ministries around the world, millions of people could die."[61] Wallace is a unique figure. His focus on the political economy of health marks a significant departure from mainstream epidemiological research, which often studies each new virus as a distinct phenomenon primarily triggered by biological and medical factors. Wallace's approach, instead, acknowledges the interconnectedness of human, animal and environmental health but also points to the larger systemic issues, including industrial farming, deforestation, global trade and international finance, that create the conditions for pandemics to arise.

Wallace's work, which underscores the need for a more radically different approach to public health, one that integrates an understanding of political, economic and ecological systems with biomedical research, did not help him in his career. Quite the contrary. The mainstream focus in university research and funding on biomedical, behavioral and biological aspects of health, rather than on the broader systemic changes that determine them, marginalized Wallace's research. In *Dead Epidemiologists: On the Origins of COVID-19*, Wallace characterized mainstream epidemiologists as "dead" because of their inability to understand the structural and systemic causes behind the emergence of new deadly pathogens.[62] Of course, Wallace was not suggesting that epidemiologists are literally deceased but rather that their approach is intellectually limited and "blind" to the deeper, underlying issues that drive pandemic emergence, such as the circuits of global capitalism and the power relations that shape national and transnational institutions. As Wallace explains in an essay published in January 2020, an epidemiologist who limits himself or herself to studying only the health effects of these structural factors, without addressing the structural factors that cause them, is like that "guy who follows elephants at the circus with a shovel ... [he or she is] busy cleaning up the messes caused by the system."[63]

The intellectual "blindness" of mainstream epidemiologists to the structural causes of pandemics largely derives from prevailing organizational processes and reward systems in academia and research institutions, which favor certain types of research over others. In essence, career paths, funding opportunities and academic recognition are structured in such a way as to discourage the examination of the complex interplay of global capitalism, neoliberal policies and ecological destruction that underpins pandemic emergence. If one's career depends on dealing or not dealing with certain issues, the choices, even if free, are inevitably conditioned. This doesn't require overt authoritarianism or coercion. No one forces researchers to deal with some topics, but some professional choices are simply more convenient than others. This system of unspoken rewards and punishments leads to freedom within a narrow framework of thought. Researchers, while believing they are pursuing objectives independently, often end up conducting research within the boundaries of what is institutionally accepted and financially supported. Often, this process of unspoken research conformism produces the feeling that there is nothing else worth pursuing other than a good career and a higher social status. This cynical attitude may promote rapid job progressions and connections in positions of power, but it can "make a person die inside." The lack of passion and ideals that can result can be compared to a chronic "professional disease" caused by the "death of one's soul." As Wallace observes, "As an epidemiologist [and social science researcher], you should aspire to put yourself out of business" to avoid being complicit in economic policies that lead to the outbreak of a pathogen that kills millions of people.[60]

Mainstream researchers who see themselves as "objective" and free from bias often accuse those who study power and the structural drivers of capitalism of being "not scientific" or "politically biased." This attitude may have helped them climb the academic ladder, but it does not make them objective or neutral. It exposes them to a specific symptom of selection bias: the specialist's illusion. This is the expectation of being able to meticulously study specific parts of the social world without examining the structural factors that shape the social world. The social sciences are not like math and physics. Studying social issues without considering power and politics is like trying to solve an equation that ignores the most important variables that affect all the other variables in the equation. If these factors are not given proper consideration, it is difficult to make sense of what happens. Of course, studying the interrelations between social phenomena in the world's political and economic context is difficult and comes at the cost of being less precise, less specific. But, the trade-off between being precise and being useful is not always in favor of the former. Indeed, a significant proportion of research in the social sciences is precise but useless, or precisely useless.

Doubtlessly, there is a significant price to be paid by those outcasts who choose to confront the contradictions of our model of global development and its multiple crises. Often, they are branded as "radicals" or "political militants" deserving ostracism and marginalization. Indeed, researchers who blow the whistle on civilisation's suicidal path have repeatedly been labeled "catastrophists," "pessimists" or "alarmists." The evidence shows that such accusations are unfounded. A survey published in *Climatic Change* found that scientists have not been "alarmist" enough. It showed that although climate scientists have studied the ecological crisis in all its specific details, they have not sufficiently addressed the large-scale threats to society and humanity that may develop as a consequence. Analyses of the existential risks inherent in the climate catastrophe, for example, have not been sufficiently taken into account in the reports by the IPCC, which instead focused on some more specific, but less collectively severe impacts of climate change, such as the effects of heat waves on the elderly or the implications of sea level rise on some populations living on Pacific Islands.[64] According to Bill McGuire, professor emeritus at University College London, while most climate change experts believe there is still a small window of opportunity to significantly reduce GHG emissions and avert societal collapse, many scientists are, in private, much more concerned about the future. They are even depressed about it. Yet, they may have sugarcoated the devastating information produced by climate science research in order to protect their careers, gain access to research funding, or "communicate in a positive style." McGuire (who is now retired) put it bluntly: "the world needs to know how bad things are going to get before we can hope to begin addressing the crisis."[65] Modern society is full of positive psychologists, but to understand why our politics and behaviour have become so dysfunctional, we need more 'collapsologists'.

Free radicals and the power of dissent

When, on October 14, 2022, a group of young activists threw soup at the bulletproof glass protecting a Van Gogh masterpiece at the National Gallery in London, mass media and public opinion reacted harshly.[66] I addressed this event during a lecture organized as part of the Sustainability Festival at the University of Padova titled "What Planet Are We Leaving to Children and Adolescents?" According to a study in *The Lancet* involving around 10,000 young people aged 16–25 in 10 countries, almost 60% of adolescents and young adults say they feel "very or extremely" worried about climate change. Almost half believe that their fears about ecological risks have already had a negative impact on their lives. Furthermore, around three out of four think the future is scary, while over half believe humanity is already doomed.[67]

Scientific literature shows that climate anxiety (as psychologists define it) of children and adolescents is often associated with perceptions of insufficient ecological actions by adults and governments, as well as feelings of betrayal, injustice, abandonment and moral damage. The concern of children and adolescents about having to face an extremely uncertain, if not dangerous, future seems to combine with the awareness of the ecological and psychosocial risks caused by procreation. In another survey on young people's eco-reproductive preoccupations reported in *Climatic Change*, 59.8% of respondents expressed being "very or extremely concerned" about the ecological footprint caused by having children while 96.5% were "very or extremely concerned" about the well-being of their existing, expected or hypothetical children.[68] Surveys on the same topic show that climate anxiety is associated with age: younger respondents are much more worried than older ones. Is it perhaps because young age is associated with an emotionally charged perception of aspects of reality that do not seem to have the same impact on adults? We don't know, and it's likely that children and adolescents interpret the world more emotionally than adults, but how can we, in the adult world, teach them any lessons as we push them toward the ecological cliff?

While the world of politics and economics seems unconcerned with the pervasiveness and urgency of the climate crisis and continues to adopt policies that barely scratch the surface of the problem, young activists in movements such as Extinction Rebellion and Fridays for Future have decided to take destiny into their own hands. They are doing everything possible to prevent the catastrophe. Criticizing and vandalizing works of art may seem useless and even counterproductive, but the question they ask is legitimate: what will we do with art on a dead planet? Mass media dismisses them as irresponsible. But who are the truly irresponsible ones here? The young activists who smashed the glass covering a Van Gogh, or anyone who has done nothing to prevent the risk of our future extinction?

Criticism and rebellion have always been important values in democracies. In the case of climate change, dissent is also existential. Never before has there been such a need for citizen movements to act as humanity's immune response to our collective suicidal psychopathology. If there is one thing we should have learned from the pandemic, it is that preventing future health crises and ecological collapse requires a radical change of direction. Being radical does not mean assaulting law enforcement officers or smashing the windows of banks and multinational corporations. It means "going to the root," or addressing the deeper causes of any social problem. In other words, if you are not "radical" enough, you are only "superficial."

Way back in 2008, I gave a talk titled "State of Cultural Calamity,"[69] in which I presented some preliminary content of a book that I published in 2013 entitled *Progress or Collapse*.[70] During the talk, I remember, making a case for rapid decarbonization of the economy and drastic political and economic changes to avoid ecological collapse. The speech, like the book, had an underwhelming impact. Now, 16 years later, I am repeating some of the very same messages. In the meantime, however, the risk of ecological collapse has significantly increased. I don't expect the outcome of this book to be radically different from the previous one, but "success" is not the motive that drove me to write it. To paraphrase a sentence often used by Pulitzer Prize–winning journalist Chris Hedges during his speeches, I do not fight for a just cause because I think I will win. I do it just because it is just.

There are rewards for the soul of those who pursue a better world. Bertrand Russell, who was thrown in prison twice for his protests against militarism and the risk of nuclear extinction, wrote that "those who live nobly ... need not fear that they have lived in vain. Something radiates their life, some light that shows the way to their friends, to their neighbors ... I find many people nowadays oppressed by a sense of helplessness, with the feeling that in the vastness of modern societies there is nothing important that an individual can do. This is a mistake. The individual, if he is full of love for humanity ... can do a lot: each of us can broaden his mind, free his imagination and spread his affection and benevolence. And it is those who do so that humanity ultimately venerates."[71]

During a moment of informal socialization at the end of one of my graduate courses at the University of Padova, a student asked me if there were any colleagues I really admired. The question was challenging and profound. My answer, more or less, was that "I admire activists and intellectuals who challenge power, especially those who risk their own status, and career to defend a just cause." Social change has always happened because a small group of determined people decided to make a difference. Those who believe that their actions and utopian ideas are useless and unrealizable have not thoroughly studied the history of social movements. It shows that change can occur even when the impact of activism seems minimal and inconsequential at first. Throughout history, the resolve and determination of brave activists have catalyzed significant change, redefining the trajectory of societies and the world at large. Initially stigmatized and disregarded as "radicals," their forward-thinking ideas often become widely accepted over time as conventional wisdom.

The facts and evidence of the ecological crisis we face are grim. But the climate science, while making useful predictions, does not predict the future. There may still be a glimmer of hope. Never before have we needed people capable of creating a new world with the same intensity with which the current economy and psychopathologies of power are destroying it. Even when we feel useless and alone, it is important to remember that both power structures and economic systems are facing a serious crisis of legitimacy. In such times, there is always some room for outcasts, mavericks and dissidents. The chances of success are not very high, but the world is always in a state of flux, and this model of progress is not monolithic. It is full of cracks, and as Leonard Cohen sang, it is through these cracks that "the light gets in."[72] Even if we feel that we are driving blindfolded at high speed towards a precipice, it is still up to us to decide where we want to go. Yet, as Howard Zinn said, "you cannot be neutral in a moving train."[73] We can either pull the emergency brake or let it go.

References

1. Gibbons A. Bonobos join chimps as closest human relatives. Science. Published online on June 13, 2012. https://www.science.org/content/article/bonobos-join-chimps-closest-human-relatives (accessed Jan 26, 2024).
2. Taylor SE. Positive illusions: creative self-deception and the healthy mind. New York, NY: Basic Books, 1989.

3. Lincoln M. Study the role of hubris in nations' COVID-19 response. *Nature* 2020; **585**: 325.

4. Cozzolino A. Papa Francesco e il Coronavirus: "Dio perdona sempre, la Natura mai". Corriere della Sera. Published online Apr 11, 2020. https://www.corriere.it/pianeta2020/20_aprile_11/papa-francesco-coronavirus-dio-perdona-sempre-natura-mai-817af4b8-7b44-11ea-afc6-fad772b88c99.shtml (accessed Jan 26, 2024).

5. Goodreads. Hubert Reeves. Quotes. "We're at war with nature. If we win, we're lost." https://www.goodreads.com/quotes/9989921-we-re-at-war-with-nature-if-we-win-we-re-lost

6. Ellingson T. The myth of the noble savage, 1st ed. University of California Press, 2001. https://www.jstor.org/stable/10.1525/j.ctt1pprf8 (accessed Jan 30, 2024).

7. Lenharo M. Morality is declining, right? Scientists say that idea is an illusion. *Nature* 2023; **618**: 441–2.

8. Kemp L, Xu C, Depledge J, *et al.* Climate endgame: exploring catastrophic climate change scenarios. *Proceedings of the National Academy of Sciences* 2022; **119**: e2108146119.

9. Kohr L. The overdeveloped nations: the diseconomies of scale. New York, NY: Schocken Books, 1978.

10. Herrington G. Update to limits to growth: comparing the World3 model with empirical data. *Journal of Industrial Ecology* 2021; **25**: 614–26.

11. Romanello M Di Napoli C Drummond P. et al. The 2022 report of the Lancet Countdown on Health and Climate Change: health at the mercy of fossil fuels, 2022;400(10363):1619–1654. *The Lancet.* https://www.thelancet.com/article/S0140-6736(22)01540-9/fulltext.

12. Costanza R, Kubiszewski I, Giovannini E, *et al.* Development: time to leave GDP behind. *Nature* 2014; **505**: 283–5.

13. Buckley J. These dolphins took a day trip up Venice's Grand Canal. CNN. Published online Mar 23, 2021. https://www.cnn.com/travel/article/venice-canal-dolphins/index.html (accessed Jan 26, 2024).

14. Pascal B. Chapter 2: the misery of man without God. In: Pensees. Maven Books, 2020.

15. Jenkinson S. Die Wise: A Manifesto for Sanity and Soul. A quote from the Iliad. Goodreads. North Atlantic Books, 2015. https://www.goodreads.com/quotes/1369173-any-moment-might-be-our-last-everything-is-more-beautiful (accessed Jan 26, 2024).

16. Su Y, Xue J, Liu X, *et al.* Examining the impact of COVID-19 lockdown in Wuhan and Lombardy: a psycholinguistic analysis on Weibo and Twitter. *International Journal of Environmental Research and Public Health* 2020; **17**: 4552.

17. Rousseau S, Deschacht N. Public awareness of nature and the environment during the COVID-19 crisis. *Environmental and Resource Economics* 2020; **76**: 1149–59.

18. McSweeney R & Tandon A. Global carbon project: coronavirus causes 'record fall' in fossil-fuel emissions in 2020. Carbon Brief. Published online Dec 11, 2020. https://www.carbonbrief.org/global-carbon-project-coronavirus-causes-record-fall-in-fossil-fuel-emissions-in-2020/ (accessed Jan 26, 2024).

19. Ritchei A & Roser M. Annual CO_2 emissions. Our World in Data. https://ourworldindata.org/grapher/annual-co2-emissions-per-country?country=~OWID_WRL (accessed Jan 26, 2024).

20. Ritchie H, Roser M. Many countries have decoupled economic growth from CO_2 emissions, even if we take offshored production into account. *Our World in Data.* Published online Dec 28, 2023. https://ourworldindata.org/co2-gdp-decoupling (accessed Jan 26, 2024).

21. Wynes S, Nicholas KA. The climate mitigation gap: education and government recommendations miss the most effective individual actions. *Environmental Research Letters* 2017; **12**: 074024.

22. Eckersley R. Is modern Western culture a health hazard? *International Journal of Epidemiology* 2006; **35**: 252–8.

23. Lu H, Zhang W, Diao B, *et al*. The progress and trend of pro-environmental behavior research: a bibliometrics-based visualization analysis. *Current Psychology* 2023; **42**: 6912–32.

24. Anthony A. From fringe to mainstream: how millions got a taste for going vegan. The Observer. Published online Oct 10, 2021. https://www.theguardian.com/lifeandstyle/2021/oct/10/from-fringe-to-mainstream-how-millions-got-a-taste-for-going-vegan (accessed Jan 31, 2024).

25. Lukacs M. Neoliberalism has conned us into fighting climate change as individuals. The Guardian. Published online July 17, 2017. https://www.theguardian.com/environment/true-north/2017/jul/17/neoliberalism-has-conned-us-into-fighting-climate-change-as-individuals (accessed Jan 26, 2024).

26. Nuga M, Eimermann M, Hedberg C. Downshifting towards voluntary simplicity: the process of reappraising the local. *Geografiska Annaler: Series B, Human Geography* 2023; **0**: 1–18.

27. Merz JJ, Barnard P, Rees WE, Smith D, Maroni M, Rhodes CJ, Dederer JH, Bajaj N, Joy MK, Wiedmann T, Sutherland R. World scientists' warning: the behavioural crisis driving ecological overshoot. Science Progress, 106(3). https://journals.sagepub.com/doi/10.1177/00368504231201372.

28. Skegg D, Gluckman P, Boulton G, *et al*. Future scenarios for the COVID-19 pandemic. *The Lancet* 2021; **397**: 777–8.

29. Global Preparedness Monitoring Board. https://www.gpmb.org (accessed Jan 21, 2024).

30. Burgio E. Ernesto Burgio: La prima pandemia dell'Antropocene. Published online Mar 20, 2021. https://www.sinistrainrete.info/societa/20025-ernesto-burgio-la-prima-pandemia-dell-antropocene.html (accessed Jan 26, 2024).

31. De Vogli R. "COVID-19 and the ecological crisis: what do they have in common?" Keynote talk. 19th Biennial European Society for Health and Medical Sociology Conference 2022 Forlì. ESHMS. 2022. https://eshms2022.wixsite.com/eshms2022 (accessed Jan 26, 2024).

32. Wallace RG, Bergmann L, Kock R, *et al*. The dawn of Structural One Health: a new science tracking disease emergence along circuits of capital. *Social Science & Medicine* 2015; **129**: 68–77.

33. Wittenberg A. Study ties environmental conservation to pandemic prevention. E&E News. Published online Feb 4, 2022. https://www.eenews.net/articles/study-ties-environmental-conservation-to-pandemic-prevention/ (accessed Jan 26, 2024).

34. Harvey F. Destruction of world's forests increased sharply in 2020. The Guardian. Published online Mar 31, 2021. https://www.theguardian.com/environment/2021/mar/31/destruction-of-worlds-forests-increased-sharply-in-2020-loss-tree-cover-tropical (accessed Jan 26, 2024).

35. Atwoli L, Baqui AH, Benfield T, *et al*. Call for emergency action to limit global temperature increases, restore biodiversity, and protect health. *New England Journal of Medicine* 2021; **385**: 1134–7.

36. Chancel L. Global carbon inequality over 1990–2019. *Nature Sustainability* 2022; **5**: 931–8.

37. Emissions due to agriculture. Global, regional and country trends 2000–2018. Food and Agriculture Organization of the United Nations. https://www.fao.org/policy-support/tools-and-publications/resources-details/en/c/1382716/ (accessed Jan 26, 2024).

38. Harwatt H, Ripple WJ, Chaudhary A, Betts MG, Hayek MN. Scientists call for renewed Paris pledges to transform agriculture. *The Lancet Planetary Health* 2020; 4: e9–10.

39. The EAT-Lancet Commission on Food, Planet, Health. EAT. https://eatforum.org/eat-lancet-commission/ (accessed Jan 26, 2024).

40. Food in the Anthropocene: the EAT-Lancet Commission on Healthy Diets from Food Systems. The Lancet. https://www.thelancet.com/pdfs/journals/lancet/PIIS0140-6736(18)31788-4.pdf?utm_campaign=tleat19&utm_source=HubPage (accessed Jan 26, 2024).

41. Harvey F. Can we ditch intensive farming – and still feed the world? The Guardian. Published online Jan 28, 2019. https://www.theguardian.com/news/2019/jan/28/can-we-ditch-intensive-farming-and-still-feed-the-world (accessed Jan 26, 2024).

42. Moving beyond capitalist agriculture: could agroecology prevent further pandemics? | MR online. Published online Aug 1, 2021. https://mronline.org/2021/08/01/moving-beyond-capitalist-agriculture-could-agroecology-prevent-further-pandemics/ (accessed Jan 26, 2024).

43. Costanza R, Kubiszewski I, Pickett K et al. After the crisis: two possible futures. The Solutions Journal. Published online Sept 1, 2020. https://thesolutionsjournal.com/after-the-crisis-two-possible-futures/ (accessed Jan 26, 2024).

44. Broom D. This is how we prevent future pandemics, say 22 leading scientists. World Economic Forum. Published online Nov 27, 2020. https://www.weforum.org/agenda/2020/11/covid-19-pandemics-nature-scientists/ (accessed Jan 26, 2024).

45. de Blas I, Mediavilla M, Capellán-Pérez I, Duce C. The limits of transport decarbonization under the current growth paradigm. *Energy Strategy Reviews* 2020; 32: 100543.

46. Researchers agree: the world can reach a 100% renewable energy system by or before 2050. *Helsinki Times*. Published online Aug 10, 2022. https://www.helsinkitimes.fi/themes/themes/science-and-technology/22012-researchers-agree-the-world-can-reach-a-100-renewable-energy-system-by-or-before-2050.html?fbclid=IwAR3MZI0OXJ5Z4I9-7P1ZCh4gDezZpJrb8B9p1W7947tDgro48b7FqqAukVc&fs=e&s=cl (accessed Jan 26, 2024).

47. Girardin C, Jenkins S, Seddon N et al. Nature-based solutions can help cool the planet—if we act now. Nature; 2021:593. Published online May 12, 2021. https://www.nature.com/articles/d41586-021-01241-2?fbclid=IwAR22NRdQiHifwPUDNLCHpkPZYtqjMl17WfY2CFKG8fMBlODQmFMR6URFAcI (accessed Jan 26, 2024).

48. Riely T. Just 100 companies responsible for 71% of global emissions, study says. The Guardian. Jul 10, 2017 https://www.theguardian.com/sustainable-business/2017/jul/10/100-fossil-fuel-companies-investors-responsible-71-global-emissions-cdp-study-climate-change

49. Climate Accountability Institute. Carbon majors: update of top twenty companies 1965–2017. CAI. Published online Oct 9, 2019. https://climateaccountability.org/wp-content/uploads/2020/12/CAI-PressRelease-Top20-Oct19.pdf.

50. Parry IWH, Black S, Vernon N. Still not getting energy prices right: a global and country update of fossil fuel subsidies. IMF. https://www.imf.org/en/Publications/WP/Issues/2021/09/23/Still-Not-Getting-Energy-Prices-Right-A-Global-and-Country-Update-of-Fossil-Fuel-Subsidies-466004 (accessed Jan 26, 2024).

51. Banking on climate chaos 2023. Banking on Climate Chaos. Published online Apr 22, 2023. https://www.bankingonclimatechaos.org/ (accessed Jan 26, 2024).

52. Friedman TL. The Lexus and the olive tree: understanding globalization, first Picador edition. New York, NY: Picador, 2012.

53. Wolff RD. Democracy at work: a cure for capitalism. Chicago, Ill.: Haymarket Books, 2012.
54. Graham-Leigh E. Forget about the "Good Anthropocene" ("The Robbery of Nature" reviewed by Counterfire). Monthly Review. Published online Sept 24, 2021. https://monthlyreview.org/press/embracing-the-good-anthropocene-a-failure-to-make-the-requisite-social-change-the-robbery-of-nature-reviewed-by-counterfire/ (accessed Jan 31, 2024).
55. Confino J. 'It is profitable to let the world go to hell'. *The Guardian*. Published online Jan 19, 2015. https://www.theguardian.com/sustainable-business/2015/jan/19/davos-climate-action-democracy-failure-jorgen-randers (accessed Jan 26, 2024).
56. Puko T. Oil, gas and coal interests swarm global climate summit in Dubai. Washington Post. Published online Dec 6, 2023. https://www.washingtonpost.com/climate-environment/2023/12/05/un-climate-conference-dubai-oil-lobbyists/ (accessed Jan 26, 2024).
57. Goar M. COP28: historic agreement in Dubai calls for 'transitioning away from fossil fuels'. Le Monde. Published online Dec 13, 2023. https://www.lemonde.fr/en/environment/article/2023/12/13/cop28-historic-agreement-in-dubai-calls-for-transitioning-away-from-fossil-fuels_6338591_114.html (accessed Jan 26, 2024).
58. Ahmed N. COP28 could phase out fossil fuels without us realising. Euronews. Published online Dec 13, 2023. https://www.euronews.com/green/2023/12/12/cop28-could-phase-out-fossil-fuels-without-us-realising (accessed Jan 26, 2024).
59. Fredric Jameson, The Seeds of Time (New York: Columbia University Press, 1994), p. xii.
60. Whalen C. The unemployed epidemiologist who predicted the pandemic. *The Nation*. Published online Aug 30, 2021. https://www.thenation.com/article/society/rob-wallace-profile/ (accessed Jan 26, 2024).
61. Wallace RG. Big farms make big flu: dispatches on infectious disease, agribusiness, and the nature of science. New York, NY: Monthly Review Press, 2016.
62. Johnjitheesh J. Rob Wallace on the political economy of pandemics. *Frontline*. Published online June 13, 2021. https://frontline.thehindu.com/cover-story/interview-rob-wallace-on-the-political-economy-of-pandemics/article34801273.ece (accessed Jan 26, 2024).
63. Wallace R. Dead epidemiologists: on the origins of COVID-19. *Monthly Review*. Published online Oct 7, 2020. https://monthlyreview.org/product/dead-epidemiologists-on-the-origins-of-covid-19/ (accessed Jan 26, 2024).
64. Huggel C, Bouwer LM, Juhola S, *et al.* The existential risk space of climate change. *Climatic Change* 2022; 174: 8.
65. McKie R. 'Soon the world will be unrecognisable': is it still possible to prevent total climate meltdown? *The Observer*. Published online July 30, 2022. https://www.theguardian.com/environment/2022/jul/30/total-climate-meltdown-inevitable-heatwaves-global-catastrophe (accessed Jan 25, 2024).
66. Zuppa su Van Gogh PS. Ma c'è il vetro, ed è una buona causa. Scienza in rete. Published online Nov 14, 2022. https://www.scienzainrete.it/articolo/zuppa-su-van-gogh-ma-c%C3%A8-vetro-ed-buona-causa/simonetta-pagliani/2022-11-14 (accessed Jan 26, 2024).
67. Hickman C, Marks E, Pihkala P, *et al.* Climate anxiety in children and young people and their beliefs about government responses to climate change: a global survey. *The Lancet Planetary Health* 2021; 5: e863–73.
68. Schneider-Mayerson M, Leong KL. Eco-reproductive concerns in the age of climate change. *Climatic Change* 2020; 163: 1007–23.
69. Il Giornale di Vicenza. Sabati culturali in Pinacoteca con Italia Nostra. Comune di Vicenza. https://www.comune.vicenza.it/albo/notizie.php/50546 (accessed Feb 1, 2024).

70. De Vogli R. Progress or collapse: the crises of market greed. London, New York: Routledge, 2013.
71. Russell B. If we are to survive this dark time–; Bertrand Russell advises us to learn, to look at things 'under the aspect of eternity'. The New York Times. Published online Sept 3, 1950. https://www.nytimes.com/1950/09/03/archives/if-we-are-to-survive-this-dark-time-bertrand-russsell-advises-as-to.html (accessed Jan 26, 2024).
72. Cohen L. Anthem (Live in London). YouTube. https://www.youtube.com/watch?v=c8-BT6y_wYg&ab_channel=LeonardCohenVEVO (accessed Feb 1, 2024).
73. Zinn H. You can't be neutral on a moving train: a personal history of our times. Boston: Beacon Press, 1994.

INDEX

Note: Pages in *italics* represent figures.

Abbasi, K. 87
Addicted to Growth (Costanza) 224
Adhanom Ghebreyesus, T. 25,
Agnoletto, V. 71
agriculture 205–209, 228–231,
    234–235, 251, 260–261
agroecology 261
Alpha variant 24, 171
Andersen, K. 202
Anelli, F. 19
Ardern, J. 49, 140
asymptomatic people 27, 43–46, 66, 98,
    162, 203
Australia 7, 108, 182, 205
Azar, A. 18

backward tracing 142
Baker, M. 140
Balakrishnan, V. 141
Baumol, W. 224
Bay, J. 144
Belgium 184
Berlusconi, S. 22, 111
Bezos, J. 186
Biden, J. 68, 168
Biebricher, T. 225
Big Farms Make Big Flu (Wallace) 266
Big Pharma 118, 161, 170
Biko, S. 187
BioNTech 117–118, 157

black swan 15
Bloomberg, M. 186
BNT162b2110 mRNA vaccine 157
Bolsonaro, J. 259
Bookchin, M. 264
Bragg, R. 206
Brazil 82, 85, 259
British Medical Association
    (BMA) 63
Bryceson, D. 231

Canceling the Apocalypse
    (Simms) 239
capitalism 225–228, 239, 250, 262,
    264–267
Centers for Disease Control and
    Prevention (CDC) 29, 44, 85, 158
Charles Koch Foundation 84
Chen Chien-jen 50, 180
Chen Shihchung 19
China 27, 39–40, 95–100, 115,
    171–172, 201–204, 207–209,
    232–235
Chomsky, N. 52, 241
Civilized Man's Eight Capital Sins
    (Lorenz) 224–225
climate change 206–213, 224, 232,
    236, 240, 253, 255–257, 260–263,
    267–269
climate endgame 250–251

Coalition for Epidemic Preparedness Innovations 120
cognitive restructuring 30
Cohen, L. 270
colding of the virus 41–42
community level, pandemic 64–67
Conte, G. 15, 63–64
Corona100m app 138
Costanza, R. 224
Costello, A. 115
COVID-19 2–3, 6–8; to children 87–89; ecological crisis 209–212, 236–237, 259, 264, 270; front line against 71–73; mortality 3–8, 47–48, 89, 94–95, 111–113, 137, 141–142, 159–160, 171–172; preventive strategies 67–71
Covid-19 Vaccine Global Access (COVAX) Facility 115–116, 121, 158
Crisanti, A. 75, 132–133, 143–144

Darwin, C. 248
Dead Epidemiologists (Wallace) 266
deforestation 205–210, 213, 229–231, 259–260
Delphi consensus method 190
Delta variant 24, 41
De Martino, G. 239–240
Democracy at Work (Wolf) 264
democratic virus 112
Dewey, J. 263
Diamond, J. 210
disinformation 41, 50, 88, 212
Draghi, M. 179
Dyer, G. 211

EAT Lancet Commission on Healthy Diets from Sustainable Food Systems 260
economic democratization 264
endemic 24, 167–169
endemicity 168–169
Espinosa, P. 212
European Center for Disease Prevention and Control (ECDC) 144
Exxon Mobil 84, 237

Farrar, J. 17, 192
Fauci, A. 68, 203
Ferguson, N. 41
financial support 182, 185, 191
Finland 7, 86, 94, 182, 187

first wave 63–64, 69, 96, 111, 132–133, 146, 148, 187
Fisher, M. 239
5G networks 38–39
flu-like 37, 39–40
Francis, Pope 249
free markets 229, 232–235, 241
Friedman, M. 185
Friedman, T. 228, 263
frontline sentinels 71–73
Fukuyama, F. 237

Galbraith, J. K. 224
Garry, R. 201
Gasparini, F. 62
Gates, B. 38, 119–122
Gavi 120
GDP growth 93–94, 96, 108, 185, 224, 229, 251, 254–256
Gelman, A. 90
geographical location 7
Germany 182
Gilbert, P. 121
Global Health Czar 18
Global Health Security Index 18
globalization 207–208, 210, 222, 229–230
Goodland (Simms) 239
Goodnow, C. 167
Gostin, L. 121
Gray, J. 223
Great Barrington Declaration (GBD) 84–86
The Great Transformation (Polanyi) 223
Greenhalgh, T. 26
greenhouse gas (GHG) emissions 209–211, 213, 230–233, 234, 259–260, 268
greenwashing 213
green wishing 213
green wishy-washy 213
Greer, S. 76
Gruyere effect 133
Guerra, R. 20–22
Gurdasani, D. 168

Ha Joon Chang 241
Hanna, M. 224
Hansen, J. 212
Harvey, D. 225
Hayek, F. v. 227
health dictatorship 38–39

helicopter money 184–185
herd immunity 76, 84–87, 90, 171
Hibberd, M. 172
Ho Chi Minh 139
Hoggan, J. 237
Hong Kong 171–173
Horton, R. 48, 112, 192
Huanan horror market 200–202, 205
hubris 249–252
Hygiene and Preventive Medicine
    74, 144
hypocrisy 99, 119

Immuni app 143–144
immunization 20, 117
Industrial Revolution 213, 220–222,
    224, 232, 262
inoculation 48–52
Institute for Health Metrics and
    Evaluation 188
International Council of Nurses (ICN) 63
International Livestock Research
    Institute (ILRI) 205
International Monetary Fund (IMF) 94,
    185, 187
Italian Association of Epidemiology
    (AIE) 73, 144
Italian National Center for
    Epidemiology, Surveillance, and
    Health Promotion (CNESPS) 21
Italian pandemic response 19–22
Italian Technical Scientific Committee
    (CTS) 21, 23, 44, 69–70
Italy 1–3, 6–7, 19–24, 29–30, 37,
    39–40, 42–43, 45–46, 50, 63,
    65–69, 73–76, 86, 88, 91, 107–108,
    111, 131–133, 142, 144–146, 148,
    179–180, 182–184, 186–189, 202,
    209, 252

Jameson, F. 265
Japan 43, 90, 108–109, 141–143, 171,
    180, 188
Jenkinson, S. 253
Johnson, B. 84, 203

Kawasaki disease 88–89
Keynes, J. M. 185, 226, 238

laissez-faire the virus 83, 87, 89, 91, 94,
    97, 167, 170–171, 228
Lantz P. M. 65
liberalization policies 119–120, 228–232

Lincoln, M. 249
Li Wenliang 202–204
lockdown 17, 19–20, 22, 29, 43, 46,
    69, 73, 82, 89–90, 93–94, 97–100,
    107–111, 113, 135–137, 141–142,
    182, 186, 252–253
Lorenz, K. 224–225
Lukacs, M. 257

Malibu surfer problem 185
Malm, A. 229
Manaus, Brazil 85
Marmolada disaster 235–237
masks 22, 26–27, 29, 42–43, 48, 68, 85,
    136, 142, 170, 182, 188
Mazza, M. 143–144
Mazzucato, M. 118
McGuire, B. 211, 268
medicalization 65
Medley, G. 84
Meloni, G. 142
Messner, R. 236
Mirowsky, P. 225
Moderna 117–118
molecular swabs 133
Montaperto, C. 92

Nacoti, M. 92
Nadeau, R. 231–232
natural immunity 162–167
neoliberalism 225–228, 231, 235–239,
    242, 255, 257, 263–264
New Zealand 6–7, 49, 99, 134–135,
    139–140
Nipah virus 206
Noi Denunceremo 66
Non-Steroidal Anti-Inflammatory
    Drugs (NSAIDs) 47
Norway 6–7, 86, 94, 108,182, 187

Oettinger, G. 223
Omicron 24, 41–42, 68, 87, 96–100,
    135, 137–142, 159–160, 167,
    169–172
One Health approach 235, 258–261
Oreskes, N. 237
Orrell, D. 241
Osterholm, M. 16, 167–168

pandemic management 17–20, 45,
    70–71, 91, 114, 131, 140, 147, 167,
    180, 188, 190–191, 203
pandemic risk 16, 204–209, 230

pan-European privacy-preserving proximity tracing initiative (PEPP-PT) 145
Pascal, B. 252
Patel, J. 181
Paxlovid (drug) 48, 118
Pence, M. 18, 68
personal protective equipment (PPE) 7, 22, 63, 191
Petherick, A. 170
Pfizer 117–118, 157
philanthrocapitalism 120–121
Pickett, K. 182
Piketty, T. 238
Pinochet, A. 227
Pinto, L. 30
Polanyi, K. 222–223, 237
Pompeo, M. 201
population density 7, 141, 208
psychodemia 110–111
Public Health Act 83
public health experts 23, 44, 46, 68, 70–71, 73–76, 84–85, 89, 117, 161, 259

Quammen, D. 16, 205

Randers, J. 264
rapid antigenic swabs 133
Reagan, R. 226–227
Rockström, J. 211, 213
Rodrik, D. 228
Rosa, E. D. 144
Russell, B. 270
Ryan, M. 24

Sachs, J. 201
Sagan, C. 202
Santa Clara study 90
Saracci, R. 75
SARS-CoV-2 1, 3, 8, 15–19, 23–27, 37–38, 40–41, 44, 46, 48, 63, 67–68, 72, 84, 88–89, 93, 98, 111–113, 120, 135, 139, 141–142, 148, 157–166, 168, 170, 187, 189, 191–192, 199–205, 207, 209, 235
scarce resources 183–187
schools 145–148
Schumacher, E. 249
SDSS project 73–74
second wave 2, 19, 23, 62, 85, 131–133
self-isolation 140, 179–182, 189
Shaman, J. 18

Simms, A. 239
Singapore 46, 134, 141, 144, 171
Singer, M. 112
Sklair, J. 121
social Darwinism 83
social murder 84–87
solidarity 170, 181–184
Soros, G. 186
South Korea 6–7, 21, 43, 46, 90, 132, 134, 137–140
Spencer, H. 83
Speranza, R. 19, 46
Sridhar, D. 46, 170
suicide 40, 107–110, 184, 252, 265
Summers, L. 185, 240
sustainability 96, 120, 131, 213, 231–232, 250, 252–258, 260–261, 263–265
Sweden 23, 85–86, 94, 108

Taiwan 6–7, 21, 27, 43, 46, 49, 93, 132, 134–137, 179
Taiwan Social Distancing App 136–137
Taleb, N. 94
tamponite 44–46
taxation 186
Taylor, S. 30
Technical Scientific Committee (CTS) 21, 23, 40–41, 68–70
Tegnell, A. 23–24, 85
test, trace and isolate (TTI) approach 134–135
Thatcher, M. 226, 237
Tool for Influenza Pandemic Risk Assessment (TIPRA) 17
Topol, E. 68
TRACE 136
TraceTogether app 141–142
The Tragic Science (De Martino) 239–240
Transatlantic Trade and Investment Partnership USA-EU (TTIP) 161–162
travel 18, 98, 135–137, 140–141, 208, 213, 258
trickle-down approach 227
Trump, D. 28, 39, 45–46, 159, 203
trust 189

United Kingdom 3, 6–7, 48, 62–63, 70–71, 76, 82, 91, 94, 100, 110, 115, 117, 135, 143, 158, 180, 182, *183*, 221, 226, *233*
United Nations Environment Program (UNEP) 204–205, 235

the United States 3, 5–6, 18, 22–24, 28,
39–42, 45, 48, 62–63, 65, 68, 71,
76–77, 82, 84, 88–89, 94–95, *95*, 97,
99–100, 108, 110, 112, 115, 117,
121, 135, 138, 141–142, *143*, 146,
158, *159*, 164, 168–169, 171–172,
180, 182, 186, 188, 203, 213, *221*,
222, 226, 229, *233*
unpreparedness 20, 74, 140
Urbani, A. 15
urbanization 205, 208, 231

vaccine/vaccination 16, 20, 25, 38, 42,
48, 70, 84, 86, 98–99, 114–121, *116*,
135, 137–138, 140, 142, 157–161,
159, 163–167, 169–170, 172, 191
Vaia, F. 209
Vargas, R. 260
Veneto 62, 73–74, 131–134
Vespignani, A. 67–68
Vietnam 6–6, 21, 49, 90, 132, 134,
138–139
Virchow, R. 193
virologist 1, 5, 20, 22–24, 29, 38–42,
45, 49–50, 65, 67, 74, 201, 203

Walensky, R. 167
Wallace, R. 173, 192, 207, 230,
265–266
Wang Guiqiang 98
The Wealth of Nature (Nadeau)
231–232
Wellcome Trust 120
white swan 15–17
Why We Will Heal (Speranza) 19
wildlife 205, 209, 258–259
Wilkinson, R. 182
Wolf, M. 237
Wolf, R. 264
Woods, N. 170
World Health Organization (WHO)
16–22, 25–29, 42–45, 51, 71, 85, 92,
96–97, 115, 118–119, 134, 137, 140,
200–201, 203
World Trade Organization
(WTO) 117

Zaia, L. 132–133, 142
zero COVID approach 96–99, 132,
134–135, 137, 139–140, 171, 232
Zinn, H. 271

For Product Safety Concerns and Information please contact our EU
representative GPSR@taylorandfrancis.com Taylor & Francis Verlag GmbH,
Kaufingerstraße 24, 80331 München, Germany

Printed and bound by CPI Group (UK) Ltd, Croydon, CR0 4YY
08/06/2025
01897008-0014